Canadian Medicine

Canadian Medicine

A study in restricted entry

Ronald Hamowy

Canadian Cataloguing in Publication Data

Hamowy, Ronald, 1937–
    Canadian medicine

Includes index.
ISBN 0-88975-062-9

1. Physicians - Licenses - Canada - History.
2. Medical laws and legislation - Canada - History.
I. Fraser Institute (Vancouver, B.C.)
II. Title.
KE2708.H35 1984   344.71'0412   C84-091302-8

Printed in Canada

Honor a physician with the honor due unto him for the uses which ye may have of him.

—Ecclus. 38:1

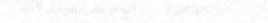

Contents

LIST OF TABLES

Preface

In 1979, the Fraser Institute published *The Health Care Business: International Evidence on Private versus Public Health Care Systems* by Professor Åke Blomquist of the University of Western Ontario. This study was mainly addressed to the demand side of the medical industry, and its main finding was that health care could be delivered with more efficiency to the Canadian public if there were a greater reliance on market-oriented alternatives. The difficulty with Canadian medical administration, it was argued, was that government-subsidized health care had set up a system of "moral hazard"; although the consumer must ultimately pay the entire medical bill (through taxes), the price he faces for any particular service is at or close to zero. This induces him to demand more than he otherwise would, leading to burgeoning health care costs.

The present study by Professor Ronald Hamowy of the University of Alberta, in contrast, is concerned solely with the supply of health care, specifically with physicians' services. As such it is a sequel to the Blomquist book. It is addressed to the questions of why medical licensing has been adopted in this country and what its economic effects are.

Two theories

Physicians in Canada have been licensed for well over a century, stretching back almost to the very birth of our nation. There are two theories that attempt to explain why doctors are licensed by government, asked to set the standards of medical practice, and urged to determine the qualifications for people entering this field.

According to orthodox theory the necessity for licensing arises from the complexity of the physician's calling, the innocence of the general public in matters medical, and the threat to health posed by unskilled practitioners. Without strict medical licensing legislation quacks would overrun the health care industry, imposing worthless and even harmful remedies on an innocent citizenry. Legitimate doctors would be powerless to stem the tide. It is widely believed by practitioners and the general public that the only way to avoid this horror is to give the men and women of medicine the power to police their own industry. Under these conditions, they will then act so as to best promote the public welfare.

The extreme version of the orthodox hypothesis maintains that regulation of the profession arises purely from a concern for the patient's welfare. In the more moderate version, while organized medicine is still viewed as primarily concerned with the medical status of the general populace, it is conceded that financial concerns about an excess supply of doctors do play a secondary role.

The alternative analysis of medical regulation reflects a very different theory of why such regulations exist. This analysis derives from the work of Nobel Laureate and Fraser Institute editorial advisor, George J. Stigler. It has formed the basis of most of the recent interest in economic deregulation, and in particular serves as the framework for the major study of economic regulation recently conducted by the Economic Council of Canada.

In whose interest?

Stigler's theory holds that whatever its stated purpose, much of economic regulation serves the interests of those who are regulated. This view runs counter to the usual interpretation of industrial and professional regulation, which sees lower prices, better quality, reduction of monopoly power, or some other aspect of the public good as the goal. But in Stigler's view, the main effect of most regulations and licensing requirements is to erect barriers against entry into the regulated industry or profession and thereby create a cartel, with all its attendant gains in income, power, and prestige. Applied to health care services, this theory implies that instead of an enhanced quality of medicine, wealth maximization is the goal of regulations touching on the profession.

Although evidence in support of this contention is gathered in the present volume, it will no doubt provoke considerable public debate. This is because while the theory of regulation has attained a dominant position within the economics profession, it is virtually unknown to the general public. There, the orthodox theory prevails. This is in part because the medical profession has supplied — on a frequent, intensive and well-articulated basis — the case for licensure of physicians.

This study by Professor Ronald Hamowy deals critically with these arguments and does not pretend to be an even-handed examination of these two opposing theories of licensure. Rather, it is an attempt to provide a counterbalance to the almost blind acceptance of the orthodox theory. Hamowy presents a careful exploration of an alternative view and it should be seen in conjunction with other evidence and other opinion.

Evidence

Hamowy has collected evidence, which he here presents, to the effect that the Canadian medical establishment at one point or another in its history has:

- banned price and other advertising for licensed doctors;
- set minimum price schedules;
- acted to prevent "overcrowding," or an oversupply of physicians by setting up a whole host of irrelevant criteria for licensing — examples include a knowledge of grammar, mathematics, Latin, history, philosophy, and other academic studies, language requirements, citizenship, etc.;
- outlawed the uncontrolled study of medicine, even for those who do not intend to practice;
- placed roadblocks against foreign doctors practicing in Canada, where they would compete with domestic physicians;
- been content with imposing entry examinations only. If the certification of quality were the true goal of these exams, they would more likely be required of practicing physicians every decade or so. For, says Hamowy, there is little guarantee — certainly not on the basis of testing — that a doctor of seventy years of age is still qualified, merely for having successfully sat an examination forty years earlier;
- fought against pre-payment contract practice, opposed doctors testifying for plaintiffs in malpractice suits, and discouraged charity work as undermining minimum fee schedules and professional prestige;
- raised medical student fees in order to increase the costs of entry into the profession;
- succeeded, from time to time, in raising physicians' income levels beyond that of other, equally skilled, professions in Canada.

These claims, and much of the data Professor Hamowy has

unearthed, are a part of the Canadian historical record with which most people, even doctors, may not be familiar. The evidence he cites will thus come as a distinct and uncomfortable surprise to most Canadians. And for good reason. This is because the typical doctor in this country is not at all involved in limiting entry into the field as a means of feathering his own nest. On the contrary the average physician works long hard hours (Winston Churchill's oft-quoted remark about "blood, sweat and tears" is a particularly apt description of medical practice), and has as his main concern the practice of his profession, not the financial exploitation of his patients.

Motivation

In this, the motivation of most doctors is not notably different from that of people involved in other callings. The average participant in the other sectors of the economy protected by government-erected barriers to entry are equally innocent of commercial chicanery. That is, airline pilots, taxi and truck drivers, safeguarded by regulations protecting their respective industries, and farmers preserved by marketing boards, are almost solely concerned with their day-to-day activities and not with the regulations which seal them off from competition.

Thus the truth or falsity of Hamowy's claims cannot be based on the experience of individual physicians who do not perceive themselves to be engaged in restricting their competitors. On the other hand, as Hamowy's research shows, the leadership of the medical profession in conjunction with well-meaning, though paternalist, bureaucrats have been doing just that for a century. Nor has the situation changed with the passage of time.

Consider the following account of a statement by Dr. Robert Gourdeau, recent president of the Canadian Medical Association:

> It's time Canadian doctors did something to end the "continuous and systematic erosion" of their territory by a horde of other allied health workers, the president of the Canadian Medical Association (CMA) warned here Wednesday.
>
> Dr. Robert Gourdeau said that for many years an increasing number of paramedical bodies—for reasons of ambition, prestige, autonomy, economics and other professional or personal reasons, not always related to the common good of the public—have been pressuring to increase their responsibility. He told a CMA gathering that doctors could face a "painful tomorrow if we do not give this problem the time and energy necessary to

develop appropriate means toward this invasion." He said medicine must ensure that those who practise the profession are appropriately trained and licensed to do so. He cited the case of Ontario psychologists who have proposed a new definition for their profession; "Professional responsibilities and authority that is tantamount to the definition of psychiatry." These people, he said, are asking the exclusive right to treat their clients according to the new definition of psychology.

There were others he said including podiatrists, a form of non-doctor foot specialist, who in some cases are practising what he feels is major surgery. Even nurses are asking for authority to perform numerous medical acts, sometimes with the support of doctors. Gourdeau warned that the requests of such groups often fall on "fertile soil" because governments, for reason of political expediency or attempts to cut health costs, are tempted to go along with them. "The financial savings often prove illusory and the quality of medical care is jeopardized," he said. He called on doctors to educate their patients "to confound those who strive to expropriate for their own profit, a greater share of our domain. . . ."

The London Free Press, June 21, 1978, p. A9, quoted in Åke Blomquist, *The Health Care Business,* (Vancouver: The Fraser Institute, 1979), pp. 46–47.

Licensure vs. certification

Crucial to the public policy analysis of health care, in Hamowy's view, is the distinction between licensure and certification. Under a system of licensure, only one agency, the College of Physicians and Surgeons (within each province) may license medical practitioners. All other people are barred from the practice of medicine. Under a system of certification, however, there would be many "certifiers of medical practitioners," each competing with the others for status in the community. This system would resemble the one in which universities at present compete with regard to the quality of their medical graduates.

Amongst physicians, those who "specialize" have acquired extra training, have passed a more rigorous series of examinations, and as a result are entitled to proclaim themselves specialists. As such, they receive the higher fee for service to which "specialists" are entitled. Doctors who specialize in a particular area—say obstetrics—but do not take the relevant examinations of the Royal College of Physicians and Surgeons of Canada, are not entitled to call themselves specialists nor do they receive the higher fee which is rendered to "specialists."

In other words, certification by the Royal College of Physicians and Surgeons of Canada is necessary if a doctor is to be able to call him or herself a specialist and to receive the higher fee. However, at the present time, a doctor may practice such a specialty without certification. (In metropolitan areas, the ability of non-certified "specialists" to operate is constrained by hospitals, which refuse to give them hospital privileges. In isolated and northern areas there are no such inhibitions and general practitioners perform what would otherwise be regarded as specialist functions.)

Increased competition

In a world of "certified" as opposed to "licensed" doctors, the public, by its decisions to buy or not buy the services of particular physicians, would decide who could successfully practice medicine. Practitioners offering a service the public wanted could obtain sufficient income to stay in business; others would not. It was the public, Hamowy suggests, that sustained the practice of chiropractic in the face of opposition by the medical profession, and in spite of the failure of state medical insurance to cover the cost. Why? Because the public valued the services of chiropractors. (These practitioners, incidentally, were certified by institutions which teach chiropractic.)

Professor Hamowy provides a detailed analysis of licensure, but he makes no specific public policy recommendations. However, it is not difficult to discern the prescriptions which follow from his study. Simply put, they would include allowing increased competition in the health care industry, and substituting certification for the present system of licensing. We know that, as a general principle, competition tends to provide a better good or service than does monopoly. For under the former system, but not the latter, if the consumer is dissatisfied with the product he receives, he can easily turn to an alternative. This in turn sets up an incentive system for all competitors to try to outdistance each other in terms of quality control, innovativeness, cost-cutting, etc. The weakest producers are forced to the sidelines, the strongest can expand the scope of their operations, to the ultimate and on-going improvement of the industry.

Although provision of knowledge to health care consumers about the skill, qualifications, experience, and general trustworthiness of doctors may not appear at first blush to be an "industry," the effects of competition would operate here as well. This is why it is important that our present system of monopoly licensing be replaced by a competitive system of medical certification.

How might it work?

It is not possible to forecast exactly how this particular market might function were government licensing regulations to be lifted. But such practices do exist in a wide range of endeavors. For example, the *Good Housekeeping* Seal of Approval is an indication of high quality for the homemaker. Private testing laboratories — in chemistry, physics, pharmacy, engineering — stake their reputations on industrial products. Consumer Union and Consumers Research are well known and highly respected guarantors of a wide variety of consumer goods. Companies such as Standard and Poor's and Moody's are world-renowned raters of bonds, including government bonds. Members of the "Big Eight" accounting firms underwrite the financial probity of the annual reports of many major corporations. Also serving similar roles are brand names, and certifying agencies such as department stores, universities, and the Better Business Bureau. These institutions have a strong incentive to maintain their reputation for reliability — for it is their main stock in trade. This is why *Consumer Reports* accepts no advertising; it must at all cost avoid even the appearance of non-independence.

How might competition work in the medical profession? Were government so minded, it could announce that at some time hence (say, ten years) it would call a halt to the present monopoly system of licensing doctors. This would usher in a competitive certification system to begin at present, to co-exist with licensing for the next decade, and to be launched out on its own at that point.

What kind of firms might undertake such an endeavor? One likely scenario would have various certification agencies — the Canadian Medical Association itself, the Royal College of Physicians and Surgeons of Canada, the several Colleges of Physicians and Surgeons of the provinces, the McGill University Medical Faculty, major insurance companies, for example — all competing with each other as to which might best be able to ensure the quality of physicians to the general public. Under such a system, according to this view, the quality of medicine and the extent of monitoring medical practice would improve, the costs of physicians' services would drop, and waiting time for doctors would decrease, to the benefit of the health care of the Canadian populace.

An objection

This public policy recommendation may seem strange to those most familiar with the debate in Canada over medical costs. It has often been put forward that the best way to reduce costs is to decrease the number of practicing physicians, not to increase them. It is argued that this occurs under our present system of medical care on the ground that there is a strong correlation between the number of doctors in a community and the medical billings presented to the government for payment. Doctors, it is claimed, can generate additional demand for their own services. They can do this by recommending further treatments, ordering extra tests, prescribing additional medicines, etc.

To a certain degree, this claim is true. (Although this phenomenon is by no means limited to doctors. Interior decorators, hairdressers and tailors, for example, cast aspersions at consumers who do not avail themselves of all their services in an effort to enhance sales. As well, there is hardly an industry or profession that does not attempt to increase the demand for its product by advertising.) However, classical supply and demand analysis teaches that, other things being equal, the greater the supply of any item (physicians' services, in this case) the lower the price it can command. If these recommendations regarding entry restrictions are implemented, this will increase the supply of physicians. Given supply and demand considerations, such a policy will force down prices. But more. Reduced restrictions on entry into the health care profession will also lead to decreased government payments under the medicare system. This is because the demand for medical services is highly inelastic; that is, people tend to increase their demand for health care to a lesser degree than any reduction in price. (For example, if the price of medical services falls by ten percent, demand might increase by only two percent or three percent.) With more doctors charging lower prices—and with additional scope for midwives, physician's assistants, technicians, and other qualified but less skilled health care professionals—and with demand for medical services increasing only by a lower percentage, total costs will have to fall.

Empirical study

So there are actually two effects. One, "the supplier-induced demand" effect, implies that as the number of doctors increases, so will total medical billings. The other, "the price elasticity" effect, suggests that with more doctors and other health care professionals offering services, the resulting lower prices will lead to falling total medical costs.

Which of these two tendencies will predominate cannot be determined from economic theory alone. But the limited empirical evidence now available indicates that the former is very weak, or non-existent, and that thus the latter effect dominates the former.[1] If so, the additional medical personnel attracted to the profession by reducing restrictions on entry will lead to decreased costs for health care. But, in any case, we must reject the facile argument that, because doctors can generate extra demand for their own product, allowing more health care professionals to practice necessarily implies rising medicare expenditures.

One possible remedy would be to dismantle the present medicare system. Blomquist, in our previous book on this subject, has argued that the Canadian medicare program gives consumers incentives to purchase more medical services than they would if forced to pay on a user fee basis (the citizens have made a lump sum payment through taxes and feel they might as well take advantage of health care services whenever possible). With the public sector middleman removed from the picture (except, perhaps, in the role of implementing a deductible system of medical "catastrophe" insurance, as recommended by Professor Blomquist) people would no longer have financial incentives to demand excessive amounts of medical services. Then the usual pattern would emerge: other things being equal, the greater the supply, the lower the price, and the less the supply, the higher the price.

Historical analysis

One final word. In some respects, the present volume is well within the tradition of Fraser Institute research. This is not, for example, the first exploration of the economic theory of regulation we have undertaken. On the contrary, the rent-seeking behavior of farmers was examined in *The Real Cost of the B.C. Milk Board* written by Herbert Grubel, published in 1977, and again in *The Egg Marketing Board: A Case Study of Monopoly and Its Social Costs,* a study authored by Thomas Borcherding and published in 1981. In addition, Professor Hamowy's book is a follow-up to Åke Blomquist's *The Health Care Business,* published in 1979, and thus the second in our health care series. However, the present study is also a departure of sorts for the Fraser Institute.

Previous Fraser Institute studies have been concerned with the analysis of economic problems as they exist in the present. Although Professor Hamowy's concerns are relevant to contemporary issues, they are primarily concerned with an aspect of Canadian history. (This is because virtually the entire corpus of legislation relevant to the licensing of physicians was in place at the beginning of the twentieth century.) Moreover, his conclusions are highly provocative. But one of the purposes of the Fraser Institute is to initiate and facilitate informed public debate on issues of economic policy—and Hamowy's findings will certainly do just that. The Fraser Institute is therefore pleased to publish Professor Hamowy's study, and thus make his findings available to the general public. Because of the independence of the author, however, the views expressed by Professor Hamowy may or may not conform severally or collectively with those of the members of the Institute.

Walter Block
August, 1984

[1] Mark V. Pauly, *Doctors and Their Workshops,* National Bureau of Economic Research, Chicago: University of Chicago Press, 1980; *The Target Income Hypothesis and Related Issues in Health Manpower Policy* edited by Jesse Hixson and Don Winslow, Washington, D.C.: Department of Health and Human Services, Public Health Service, H.R.A. 80-27, 1980; Jerry Green, "Physician Induced Demand for Medical Care," *The Journal of Human Resources,* Volume XIII, Supplement, 1978, pp. 21-34; L. J. Brown, Jesse S. Hixson and Gerry L. Musgrave, "Implications of the Expanding Supply of Physicians for Geographic Distribution" in *Contemporary Policy Issues,* Eldon Dvoric, ed., Huntington Beach, California: Western Economic Association, 1984; Gerry L. Musgrave, *Potential Impact of Increased Numbers of Physicians Upon Physician Behavior, Access to, and Costs of Medical Care,* U.S. Government Printing Office, Rockville, Md: Health Resources and Services Administration, H.R.A., #232-82-0023, 1984.

Summary and Acknowledgements

The following essay is the outgrowth of a long-standing interest in the history of legislation in North America, and particularly that aspect of legislation touching on the medical profession. The subject thus narrowed is, in its entirety, still vast, encompassing the licensing of health personnel, the introduction of bureaus of public health, pure food and drug laws, regulations affecting the sale and distribution of alcoholic beverages, tobacco, pharmaceuticals, and a host of other substances; in fact, this topic embraces a substantial portion of the statutory enactments and regulations associated with the modern welfare state. Additionally, it bridges the legal history of two distinct and widely differing societies, the United States on the one hand, and Canada on the other.

This particular monograph does not, of course, attempt anything as ambitious as a treatment of the whole spectrum of such regulations in the two countries. Rather, it confines itself solely to an analysis of the historical development of legal restrictions on entry into medical practice in Canada. This essay covers the period from the introduction of medical licensing laws at the end of the eighteenth century through the first decades of the twentieth century. The study closes with the introduction of dominion reciprocity immediately prior to World War I and the enactment of legislation limiting the practice of drugless healers in the 1920s, at which point the organization of the medical profession and the legal arrangements respecting the right to practice essentially took the form they currently have.

In analysing the history of the professionalization of medical practice in British North America, I have tried to bring to bear, where pertinent, the findings provided by a growing body of literature in economics and sociology relating to occupational licensing. Because of the weaknesses inherent in earlier treatments of the Canadian medical profession, it has been particularly important to rely as much as possible on primary material, that is, on the statements of physicians as they appeared in the speeches, articles, and editorials published in the medical press during the period under consideration. Consequently, this monograph quotes extensively from the medical journals published over the course of the nineteenth century.

Because of the poor typography from which most of these journals suffered, I have corrected most typographical and grammatical errors that appeared in the original, except in those instances where American and British spellings were used randomly, in which case they are reprinted unaltered. It was an unfortunate habit of the nineteenth century medical press to use identical titles for a host of comments appearing in different issues of a journal or, indeed, in several different journals. Thus, "The College of Physicians and Surgeons" might be the title of dozens of editorials, articles, and comments published by a number of periodicals about a variety of different subjects and spanning a number of years. Consequently, citations, including journal title and date, are given in full for all articles appearing before 1935. I have employed the term "*ibid.*" for the journal name itself where the same journal is cited in the note immediately preceding or where there is no possibility of confusion. Finally, the laws of the various provinces, territories, and the federal government are cited by regnal year throughout, but in all cases the year of passage has been provided.

I should like to thank Douglas R. Owram and R. C. Macleod, both of the History Department of the University of Alberta, and J. C. Smith of the Law School of the University of British Columbia, all of whom were kind enough to read the manuscript and who offered a number of helpful suggestions. I am especially indebted to William M. Bartley and Doris Bergen, also of the University of Alberta, whose research and editorial help have proved invaluable throughout the period during which this monograph was written. Nor would this book have been possible without the amiable assistance of the staffs of the law libraries of the University of Alberta and Stanford University. Above all, I wish to acknowledge the unfailing cooperation and patience of the staff of the Lane Medical Library at Stanford University, whose collection of Canadian medical periodicals is one of the best in North America. The generosity with which its librarians gave of their time and effort in dealing with my many requests has made working there a truly pleasant experience.

RONALD HAMOWY
Edmonton, Alberta
July, 1984

About the Author

Ronald Hamowy did his undergraduate work in history and economics at Cornell University and at the City College of New York, where he received his B.A. in 1960. He then went on to do graduate work in the history of social and legal theory at the University of Chicago, where he worked under F. A. Hayek on the Committee on Social Thought, from which he received his doctorate. Mr. Hamowy has studied at the Faculty of Law at the University of Paris and at Oxford University, where he was a student of Sir Isaiah Berlin. He has been awarded fellowships by the University of Chicago, the University of Paris, and Balliol College, Oxford.

After serving for one year as a lecturer in modern European history at Brooklyn College, New York, Mr. Hamowy became an instructor in the history of western civilization program at Stanford University, where he remained for four years. In 1969, he took up the position of assistant professor of intellectual history at the University of Alberta, where he currently holds the rank of professor. From 1975 to 1977, he was visiting associate professor of political theory at Simon Fraser University.

Mr. Hamowy has published a number of articles in the area of social and legal theory. Among the journals in which they have appeared are *Economica, Il Politico,* the *William and Mary Quarterly,* and the *Canadian Journal of History.* He is the author of "Preventive Medicine and the Criminalization of Sexual Immorality in Nineteenth-Century America," in Randy E. Barnett and John Hagel III, eds., *Assessing the Criminal: Restitution, Retribution, and the Legal Process* (Cambridge, Mass: Ballinger Publishing Co., 1977): 35-97. He is currently editing a collection of essays on the history and economics of medical licensing in the United States.

Introduction

What follows is an account of the development of medical licensing legislation in British North America from its inception through the first decades of the twentieth century. I have attempted to analyse the history of legal restrictions on entry into the medical profession in terms of the forces working towards the enactment of such legislation. That it was not the consumers of physicians' services but medical practitioners themselves who sought the statutory protections they now enjoy has never been denied. However, the motives behind the profession's unceasing appeals for more stringent legislative controls over entry into medical practice are somewhat more obscure. Histories of the medical profession in Canada—traditionally written by and for physicians—have continually stressed the selfless nature of these demands.[1] And this view, so often reiterated by medical practitioners and medical organizations throughout the Dominion, has managed to find its way even into studies of the profession authored by non-physicians.[2]

Now, all historians possessing even a modest familiarity with the economic literature of professional monopolies are aware that barriers to entry act to the economic advantage of those already in practice at the time the barrier was erected.[3] Thus, members of a protected profession have a continued interest in exacting progressively more severe qualifications for new entrants. In addition, there is strong evidence to suggest that these restrictions on entry have resulted in greater than competitive earnings to physicians, even to those practitioners entering the profession after the imposition of the more stringent requirements. Or, put in slightly different terms, simply being admitted to a medical school has an economic value greater than zero.[4]

Increased costs of entry

It does not take a sophisticated knowledge of economic theory to know that such policies as increasing the costs of entry into the profession, limiting the number of new entrants, restricting advertising, discouraging price competition, and defining the ambit of professional practice so as to restrict the availability of substitute services, all redound to the economic benefit of members of a profession. And it is absurd to suppose that these simple economic facts, known even to the medieval craft guilds,[5] were a mystery to physicians in the nineteenth century or that they played a negligible role in determining their actions. Indeed, evidence contained in the medical journals and in the statements of Canada's leading practitioners shows that the Dominion's physicians were keenly aware that the legislation they sought served their own financial interests. All their claims about the public welfare notwithstanding, every policy legislated by the profession, every statutory enactment for which they lobbied, had as its objective maximizing the incomes, status, and prestige of the profession's members, even when such legislation conflicted with the wishes of the nation's consumers of health services.

Physicians sought to cartelize the profession for the same reason the medieval guilds sought monopolies and, in turn, justified their demands for privileged status on similar grounds: to safeguard the public from incompetent practitioners and thus to ensure the quality of the good or service offered. Without such a rationalization, it would be next to impossible to mollify consumers, who have no incentive to acquiesce in the higher prices they would be required to pay. Public interest defenses of licensing, however, are of doubtful merit. In his essay on occupational licensure in Canada, David Dodge notes:

> Three reasons are generally advanced to provide a social justification for the licensing of occupations:
>   (1) to provide information for the consumer who is not able to judge the competency of the professional rendering the service:
>   (2) to prevent the rendering of "misservices" to the consumer in cases where the social costs of "misservice" may exceed the private costs; and
>   (3) to ensure the rendering of services that society feels ought to be rendered because society is a better judge of what is good for the individual consumer (and society) than he himself is.[6]

To these arguments, Dodge responds:

> These justifications for licensing are not supported by logical argument or appeal to the evidence, however.
>   First, licensing (as normally implemented) only provides evidence that a practitioner met certain standards when he entered the profession but provides no information about his current competence. Moreover, information may be provided through voluntary certification of practitioners without the necessity of incurring the cost of loss of choice of practitioner by the consumer.
>   The second justification for licensing implies that the social

cost of improper service... is greater than the social cost arising from failure of individuals to have the service performed at all by a licensed practitioner because of a greater price of the service after licensing. This assertion is not a logical necessity, but rather a subject for empirical verification. To my knowledge it has never been empirically verified.

While the third argument has the virtue of logical consistency, it is not supported by an appeal to the evidence.[7]

Licensing and quality of service

As Dodge suggests, it is not even clear that the quality of the service offered the public is improved by licensing its practitioners. "It should be noted," concludes a leading student of the subject,

> that, while licensing causes the mean quality of legal practitioners to rise, by excluding those at the lower part of the qualitative range who could have practiced legally in the absence of a licensing statute, it does not necessarily cause the mean quality of the relevant service to rise. Whether it does or not turns on the behavior of consumers of the service after the trade has been licensed, who in the absence of licensing would have employed the qualitatively low tradesmen who sold their services at correspondingly low prices. If consumers substitute for low-quality barbers, who are now not permitted to practice, the haircutting services of their (own) wives, the qualitative mean falls; if they substitute the services of higher-quality barbers, the qualitative mean rises. If both occur, as is likely, the outcome is an arithmetic consequence of the magnitudes of opposite movement.[8]

And, with specific reference to the licensing of physicians, one noted economist has written:

> It is of course a well known axiom that an increase in quality requires an increase in price. And an increase in price implies an increase in efforts to economize on a resource that has become more scarce. Hence, an increase in quality implies a greater effort to economize on physicians' services. What this means specifically is that people tend to substitute self-diagnosis and treatment for the services of a physician. This tendency manifests itself at the onset of an illness or suspected illness, and going to a physician is deferred until the symptoms become alarming. Consequently, increasing the quality of physicians does not necessarily mean that

the quality of medical care that the public as a whole receives also increases, since the public receives a mixture of professional attention and self-treatment. . . . The argument that restriction on entry and licensure has raised standards of medical practice has great appeal and acceptance. Unfortunately, there does not appear to be any empirical study available to support this view, and it is striking that organized medicine has not investigated the effects of licensure on the quality of care of the community.[9]

All this is not to suggest that all, or even most, physicians were aware that the cartelizing policies they espoused worked to their economic advantage at the expense of harming the public. Doubtless many practitioners believed that professional licensure would raise the quality of medical care offered the public while at the same time financially benefitting the profession. Indeed, so great is the capacity of individuals to identify their private interests with those of the public, despite the absence of evidence to support this conviction, that it would be surprising if physicians did not embrace the belief that restricting entry into the profession protected a befuddled public from the depredations of incompetents and purveyors of poisons. If the interests of the community were consistent with those of the profession, so much the better! But the evidence does not support the conclusion that what lay at the root of physicians' efforts to cartelize the profession was concern for the welfare of a helpless citizenry. Such selfless motives were inconsistent with the profession's insistence on grandfathering in all existing practitioners when stricter standards for licensure were imposed or in making licensure a grant of lifetime tenure, without any proof of continued competency. Nor is the concern for the public welfare compatible with such policies as restricting advertising or fixing schedules of fees.

Professionalizing an occupation

Analysis of the historical evidence regarding the medical profession in Canada supports the findings of current sociological theory, that monopoly control and lack of public accountability are historical attributes of professionalizing an occupation and that this process is initiated and brought to fruition, not by the lay public, but by the members of the profession themselves.[10] In sociological terms, the privileged economic and social status that followed upon licensing legislation marked the transition of North American medical practice in the period from 1880 to 1910 from a trade to a profession. Profession status was intimately associated with success in limiting access to medical education which, in turn, lent credibility to physicians' claims to a monopoly of scarce knowledge and skills. The fact that only a select group possessed medical expertise provided the basis for demands that practitioners be granted professional autonomy. One sociologist has explicated this process in the following manner:

> A basic component [of current sociological theory on the nature of professions] is the monopolization of knowledge, achieved through limitation of access to university training and mystification of the public about how esoteric that knowledge is. Licensing procedures are mechanisms against alternative claims to knowledge by interlopers and help to guard the monopoly. . . .
>
> Claims to esoteric knowledge and unselfish service have an important result, namely authority and autonomy in dealing with clients, two aspects of the crucial power dimension of the professional role. It has been suggested that it is this third dimension which really distinguishes professions from other occupations. Power, when it is accepted as legitimate, becomes authority, the *right* to direct activity of others and to be obeyed. Authority in the professional context in turn implies work autonomy, the right not to be subject to direction by others in carrying out tasks. Since the element which legitimates power as authority is monopolized knowledge not available to the lay clientele, the implication is that practitioners are not subject to external controls either; that is, they have the right to use their specialized knowledge in the manner which their training and experience indicate as most appropriate, free of supervision. . . . Only fellow practitioners realize the shortcomings of knowledge and the uncertainty of outcomes, and can be trusted to make fair and informed judgments of their colleagues' job performance.
>
> From the perspective of the sociology of work, this theoretical model of professional self-regulation provides a rationale for rejection of any accountability except to peers and explains public willingness to accede to this arrangement, at least to the extent that it still does.[11]

Economic implications

Whether within the context of sociological theory or not, no book-length history of Canadian practitioners has touched on the economic implications of legislative restrictions on entry into the profession.

Indeed, to the extent that these restrictions are chronicled at all, they are almost invariably hailed as evidence of the profession's ongoing altruism towards a fractious and ungrateful public. This naiveté becomes nothing less than disingenuousness when the writer has had access to the primary material in the field, as have most historians of the Canadian profession. The historiography of Canadian medicine has had a long and undistinguished career. Consisting in the main of a series of tedious, often banal, works, these histories have commonly been authored by physicians, who appear to have had little or no interest either in analysing or interpreting the events which they chronicled.[12] Their accounts tend to be only minimally informative and suffer from the worst form of special pleading. Orthodox physicians are invariably portrayed as singlehandedly protecting medical science and the quality of medical care against the incursions of countless quacks and charlatans, while the profession's unrelenting demands for strict licensing legislation are presented as the product of a humanistic concern that the public be protected from incompetents. Homeopathy and eclecticism — the two major heterodox therapies of nineteenth-century medicine — if they are mentioned at all, are dismissed as unscientific nonsense, their practitioners amateur bunglers who preyed on the credulity of ignorant men and women.[13]

Intentional obscurity

The faults of Canadian medical historiography are more than simply limitations. The orientation adopted by those writers who have attempted to recount the history of the profession has been such as to intentionally obscure the real motives behind much of the activity of organized medicine.[14] As just one example, consider the historical treatment given the ongoing efforts of established practitioners to gain enactment of legislation raising the educational requirements for licensure. If these efforts are discussed at all, they are assumed to issue exclusively from the profession's concern with the quality of care available to the public. The minutes of the various provincial boards, however, show with pristine clarity that the motive behind such lobbying was the wish to restrict the number of prospective physicians entering medical practice and thus to reduce "overcrowding" in the profession. Instead of providing a coherent account of the evolution of medical practice that takes account of these facts, however, Canadian medical histories have traditionally subjected their readers to the most partisan narrative of legislative and institutional developments. The value of these works is even further reduced by the inclusion of count-less biographies of physicians of no historical import, by lists of presi-dents and members of some society, board, committee, association, or another, and by lengthy discussions of totally irrelevant events. It is, in fact, no exaggeration to conclude, as has one current medical his-torian, that if "European medical historians 'are more than a genera-tion ahead of their American counterparts,' the state of the art in Canada has barely left the list-compiling Dark Ages."[15]

Medicine as a case study

The inadequacies of medical historiography in Canada make a study of the development of legislative restrictions on entry into the pro-fession that much more imperative. The politicization of medicine, that is, the organization of the profession into a self-governing body endowed with police powers, serves as a particularly useful case study of the abandonment of a reliance on market forces in favor of govern-ment intervention. How this came about and who benefited by it are questions worthy of detailed investigation not only for their own sake but also for the implications they have on why this process has con-tinued unabated—indeed, accelerated—over the last hundred years. What is especially noteworthy about the transformation of the medi-cal profession into an arm of government is the fact that this change was initiated in the face of substantial public opposition. Just as prac-titioners knew that erecting barriers to entry into medical practice served their economic interest, so were many consumers aware that the effect of such policies would be to raise the cost of physicians' ser-vices and to limit the range of therapeutic techniques available to them. But so strenuous and systematic were the efforts of physicians in the various provinces to gain enactment of the desired legislation, so unorganized the resistance to these laws, that practitioners were successful in achieving total cartelization of the profession by the beginning of the twentieth century.

Economic self-interest a significant factor

The following study attempts to offer an account of these efforts. Its conclusions dispute the widely held belief that the various statutes and regulations raising the requirements for medical licensure were, in the first instance, enacted to protect the public from so-called incompe-tents. The historical data provide substantial evidence that the profession's motives in raising the standards of entry into medical practice and in instituting policies that prohibited advertising or any sort of price competition were almost purely ones of economic self-interest. It is a tribute to the reputation physicians have managed to attain among their fellow citizens that many educated people today would find this conclusion barely credible. Yet this fact should come as no more of a surprise than would an equivalent statement about barbers or architects. Physicians are neither greater nor lesser mortals than are other men. It is foolish to suppose that their occupation exalts them above using the means at their disposal to act in their own private interests.

Needless to say, the position of the various provincial Colleges of Physicians and Surgeons was, and continues to be, that they have never sought legislation or acted for selfish ends. The following statement of the Ontario College, contained in a brief issued in 1967, is typical:

> In no sense is the College a guild or union of medical practitioners, nor is it any part of its purpose to serve the self-interest of the profession. The record of the past century bears out that its dedication is to the public interest.[16]

As this study will show, the facts of the matter belie this. And it is a reflection on the quality of Canadian medical historiography that few, if any, writers have questioned the official view. If the following monograph contributes to a more realistic assessment of the causes and events that led to the current organization of the medical profession, it will have served the purpose for which it was written.

Chapter 1

Medical Licensing in Canada in the Period to 1840

LICENSING IN THE EIGHTEENTH CENTURY

Medical licensing in Canada predates the conquest of Quebec by the British and appears to have been sought by the same group ultimately responsible for all future restrictive medical legislation in the country; those physicians[1] with established practices. In 1750, the Intendant of New France enacted a bill forbidding all ship's surgeons and surgeons from whatever country "other than those who are established in the cities of this country and its coasts" to practice medicine or surgery in any form without first having submitted to a "serious preliminary examination in the art of surgery and having been judged capable of exercising it," under penalty of a fine of 200 *livres*.[2] The reasons for instituting this measure are contained in the preface to the bill:

> From information we have received it appears many unknown individuals coming from Europe and elsewhere have engaged in surgery as much in the cities as in the country districts of this colony, without any permission; that these strangers whose ability is unknown treat the sick with little care and without giving them relief; distribute worthless remedies which give unsatisfactory results, not having all the experience necessary, and leading as a final result to abuses which are prejudicial to the well-being of the subjects of the King, . . . [3]

The information to which the Intendant refers doubtless originated in the complaints of established practitioners that comparatively large numbers of new physicians were establishing themselves in the communities of New France by the mid-eighteenth century. Either educated through an apprenticeship system or armed with easily available Letters Patent from the King,[4] they represented an unwelcome competitive force to the older practitioners who, for the most part, were no less nor no better able to treat their patients than were the new physicians.[5] Indeed, in writing of the medical profession in New France, John J. Heagerty notes the unrestricted nature of medical practice that prevailed in the colony up to the passage of the ordinance of 1750:

The surgeons of Canada of those early days had no degree. Surgery occupied a very inferior status socially and scientifically; the surgeons. . . had for their associates barbers, and they practiced conjointly with them and performed bleeding and minor operations. This fraternity was sanctioned by Royal assent and Letters Patent in 1613. It was not essential that one be apprenticed to a surgeon or that one obtain degrees; it sufficed that one settled in the country to enjoy the privilege of the practise of any of the professions.

The King decreed, when establishing the colony of the Hundred Associates, that any artisan who went to New France and practised his art for a period of six years would, on returning to France, be considered a master in his work and could open shop of his own.[6]

By far the larger number of physicians practicing in New France, particularly during the seventeenth century, as Heagerty earlier points out, were originally ship's surgeons, either temporarily or permanently settling in the colony.[7] They were eventually augmented by doctors who received their training through an apprenticeship system in Quebec itself.[8] These factors appear responsible for keeping the colony well supplied with much needed physicians[9] and also accounts for the pressure that was eventually brought to bear on the government of New France to limit continued free entry into the profession.

The British regime

The British conquest of Canada in 1759 put an end to all French regulations respecting the profession in the colony.[10] With the success of the American Revolution some two decades later, numbers of English-speaking loyalists and disbanded soldiers entered Quebec, many settling in the territory that today forms part of the province of Ontario.[11] There appears to have been a dearth of medical men among those who emigrated north into the wilderness of the western portions of Quebec; of the physicians remaining loyal to the Crown after the Revolution, most of those banished from the United States settled in New Brunswick and Nova Scotia.[12] In the absence of constraints against entering practice, however, many persons possessing some qualification from Great Britain offered themselves as physicians to meet the medical needs of the new settlers. This group was soon augmented by Americans, some of whom held degrees from American medical colleges. Sharing a common mother tongue with the loyalists, they set up comparatively lucrative practices in the newly-settled areas.[13]

With the influx of new entrants into the profession, pressures for the reintroduction of restrictive legislation once again emerged. Physicians who were degree-holders from medical schools resented the competition of those who received their training either through an apprenticeship system or from experience alone. As a result, in 1788 a medical act was passed in the colony, forbidding any person "on any pretense" whatever to

> sell, vend, or distribute medicines by retail, or prescribe for sick persons for gain, or practise physic or surgery within the Province, or practise midwifery in the towns of Quebec and Montreal, or the suburbs therof, without license first had and obtained from His Excellency the Governor, or the Commander-in-Chief of the Province, for the time being, which license shall not be granted but upon certificate of the person applying for the same, having been examined and approved by such persons as the Governor or Commander-in-Chief, for the time being, may have appointed for the purpose of examining and inquiring into the knowlege of such persons in physic, or skill in surgery, or pharmacy, or midwifery, ...[14]

The penalties for non-compliance were absurdly severe: a £20 fine for the first offense, £50 for the second, and £100 and two-months' imprisonment for each subsequent offense. Most significant, the ordinance exempted from examination "such persons as shall have taken a degree in any university, or who have been commissioned or warranted as surgeons in His Majesty's army or navy."

The syphilis epidemic

The ostensible reason for passage of this bill was the inability of unqualified practitioners to adequately minister to the population of Quebec during the syphilis epidemic that ravaged the province between 1775 and 1786.[15] The epidemic was so widespread that it is estimated to have struck at least three to four thousand persons, out of a population of less than 120,000.[16] The orthodox treatment consisted in the administration of massive doses of corrosive sublimate to the stricken patient, which was almost certain to cause mercury poisoning and death. Dr. Philippe Badelard, ordered by the Governor, General Carlton, and by his successor, General Haldimand, to repair to the parishes where the disease was most common to treat its victims, boasted that he insisted on "the strongest dose of corrosive sublimate." In his report to General Haldimand, in which he claims a remarkably high success rate, Dr. Badelard noted that his unfortunate patients were forced to consume

> during 10, 15, 20, or 30 days a grain of corrosive sublimate a day, washed by at least three pounds of an infusion of mallow, barley or rice. One always added when one could a quart of milk. One could, to remove the aversion of wheat brandy, melt in a little of this liquor the dose of sublimate finely powdered; and add a pound and a half of infusion of mallow, barley or rice. This pound and a half of liquor in which are placed the fifteen grains of sublimate, which I have given without accident, to the most advanced case, contains 48 soup spoons, which at three a day make 16 days.[17]

We are cautioned that "cramps sometimes take place and a flux of urine," and that the physician then "must stop for a couple of days and purge with rhubarb."[18]

Under this regimen, it is no wonder, as a medical committee reported to the Grand Jury of Montreal, that, "although there are several who have been perfectly cured of it, the numbers of these bear too small a proportion to those who are infected as to be little or no hindrance to the spreading of the disease."[19]

The mortality rate from the disease and, equally commonly, from its treatment by the colony's most respected practitioners, was seized upon by them as sufficient reason for the passage of legislation limiting entry into medical practice. A letter from Dr. Charles Blake to the colony's Committee of His Majesty's Council on Population is indicative. Dr. Blake writes:

> It cannot have escaped your notice the very great nuisance that prevails in this country, and which for a long time has cried loudly for a remedy; it is the imposition the community at large suffers from inexperienced and illiterate men practicing the art of physic and surgery. The destruction attending mankind in these parts by those wicked pretenders is shocking to humanity. All ranks of people join in one voice to beg that His Majesty's Council will so far interest themselves for the public good, as to put a stop to these gross misdemeanours;[20]

Blake then proceeds to offer us two cases of malpractice so blatant as to be humorous and to outline proposals for regulating the profession in the province.[21] Heagerty informs us that such complaints eventually induced the government to enact its ordinance of 1788.

EARLY ATTEMPTS AT LICENSURE IN UPPER CANADA

In 1791, the United Empire Loyalists proved successful in their petition for autonomy for Upper Canada, and in March of that year the Imperial Parliament divided the province of Quebec into two autonomous areas—Upper and Lower Canada—each with its own governor, legislative council and house of assembly.[22] The first Lieutenant-Governor of Upper Canada, Colonel John Graves Simcoe, took office in July, 1792, and the first session of the province's parliament was held that September.[23]

Attempts to license physicians in Upper Canada began immediately; on the 24th of September, 1792, the Assembly struck a special committee to determine "the most effective means of preventing persons not duly qualified from practising physic."[24] The lobbying efforts of physicians seem to have done little good at this juncture, since the committee took only one evening to determine that no attempt should be made to restrict the practice of medicine in the province. Established practitioners appear to have had greater success two years later. In 1794, the Assembly passed a measure regulating the practice of medicine and referred it to the Council, and it was only due to inaction on the part of the Council that the bill lapsed.[25] The following year, however, a similar bill, having passed both houses, became law.[26] The 1795 act was modeled on the medical ordinance of 1788 and prohibited any person to

> practise physic, surgery or midwifery within the Province, for profit, until such person or persons shall be duly examined and approved of by a board of surgeons, who shall be constituted and appointed ... with full powers to grant licenses for the practise of physic, surgery and midwifery within the Province, and has received a license under the hands of and seal of the President of the said Board and such members thereof as may be present at his or their examination.[27]

The penalty for non-compliance was set at £10 and, in order to encourage the population to turn in illegal practitioners to the authorities, a half of each fine collected was to be given to the informer. The law exempted from its provisions holders of degrees from universities within the British Empire and those commissioned as surgeons in the British armed forces. The bill thus discriminated against graduates of American medical schools — of educated practitioners, those most likely to settle in Upper Canada to tend to the province's growing population. Additionally, all persons who had been in medical practice in Upper Canada before 1791, regardless of their credentials or competence, were exempt from examination. This grandfather clause was doubtless included to win the support of many of the practitioners then operating in the province, but despite the provision rewarding informers, the act does not appear to have been enforced, nor is there even any record indicating that an examining board had been organized.[28]

Midwifery

Certainly limiting the practice of midwifery to licensed physicians was totally unworkable[29] and likely contributed to the repeal of the act in 1806.[30] It is interesting to note the reaction of a contemporary layman to this law. Robert Gourlay, an outspoken opponent of Upper Canada's loyalist oligarchy,[31] wrote of the medical act in 1795 in his Sketch Book:

> Now the fact is that few men who could stand the examination of such as were regular-bred and well educated, and fewer still had received a degree at a university, *would* practise. Nobody above the rank of a common cowherd would travel round a circle of forty or fifty miles in the wilderness for the pittance which could be collected long after this law was made; and save in the larger villages — Kingston, Niagara and York — nothing like a genteel subsistence could be obtained. How absurd then, to think of preventing the remotely scattered people from choosing whom they liked to draw their teeth, bleed, and blister them! How absurd, how cruel, how meddling that a poor woman in labour could not have assistance from a handy, sagacious neighbour, without this neighbour being liable to be informed upon and fined! This absurdity was not sufficiently perceived for ten years, and then the Act was repealed in 1806.[32]

The repeal of the 1795 act does not seem to have long discouraged the medical fraternity from working for the passage of a substitute law. The unrestricted nature of the trade continued to attract practitioners into Upper Canada[33] and, in 1808, a similar bill was introduced into the provincial legislature, but it failed to pass.[34]

Physicians were to have better luck in 1815, when a statute similar in its provisions to that of 1795 was enacted.[35] The only changes made were that female midwives were added to the list of those exempt from the law and the penalty for practicing without a license was increased to £100. The act appears to have been as difficult of enforcement as its predecessor, despite the draconian penalty attached to violation of its provisions, and it too was repealed with the passage of a new and more effective medical licensing law three years later. MacNab suggests several reasons why the 1795 and 1815 acts were such failures:

> Both these Acts were administratively and politically impractical. In the first place they did not suggest how they should be carried out. While the appointment of a Board of Examiners was provided for, no provisions were made concerning its size, when and where it should meet, or how it should conduct its examinations (i.e., how applicants should apply, and how often examinations should be held). Further, no exemption from the licensing provisions was allowed for those who had started to practise after 1791, and these men formed a small but politically powerful group. Finally, the problem of a scattered population and an inadequate supply of qualified doctors still existed.[36]

A shortage of doctors

There seems to be no question that an adequate supply of physicians who could meet the standards demanded by the statutes of 1795 and 1815 simply did not exist in Upper Canada at the time. Canniff calculates that, after passage of the 1815 act, the number of doctors possessing the requisite credentials in the province did not amount to more than thirty-six to forty.[37] The population of Upper Canada was then almost 100,000,[38] allowing, at best, for a ratio of one physician to each 2,500 inhabitants. And even these figures are inflated since the better-educated physicians tended to cluster in the larger towns. Thus, as one authority has noted, when the fact that settlers were scattered over a vast area of mostly uncleared countryside is taken into consideration, the paucity of "qualified" physicians is even greater than the raw figures suggest.[39]

Given the conditions that then prevailed, it is little wonder that large numbers of people who lacked regular training or possessed only a modicum of formal medical education set up practice in the province. The established practitioners appear to have been fully aware that the 1815 statute was enacted more for their own benefit than that of the general public, many of whom, had the law been strictly enforced, would have been effectively deprived of any professional medical help whatever. But the profession was intent on seeing to it that the provisions of the law were fully observed. Canniff quotes the following notice circulating in Kingston in mid-1817 by one James Scott, M.R.S.C., Dublin, "late Surgeon of His Majesty's Ship *Montreal*" as an example:

> Notice to all unlicensed Practitioners of Medicine and Quacks in and about Kingston:
> Doctor Scott will indiscriminately and impartially make known to the Attorney-General's Office, in this province, and prosecute with the utmost rigour of the law, all and every person whom he may hereafter discern practising any branch of the medical profession under the above denomination.[40]

Indeed, even those non-physicians who supported restrictive legislation recognized the brute fact that the established profession had much to gain from passage of the medical act. Thus, a letter appearing in the Kingston *Gazette* in 1815 by someone signing himself "W" ("Not of the profession") notes that "the Parliament of this province, during the last session, provided, in part, against the imposition of empirics in medicine. This was not more necessary for the safety of the diseased than the reputation of the faculty."[41]

Restricted entry and anti-Americanism

Thanks to the efforts of both the established profession and the civil authorities, the movement to restrict entry into the medical profession had, after the War of 1812, become intimately linked in the mind of the educated public with anti-American sentiments. The great majority of practitioners in Upper Canada came from the New England states,[42] including large numbers of physicians who would have been incapable of meeting the standards established by the 1815 act. The aversion to practitioners emigrating from the United States eventuated in all poorly educated medical men being labeled "Yankee loafers" by the establishment.[43] A good example of this anti-American bias, predictably coupled with a plea for more effective enforcement of the statute, emerges in a letter to the Kingston *Gazette* of May 25, 1816:

> Sir, — It is a subject of deep regret to many that the executive or magistracy should show such a sluggishness in enforcing the laws of the Province. It is particularly to be deplored so far as those laws relate to persons calling themselves doctors; not only our fortunes, but also our lives are in the hands of those despicable quacks. How does it happen that an Act of the session of 1815 is not acted upon? Is it because that Act is unwise, or is it because the executive does not think it of sufficient importance to put it in opperation [*sic*]? If the first, why not expunge it from the laws of the Province? If the latter, what is the use of a house of assembly at all?
>
> Perhaps, Mr. Editor, you and other respectable gentlemen living in town, who have access to, and knowledge to value the merits of those practising medicine, may not feel so much as I do the miserable situation of the country; but, Sir, if the health of the subject is not a matter of sufficient importance to rouse the morbid sensibility of those whose duty it is to administer the laws, I should imagine that in a political point of view it would be a matter of great importance to look after those quack spies who are daily inundating the Province. Those men (most brutal, generally speaking, in their manners, and in their conduct immoral in the highest degree) go from house to house like peddlers, dealing out their poisonous pills and herbs, and holding out to the gaping ignorant the advantages of a republican government.
>
> . . . .
>
> To conclude, Mr. Editor, the consequences of the present system will be, in the first place, to prevent native merit entering into the profession; secondly, those few respectable and regularly educated men whom we have amongst us will either leave the Province or get a miserable subsistence if they remain; and, lastly, though not the least, the Province will be in some degree revolutionized by those emissaries of a licentious republic.[44]

The letter is signed "Veritas," but there seems little question that its author was a physician.[45]

A stronger statute

The 1815 law was too "anemic"[46] to long remain on the statute books and it was repealed in 1818, at which time it was replaced with a more workable restrictive statute. The act of 1818[47] created a board of examiners to consist of five appointed physicians, who were to meet twice yearly at York for the purpose of conducting examinations in medicine. A certificate indicating that the applicant had successfully completed his examination, when presented to the Governor, entitled the holder to a license to practice in the province — "if the Governor be satisfied of the loyalty, integrity and good morals of the applicant." The penalty for violation of the act's provisions remained at £100 and, as was the case with previous licensing legislation, one-half of the fine was to be paid over to the informer. Once again, holders of degrees from any university within the British Empire and military surgeons were exempt, as were female midwives. In addition, the act provided that all physicians who had been practicing in the province prior to 1812 were to be given twelve months' notice of the time and place where examinations were to be held before being required to undergo an examination.[48]

The Medical Board established by the act duly convened at York in January, 1819, and immediately proceeded to examine and reject candidates. Of the sixteen applicants appearing for examination in its first year of operation, the Board failed eight.[49] The Board appears to have been even more exacting in its second year when, of twelve candidates, only four were passed.[50] By its third year of operation, only one person presented himself for examination, and he was rejected.[51] Such a policy during a period when there existed a pressing need for medical practitioners in the rapidly growing province[52] apparently led to much dissatisfaction with the unrealistic standards of the Medical Board.[53] In October, 1825, of the five candidates rejected, four were found deficient not only in pharmaceutical chemistry — a subject that could barely be regarded as necessary to the active practicing physician at the beginning of the nineteenth century and one which remained a mysterty to most — but also in classical education![54] During the five years between 1822 and 1826, according to the Board's minutes as they appear in Canniff, only nineteen applicants were accepted for practice.[55]

The Medical Act of 1827

In 1827, Upper Canada's medical act was revised and the Medical Board's compass considerably expanded. Under the terms of the new statute,[56] all prospective practitioners—except female midwives and those practicing in the military—were required to receive a license before practicing in the province. Holders of degrees from a university within the British Empire, licentiates of the Royal College of Physicians and the Royal College of Surgeons in London, and physicians who had held commissions as surgeons in the armed forces, were permitted to apply to the Governor for a license without examination. All others were required to sit the Medical Board's examination. A provision so tortuous as to be nearly impossible of fulfillment, was provided doctors who wished to avoid examination by the Board and who had been practicing in Upper Canada prior to 1812. They were required to present a certificate to that effect, signed by a magistrate, by the chairman of the quarter-sessions, and by the clerk of a district in the province. Finally, the practitioner was obliged to offer testimonials from three licensed physicians within the province, stating that the applicant was personally known to them and that he was a competent doctor.

The 1827 statute also revised the penal provisions associated with illegal practice. The maximum penalty was reduced from £100 to £25 and/or six months' imprisonment with a statute of limitations of one year. However, a reverse-onus clause was added, placing the burden of proof respecting his right to practice on the defendant.

Armed with these broader powers of examination, the Board continued to reject many of the applicants appearing before it. In October, 1831, one applicant who had two years' medical training at Dartmouth College and a diploma from the Medical Society of Jefferson County was rejected as being "deficient, so much so as not to be competent to translate a sentence from the London Pharmacopoeia."[57] A second candidate, who also had attended two years' of lectures in medicine and possessed a diploma in the subject was rejected as well.[58] The minutes of the Board for April, 1832, note that one applicant was interviewed, "but from his total ignorance of the Latin language, so highly necessary in the profession, could not proceed in his examination. The Board admonished him and recommended further study preparatory to his coming before them at any subsequent sitting."[59] Yet another applicant, possessed of a diploma from Apothecaries' Hall, was rejected, the Board finding that he was "deficient in classical knowledge and ignorant of Chymistry and Pharmacy."[60]

Latin required

In April, 1832, a circular issued by the Board specifying the requirements it would impose on prospective applicants includes the following:

> The Board . . . must hereafter require that each candidate at the commencement of his examination shall translate into English some portion of a Latin author, that they may be satisfied he has acquired a competent knowledge of a language in which the formula of medical authors and extemporaneous prescriptions of practitioners are written and from which are derived so many terms used in all the sciences with which he must be conversant.[61]

That it was serious in its unrealistic demand that practitioners know Latin is evidenced by the fact that over the following five and a half years (through 1837), fourteen candidates appear to have been rejected for no other reason than their being deficient in either a knowledge of Latin or classical knowledge in general.[62] Of these, one applicant held "a doctor's degree in medicine after four years' study"[63] and another, who "exhibited a total ignorance of the Latin language, and seemed to be as uninformed of English Grammar," was educated at the Universities of Maryland and Pennsylvania.[64] A third, from the Royal College of Surgeons, Edinburgh, was rejected because of his inability to construe a prescription written by a member of the Board.[65] Additionally, since only licentiates of the Royal College of Physicians and of the Royal College of Surgeons of London were exempt from examination to practice in Upper Canada, the Board took it upon itself to reject the applications of several candidates holding diplomas from the College of Physicians and Surgeons, Glasgow,[66] failed another applicant who was a member of the London College of Medicine and of the London Vaccine Institution of the Royal Jennerian Society,[67] and yet another applicant who held certificates from both Glasgow and Edinburgh.[68]

In an appendix to a letter directed to the Lieutenant-Governor and dated November 12, 1837, the Board summarized its activities since the beginning of 1830. It there claimed to have examined 164 candidates through October, 1837, of which 64 were rejected.[69] But, if Canniff's transcriptions of the Board's minutes are correct, these figures are deceptive. The Board did not count among those candidates rejected, applicants who were seen but whom it refused to examine further after finding some deficiency, such as a poor knowledge of

Latin. A careful analysis of the minutes indicates that, during that period, only 91 applicants passed their examinations, while the Board rejected 75. From its inception in January, 1819, to the end of 1837, the Upper Canada Medical Board considered 233 applications, rejected 111 of them, and passed 122. During that time, the population of the province increased from approximately 110,000 to almost 400,000.[70] The Board had legally licensed, at best, only one physician for each 2,400 new residents.[71]

UNLICENSED PRACTICE AND THE RISE OF HETERODOX MEDICINE

The Medical Board's onerous standards,[72] so far out of touch with the reality of conditions then prevailing in the province, only served to encourage the illegal practice of medicine. Unlicensed practitioners abounded, especially in the outlying areas,[73] where licensed doctors were either not available or could be had only at prohibitively high fees. Difficulties in enforcement were exacerbated by the unrealistic penalties associated with unlicensed practice. The £100 fine attached to violation of the medical acts of 1815 and 1818 were regarded by the more sensible as outrageous, given the nature of the "crime" committed.[74] Indeed, MacNab points out, "often no one would prosecute the offender, and if he was charged, generally he was found not guilty."[75] It was in part to encourage successful prosecutions that the penalty for illegal practice was altered in the 1827 statute to a maximum fine of £25 and/or six months' imprisonment. This change seems to have done little to discourage unlicensed practice. One historian has noted of this period that

> there are few records of any prosecutions for illegal practice, as cases would have been tried in local courts and were not recorded in any Law Registers. The colony... made many efforts to suppress quackery with legislation, but found the same difficulty in enforcement of the law. It was cheaper and easier to self-dose or go to a friendly quack, than go to a licensed doctor, who had a monopoly over prescribing. The unlicensed continued to ply their trade.[76]

Unauthorized practice

The regular profession was predictably outraged at the large number of unauthorized practitioners with whom they had to compete. Writing in the *Western Mercury* in 1832, one anonymous physician deplored the current state of the profession and called for more vigorous enforcement of the law:

> No greater imposition exists in Upper Canada than Quackery — its every-day use makes it appear tolerated by the laws of the land; it is an existing evil under which this Province has long groaned, but to which public attention should be directed. The regular practitioner meets it in every day's travel, is perplexed with its impudence, and with horror views its ravages and its influence.
>
> The character of the real Quack is the same in all countries. These persons have generally been so degraded by their views as to render themselves odious to society, or too ignorant and indolent to gain a living by any honest means....
>
> Another sort of practitioners [sic] are what may be denominated Licensed Quacks; these are men who have studied but one part of the profession and have obtained license to practise that part only. These men are generally the most impudent, and set up for the great doctor! They practise all parts of the profession without distinction, and thus the Licensed Quack grows rich by imposition and a knowledge of a small part of his profession. He will gravely tell you that 'he has his license,' and people not acquainted with the deception will take it for granted he is regularly authorized to practise physic, surgery and midwifery, when he has been licensed to practise one of these branches only.
>
> If these things are known and not remedied, we shall, ere long, be overrun by such men. The student may study a favourite branch, and in one or two years may become the *great doctor!* whilst the honest man who has devoted all his time and most of his money to obtain the necessary information, is doomed to endless defamation, indigence, and an humble walk in life. Thus impudence and ignorance triumphs over humility and education, whilst vice and roguery tramples under feet virtue and honesty.
>
> Will the public any longer allow such gross impositions? Or, will honest men suffer their rights to be thus invaded? I trust not. Would some gentleman of the law confer a favour by making known to the public by what means and with what expense we can detect these impostors and bring them to justice. For one, I am not content to acknowledge a Quack my superior or contend with him for my bread, but will, if possible, make an example of the nearest when the necessary information is obtained to accomplish it.[77]

A similar sentiment is contained in a letter to the Attorney-General of Upper Canada dated the same year and signed by three of the leading physicians of Niagara:

> Physicians of proper attainments were seldom to be met, being thinly scattered about the country surrounded by empirics (licensed or not) who generally succeeded better than the former in obtaining practice, because they would adopt habit and cunning that respectable men could not think of; that these were, and continue to be facts, we at present barely assert, but if proof be required we are ready to furnish it abundantly.
>
> We could not any otherwise account for this state of the profession than by attributing it to a defect in the Laws, and much reflection since has confirmed us in the opinion.[78]

The authors then proposed the replacement of the existing statute with one creating a College comprising all licensed physicians in the province to both enforce the law against unlicensed practitioners and to discipline its own membership for acts "derogatory to the profession."[79]

Orthodox therapy

Regular physicians indeed had cause to worry. The problems they faced had, by the 1830s, extended beyond the unwelcome competition of unlicensed practitioners to encompass heterodox theories of medical therapeutics. The established profession relied extensively on symptomatic treatment consisting, in the main, of massive bloodletting,[80] blistering, and the administration of purgatives and emetics. The most common of these, calomel (mercurous chloride)[81] and tartar emetic (tartrate of antimony), both mineral poisons, were prescribed in large doses to "cleanse the stomach and bowels." If the patient survived this regimen, the regular physician commonly dispensed arsenical compounds and opium to the debilitated victim, which, it was thought, acted as tonics.[82]

An instance of treatment

The following extracts from the diary of Jonathan Woolverton, a licensed physician practicing in Upper Canada from 1834 until his death in 1883, offer some indication of the therapeutic regimen in vogue in the 1830s among the better-educated orthodox physicians.[83] In treating a case of diarrheal infection, diagnosed by Dr. Woolverton as dysentery, he recommends that:

> Upon the first coming on of the disease, give a mild Emetic of Ipecac; to cleanse the stomach, and obviate if possible the irritability of this organ; after this exhibit a large dose of calomel to open the bowels; when the operation of the calomel was over, I would give antiseptics, and the best perhaps that we can exhibit is the burnt cork, as it not only answers all the ends of the common charcoal, but from its levity and pliability must be very congenial to the bowels; what would give us the most reason to expect beneficial results from the employment of these antiputrescent substances is that the blood which they void by stool appears to be in a dissolved, putrescent state, and after death takes place, the body in a few hours becomes gangrenous, and runs shortly into putrefaction. As the liver appears also to be disordered, I would give also in conjunction with the antiseptics, small doses of an alternative medicine in combination with opium.[84]

And for a child suffering from "Hydrocephalus" — the symptoms described are, in fact, similar to those of tuberculous meningitis — Woolverton noted: "Blisters, tort ointment [sic], mercurial ointment, drastic purgatives, were the remedial measures."[85]

In opposition to the therapeutics of orthodox medicine — known as "heroic therapy" — there arose in the first half of the nineteenth century two competing sects, eclecticism and homeopathy, whose increasing popularity was assured as long as regular practitioners continued to kill far greater numbers of their patients than they cured.[86]

Thomsonianism

The principal theoretician of eclectic medicine was Samuel Thomson, originally a New Hampshire farmer who early developed an interest in botanical medicine. In 1813, Thomson developed and patented a system of medicine, which he published in book form in 1822 under the title *New Guide to Health*. Thomsonian therapy totally repudiated the therapeutic arsenal of heroic medicine, attacked bleeding, blistering and the administration of mineral poisons as "instruments of death," and offered in its place a therapy relying exclusively on botanical remedies, steam baths, and bed-rest. Thomson's therapeutics injected much common sense into the care of the sick and ailing and provided a salutary alternative to orthodox medicine. An edition of his book was published at Hamilton in 1832,[87] and his system, easily understood by the public, appears to have become quite popular in Canada.

Canniff, at one time dean of the medical faculty at the University of Victoria and President of the Canadian Medical Association, devotes several pages of his history of the profession in Upper Canada to Thomson and his therapeutic system, in which he displays his characteristic disdain towards any method of practice deviating from the most rigid orthodoxy. He writes at one point:

> Thompson [*sic*] was, we believe a subject of the United States; but he found in Canada a somewhat fruitful field for the practice of his peculiar views of medical science, and in time, had a considerable number of followers. They were known as "Thompsonians." Not a few young Canadians, disinclined to do manual work, as their fathers had done, cast aside the home-spun clothes, donned a broadcloth suit and kid gloves, hung up a shingle and announced themselves to be "Doctors" according to the doctrine of Thompson. Little or no preparation was required for this change of occupation, and money was generally made by the change. For many years the Thompsonians practised without a license and in defiance of law. But later on they assumed the name of "Eclectics," and commanded sufficient influence to secure from Parliament the right to grant licenses to practise medicine.[88]

Homeopathy

The other sect that represented a serious threat to orthodox medicine — or allopathy, as it was called by many irregular practitioners — was homeopathy, the creation of the German physician Samuel Hahnemann.[89] Hahnemann, unlike Thomson, had a formal and rigorous medical education. Distrustful of the therapeutic benefits of bleeding, blistering, and the administration of purgatives, Hahnemann's researches led him to the novel conclusion, that the most efficacious remedy for any illness consisted in the administration of a drug that, when tested in a healthy person, produced those symptoms most closely approximating the symptomology of the ailment to be cured. This law, *similia similibus curantur,* became the foundation of homeopathic therapeutics.[90]

Far more revolutionary in its impact on the development of medical therapy was the homeopathic theory of optimal dosage. It had become a commonplace among regular physicians that prodigious doses of a medication were more effective than were smaller ones, especially in severe cases of disease. Hahnemann, on the other hand, argued that extremely attenuated doses were superior; indeed, the more attenuated, the better. He went so far as to recommend dilutions to the one-decillionth drop of the original medication. Perhaps the most significant contribution of the homeopathic system to nineteenth-century medicine, however, was its stress on the recuperative powers of the organism itself. Homeopaths advocated fresh air, proper diet, sunshine, bed rest, and personal hygiene during a period when the regular profession saw these as of little or no value. As one commentator has observed: "In his eccentric fashion, Hahnemann made one of the great discoveries of his time; he established that, given the existing state of medical knowledge, the absence of therapy was vastly superior to heroic therapy."[91]

Homeopathic medicine in North America

Homeopathy was brought to North America by a German physician, Hans Gram, in 1825. Gram, who settled in New York City, was followed by Constantine Hering, one of Hahnemann's students, and a number of Hering's colleagues a decade later.[92] The sect soon had a considerable following in the United States and became the subject of a number of attacks by leading American medical theorists. The first homeopathic physician in Ontario is reputed to have been Joseph J. Lancaster, a native Canadian who had studied allopathic medicine but became a staunch supporter of homeopathy upon becoming disillusioned with the failures of conventional therapy.[93] He was quickly joined by numbers of other homeopathic practitioners and the sect appears to have achieved a fair degree of popularity in Canada.[94]

Homeopathy was considered by many as a serious alternative to orthodox treatment, as indeed it was, and separate homeopathic boards were at one time created in both Ontario and Quebec.[95] It was assailed by the regular profession unceasingly as a particularly pernicious species of quackery and as its acceptance became more widespread, the virulence of these attacks, both upon the theory and upon its adherents, intensified. To discredit them in the eyes of the public, it was not uncommon to force homeopathic practitioners, including Dr. Lancaster, to defend themselves against charges of manslaughter, "a frequent manoeuvre on the part of the allopaths," we are told.[96] There seems no question that these attacks were motivated, in the words of one writer on Canadian medicine, "by the fact that the homeopaths were making real inroads on the earning ability of the allopaths."[97]

Increased competition

The introduction of rival therapeutic systems added to the competitive pressures faced by the established profession throughout British North America. Not only were many of the unlicensed practitioners Americans who crossed the border to set up practice in competition with licensed physicians,[98] but eclecticism and homeopathy, which were gaining in popularity, were also importations, either direct or indirect, from the United States. Additionally, Canadians studying medicine in America were doubtless struck by the situation which prevailed there. Medical schools, the great bulk of which were privately owned and operated, abounded,[99] and the prospective medical student could gain admission to even the best of them without great difficulty. Tuition was cheap and entry into the profession unrestricted, the exigencies of the marketplace alone determining which physicians would prove successful and which not. As a result, medical care — such as it was in that period — was both inexpensive and readily available throughout the United States.[100]

Large numbers of the regular profession in Canada, joined by elements of the civil administration, feared that Canadians studying medicine in America, once having witnessed the absence of restrictions that existed on its practice there, would, on returning home, be less tolerant of the licensing authorities and more sympathetic both to unlicensed practitioners and to heterodox medical theories.[101] There was a general apprehension that English-speaking Canada was a fertile breeding-ground for American principles of government from which it was necessary to protect the populace. This concern was especially strong throughout the first half of the century and was aggravated by the rebellion of 1837. In the medical profession, anti-Americanism was associated with support for the licensing authorities and the government they represented.[102] It was felt that the establishment of Canadian medical schools would do away with the need for Canadians to study medicine in America while at the same time allowing the licensing boards to demand of their applicants more rigorous training than could be acquired through an apprenticeship system.

Medical education in Upper Canada

Thus, John Strachan, that implacable antagonist of everything American and steadfast enemy of all uncoerced relationships wherever they might appear, wrote the Lieutenant-Governor in 1826 on the subject of medical education in Upper Canada:

> In regard to the profession of Medicine, now becoming of great importance in the Province, it is melancholy to think that more than three-fourths of the present practitioners have been educated or attended lectures in the United States; and it is to be presumed that many of them are inclined towards that country. But in this colony there is no provision whatever for attaining medical knowledge, and those who make choice of that profession must go to a foreign country to acquire it.[103]

A similar sentiment was expressed by the Upper Canada Medical Board in a memorial forwarded to the Governor-General in his capacity as chancellor of the University of King's College in 1842:

> Among the numerous classes of young men whose preliminary education has been completed in that excellent institution, Upper Canada College, many of course are destined for the learned professions. In those of law and divinity no difficulty exists in following out the full completion of the necessary studies at home. But in the profession of medicine it is different; the student must resort to a foreign country to obtain his object, and unfortunately the neighbouring United States affords the only opportunity within his reach of acquiring the necessary information with economy. There, it is admitted, he may attain all the knowledge that is desired, but surely the necessity of resorting to such a source of instruction is to be deprecated, for no other result can be anticipated than the acquirement of those democratic principles which are so interwoven with the system there pursued.[104]

The rebellion of 1837 exacerbated the fear of American influence, both on the profession and on the public as consumers of medical care. At the same time, renewed efforts were made by the regular profession for passage of a stronger medical act.[105] In October, 1838, the Medical Board drafted a petition, which was then circulated to the profession, calling on the provincial parliament "to cause such enactments to be made as in your wisdom may seem best fitted for placing the profession upon a more honourable and favourable footing than it has hitherto stood in this Province."[106] The anxieties of the government respecting the large numbers of Americans practicing in Upper Canada in defiance of the law were certain to have been aroused by the petition's opening paragraph:

The petition of the members of the Medical Board, and of certain other licensed practitioners of medicine, humbly shewth:

That the law now in force in this Province, regulating the practice of the medical profession, and for the prevention of persons practising without license, has been found very inadequate. That of late years the number of persons practising without license or qualification has much increased, chiefly by the influx of empirics from the neighbouring States, causing great danger to the health of the community, and in some instances the loss of valuable lives; being alike detrimental to the peace and tranquility of the country, and degrading and humiliating to the honourable and useful profession of medicine.[107]

Medical practice and politics

The link between illegal practice and radical politics was made explicit by the Toronto *Patriot,* in its issue of October 12, 1838. The profession's petition was there reprinted and the paper editorialized:

Quacks are an intolerable nuisance in any and every country, but especially in this, where empiricism and radicalism go hand in hand. It is a monstrous grievance that our Government should allow the Province to swarm, as it does, with these pestilent vagabonds, every one of whom is a Yankee loafer, and makes his occupation a cloak for inculcating Jacobinical principles. All know how numerous have been the self-styled 'doctors' implicated in the rebellion, but perhaps all may not know that they were almost one and all Yankee Quacks. We are truly glad to see that the Medical Board are active in setting about means to annihilate the dirty birds, nest and all; we trust the Legislature will second their efforts.[108]

The Board's petition had the desired effect;[109] in 1839, a new and far-reaching medical law, placing full powers to govern the medical profession into the hands of the profession itself, was enacted to replace the act of 1827.

LOWER CANADA'S MEDICAL ACT OF 1831

Upper Canada, of course, was not the only area of British North America to attempt to impose restrictions on the practice of medicine. Lower Canada had inherited the medical act of 1788, and district medical boards appointed by the governor were eventually established under its terms at Quebec and Montreal. The standards applied by these boards to candidates appearing before them, although stringent enough to act as an effective restraint on large-scale entry into the profession, do not appear to have been as strict as those applied in Upper Canada.[110] One physician, decrying the licensing policies of the province's boards, complained of being forced to witness

> the health and lives of the inhabitants of many of the most populous and wealthy sections of the province, generally at the mercy of a sordid class of men, totally devoid of education, German Felchers (dressers and barbers, formerly attached to the Hessian troops and their descendants) and other nondescript M.D.'s from the cheap colleges of our neighbours, wholly unacquainted with the most obvious principles.[111]

The boards' criteria for licensing were apparently somewhat looser with respect to those applicants intending to practice in the rural areas of the province:

> But this deplorable deficiency in medical qualifications may, in a good measure, be attributable to the three or four antiquated gentlemen then constituting a Board of Examiners (I allude particularly to the then capital, Quebec), who, in the plenitude of their wisdom, only exacted inferior professional acquirements in the candidates for country practice! as if the lives of Her Majesty's subjects in the rural districts were not as valuable as those in cities and towns.[112]

Yet, despite the profession's complaints that the licensing requirements were lax, a great deal of unlicensed practice continued to prevail throughout Lower Canada.[113]

The profession in Quebec

In 1823, at the suggestion of Dr. William Robertson, the governor, Lord Dalhousie, in an effort to improve the quality of the province's examiners—and to further consolidate the dominant position of the English-speaking profession in Quebec—reconstituted the Montreal medical board to comprise five members, all on the staff of the Montreal General Hospital and founders of the newly-created Montreal Medical Institution.[114] The established profession had unsuccessfully attempted to replace the 1788 law in 1820 and again in 1822, and demands to modify the act increased after the restructuring of the Montreal board in 1823.[115] A substantial portion of the French-speaking profession and certain members of the public objected to the fact that the membership of the Montreal licensing board and the staff of the province's only medical school were one and the same.[116] Additionally, pressures for reform were brought to bear by the profession in Quebec City, which had organized itself into a formal association in 1826. In November of that year, a general meeting of the established profession in Quebec City was called for the purpose of creating what was to become the first medical society in Canada.[117] Heagerty reports that "from its inception, active steps were taken by the Society to standardize the practice of medicine in Canada."[118] Thus, in 1830, the Quebec Medical Society petitioned the government of Lower Canada for a new law that would more effectively restrict entry into the profession and more adequately deal with the large number of unlicensed physicians practicing in the province. The petition stated in part

> That experience has fully shewn that, the existing Laws, with respect to the practice of Physic and Surgery in this Province, are totally inefficient to repress the abuses which in defiance of the Laws, to the great injury of the Public, and the prejudice of the Profession, are increasing to an alarming degree.[119]

The result of this agitation was passage of the Medical Act of 1831.[120]

Provisions of the 1831 act

The provisions of the 1831 act were somewhat more extensive than those of its predecessor. It called for the establishment of boards of examiners, each comprised of twelve physicians, to meet in both Quebec and Montreal. Examiners were to be elected by the province's licensed physicians resident in Quebec and Montreal and meeting for that purpose in each of the cities.[121] The boards were empowered to examine all candidates for a license to practice. Physicians and surgeons commissioned in the armed services, holders of medical degrees from any college, university, or other institution teaching publicly—provided the course of study undergone was at least five years—and all physicians previously licensed in the province, were exempt from sitting the examination, but were required to have their credentials certified by the board. All other candidates had to undergo an examination after having satisfied the board that they were at least twenty-one years old and had undergone at least five years of medical study, either as an apprentice to a licensed physician in Lower Canada or as a student in some medical school. Additionally, prospective students of medicine were obligated under the act to undergo a preliminary examination indicating they knew Latin and that they were qualified to begin the study of medicine. The governor was empowered to grant a license upon the examining board's certification of the applicant's medical credentials. Female midwives were exempt from the law. Practicing without the requisite license was punishable by a fine of £10 for the first offense, £20 for the second, and £30 for each subsequent offense.

Strict interpretation of the statute

The behavior of the licensing boards created under the new act was occasionally highly arbitrary. The Montreal board immediately proceeded to interpret the statute with an inordinate degree of literalness. Thus, section five of the act, which required applicants who had studied medicine under an apprenticeship system to have "performed a regular and continued apprenticeship of at least five years," was used by the board to reject the credentials of a candidate who had interrupted his apprenticeship for one season. The board interpreted the law as barring from consideration any candidate whose studies had been at all interrupted![122] Section six was similarly construed; it provided that graduates of any university or college of surgeons or of any medical school or institution providing public instruction were exempt from examination. This, if the candidate's degree were obtained "after a course of Medical study, performed in such University, College or Medical Institution, in conformity to the rules thereof, and after five years study at least." The Montreal board rendered this passage to mean that the applicant must have spent all five years in the same institution.[123] One candidate who had begun his studies at the Montreal Medical Institution and completed them at the University of Vermont — the Montreal Medical Institution, which in 1829 became the medical faculty of McGill University, was not yet empowered to grant degrees — refused to submit to an examination and consequently was not awarded a license to practice. To confuse matters further, the same candidate then appeared before the Quebec board and was granted a license to practice forthwith.[124]

McGill's first graduate

This situation reached a ludicrous extreme with respect to the first graduate of the McGill medical faculty.[125] In late 1831, the faculty had petitioned the governor, Lord Aylmer, for authority to grant degrees, noting that, as things then stood, candidates for degrees in medicine had either to travel abroad, "an expense too great to many, or to the United States, where they are in danger of imbibing principles inimical to our Government and our Institutions."[126] The petition, designed as it was to appeal to the political fears of the government, was quickly granted, and in July of the following year the medical faculty was empowered to confer degrees.[127] In 1833, William L. Logie was duly awarded Canada's first degree in medicine, having studied at the Montreal Medical Institution both before and after its transition to the medical faculty of McGill.

When Logie applied to the Montreal board in July, he was refused a license on the basis of his degree and was ordered to undergo an examination, despite having completed five years of study and been awarded a degree in medicine. Logie refused to sit the examination and appealed to the courts. It was only after much litigation that the board was ordered to grant Logie a license to practice in October, 1834. Rather than bring themselves to comply with the court's decision to license a graduate from a school that had technically not remained the same institution during Logie's years of study, the board skipped its regular meeting of January, 1835, and postponed its April meeting to May. At that point, it finally capitulated and began granting licenses to graduates of McGill without examination.[128]

Section twenty-six of the 1831 act provided that the statute was to remain in force only until May 1, 1837. It was not renewed and, despite the fact that the 1788 statute had been repealed by its preamble, the provisions of the old act once again came into force in the province.[129] The 1788 act remained in effect in Lower Canada until 1847. In any case, the boards established under both the 1788 act and its successor do not appear to have been effective either in enforcing the provisions against unlicensed practice or in restricting the number of practitioners in the province to the degree desired. Dr. von Iffland was only echoing the complaints of most regular members of the profession when he wrote in 1845 that if the old boards added little to the respectability of the profession in the rural districts, the elective ones contributed largely to increase the number of its members, and so far provided the seignorial parishes with practitioners as to endanger the subsistence of both the licensed and *unlicensed idols of the habitans* [*sic*].[130]

THE PROFESSION IN THE MARITIMES

Unlike Upper and Lower Canada, neither Nova Scotia nor New Brunswick had seriously attempted to restrict entry into the medical profession until the second half of the nineteenth century. New Brunswick had enacted a licensing law in 1816,[131] and Nova Scotia in 1828,[132] but the only penalty associated with practicing in violation of these statutes was that the practitioner was prohibited from suing for the recovery of fees.[133] Indeed, the New Brunswick law appears to have been taken so lightly that even those physicians composing the examining board appointed by the Lieutenant-Governor did not bother to take out licenses.[134]

It is possible that the medical profession in the Maritimes, originally comprising such a large proportion of American loyalists,[135] was less fearful of the possibilities of competition. The population of these areas remained small enough to act as a natural market barrier to the influx of large numbers of physicians emigrating from the United States.[136] Additionally, the loyalists had early secured a social and economic ascendancy and an informal monopoly of the professions in the major centres of population[137] that probably made restrictive legislation unnecessary. To the extent that practitioners lacking a formal education operated in the area, they seem to have confined their operations to the sparsely-populated sections of the country.[138] Finally, anti-American sentiment in the Maritimes was far less intense than in either Upper or Lower Canada, and American institutions and habits of mind were occasionally held up as models for emulation rather than as threats to established authority.[139]

The American example

These factors all appear to have contributed to the fact that both New Brunswick and Nova Scotia followed the pattern set in the various American states that had attempted to regulate the practice of medicine. Although twenty states and the District of Columbia had some form of licensing prior to 1850, these laws were poorly enforced and short-lived. Five states, including Maine, attached no penalty to practicing without a license, and six others, including Massachusetts, provided that, at worst, unlicensed physicians could not sue for the recovery of fees. Where stiffer laws were enacted, they appear not to have been enforced at all.[140] It was not until the last quarter of the century that the medical profession in the United States was successful in moving towards effective legislation to restrict entry into the profession.[141]

The American example was, of course, never followed in either Ontario or Quebec. Sir William Osler, in attacking the notion that the practice of medicine should be left to the exigencies of the market, noted some years later that the model for the regulation of medical practice in Canada was the system that traditionally prevailed in Great Britain.[142] Leaving aside the truth or falsity of this claim, certainly the model described by Osler did not apply to the Maritimes, which patterned its legislation after that of the American states until well after Confederation.

CREATION OF THE COLLEGE OF PHYSICIANS AND SURGEONS OF UPPER CANADA, 1839

Established physicians in Upper Canada were fortunate in their endeavors to gain passage of a comprehensive statute governing the medical profession in 1839. In that year, the provincial legislature enacted a law creating a College of Physicians and Surgeons of Upper Canada.[143] The College, comprising all licensed physicians in the province, was to be directed by its fellows—the first of whom were stipulated in the act as consisting of the same group of physicians as had composed the medical board that it replaced. All physicians wishing to henceforth practice in Upper Canada were required to sit an examination set by the fellows of the College, excepting holders of diplomas from universities within the British Empire, members and licentiates of any college or faculty of physicians, or of surgeons in the United Kingdom,[144] and physicians possessing a military commission. A pass on the examination or proof of one's credentials entitled the holder to a license to practice and to membership in the College.

More significant were the penal provisions of the statute, whereby the procedures for prosecuting unlicensed practitioners were greatly simplified. The act provided that trials could take place before any justice of the peace and conviction was obtainable on the basis of the

testimony of one witness only. The fine for illegal practice was reduced to the more realistic but still substantial sum of £5, which was
payable to the College. Female midwives were exempt from all provisions of the act.

The profession was delighted with the statute. The law was interpreted to entitle the College to legally take upon itself the prosecution
of unlicensed physicians and to appropriate any portion of the fines
received, or any other of its funds, to prosecuting offenders.[145] The
fellows of the College lost no time in formally thanking Mr. Henry
Sherwood, a member of the provincial legislature, for his tireless
efforts in gaining passage of the bill.[146] Beyond a vote of thanks, Mr.
Sherwood was soon thereafter rewarded with the position of solicitor
for the College.[147]

Establishment of a degree-granting medical school

The College proceeded almost immediately to agitate for the creation
of a degree-granting medical school in the province. The advantages
of a school located in Upper Canada with the power to grant degrees
in medicine were several. Both the preliminary requirements for entering upon the study of medicine and the length, composition, and level
of difficulty of the medical curriculum—even, to some extent, the size
of the entering class—would be under the direct and immediate
control of the established profession in Upper Canada; indeed, under
subsequent medical laws enacted in the various provinces, such decisions were placed directly under the statutory control of the various
boards of medical examiners. The province's licensing authorities
would thus be provided ample excuse to reject the graduates and licentiates of other schools and licensing bodies if they were judged as not
measuring up to the standards operating within the medical schools of
the province. The establishment of an institution providing instruction
in medicine over which the local profession had control became an
extremely effective method of restricting the number of licenses
granted to graduates of out-of-province schools, and of limiting the
number of practitioners in the province.

Undoubtedly mindful of the value of a provincial degree-granting
school of medicine,[148] the College petitioned the governor in May,
1839, for the establishment of a faculty of medicine at King's College.
It invoked the honor of the profession, and included the obligatory
warning respecting the danger to Canadians forced to undertake their
studies in the United States.[149] So strongly did the College—"the
guardians of the medical profession in Upper Canada," as it referred

to itself [150] — support the creation of a medical school in the province that it offered to defray the costs of a medical faculty conjointly with the Council of King's College.[151]

Suppression of unlicensed practice

The establishment of a medical faculty in Upper Canada was not the only occupation of the College, however. It put great effort into attempting to suppress the activities of unlicensed practitioners in the province, going so far as to designate one of its officers as "collector of the College" with the duty

> to collect evidence and lay information before the proper authorities against all persons practising any branch of the profession who have not been legally licensed.... The said officer shall receive the sum of £2 [s]10 as a remuneration for his trouble, on all convictions arising from his information, and... he shall receive the sum of one and a half per cent. on all other fines collected.[152]

In addition, it ordered its secretary to inform the Mayor of Toronto that unlicensed practitioners were operating within the boundaries of the city and to request that proper steps be taken to suppress these physicians.[153] The College even went so far as to complain of the appointment of surgeons of militia who had not been properly licensed. In July, 1839, it resolved:

> That as several instances of the appointment of persons not qualified by law to practise the profession of medicine, to be Surgeons and Assistant-Surgeons of Militia, has come to the knowledge of the College of Physicians and Surgeons, the Secretary be therefore requested to inform His Excellency the Lieutenant-Governor through his Civil Secretary, of the fact, that such steps may be taken by His Excellency as may be necessary to prevent the continuance of a practice alike derogatory to the profession and injurious to the public service.[154]

One thing the College does not seem to have done with any great avidity is license new physicians. Between its first meeting of May 13, 1839, and its last, in January, 1841, the College admitted no more than seventeen new members,[155] thirteen of them by examination. Of these thirteen, three were diplomates of the Royal Faculty of Physicians and Surgeons, Glasgow, one, a member of the Royal College of Surgeons, London, and another, a diplomate of the Royal College of

Surgeons, Edinburgh.[156] Four applicants were found unqualified and two others, both diplomates of the Royal College of Surgeons, London, in the one case refused to sit, and in the other, failed, the examinations given them in medicine, and declined their licenses in surgery.[157] During that period, the population of the province increased by approximately 35,000.[158]

Disallowance

To the great consternation of the established profession in Upper Canada, the medical act of 1839 proved to be short-lived. Indeed, the College's treatment of British licentiates contributed substantially to its demise. In 1840, the Royal College of Surgeons, London, petitioned the Imperial government to disallow the act and they were joined in this view by the British Solicitor-General.[159] The minutes of the provincial College contain a summary of the arguments for disallowance prepared by a committee of the College struck to consider the issue:

> Your Committee find that the proposed disallowance of the Act of Incorporation of this College has been founded on the following grounds:
> 1st. A petition from the Royal College of Surgeons of London, which recites that part of 18th George II, cap. 15 [1745], which confers on the members of that body the right to practise freely and without restraint the art and science of surgery throughout all and every part of His Majesty's dominions.
> 2nd. This petition represents that this Act (of Incorporation) confers on the College powers greater than any ever granted to any existing body or college, that such powers are not clear and defined, and that several clauses of the Act infringe the rights and privileges conferred by the Charter of the London College of Surgeons.
> 3rd. The opinion of the [British] Attorney and Solicitor-General, viz., that several provisions of the Act encroach on the privileges of the College and of several other bodies in this country [Great Britain], and have a tendency to establish a monopoly which might be found highly inconvenient to the inhabitants of that Province.[160]

The College's response

The provincial College immediately responded to these objections in great detail. Of some interest is their reply to the fears expressed by the

Attorney and Solicitor-General respecting the dangers inherent in the
1839 act of creating a monopoly of physicians' services within Upper
Canada. There are few instances of such bald disingenuousness and
evasion as are contained in the College's rejoinder to these charges:

> Section 3. The opinion of the Attorney and Solicitor-General,
> which may be divided into two parts: ...
> 2nd. That they 'have a tendency to establish a monopoly in
> Upper Canada, which might be found inconvenient to the inhabi-
> tants of that Province.'
> Your Committee can hardly imagine that this idea could have
> entered into the mind of any person who had looked into the pro-
> visions of the Act.
> If this College had a discretionary power of withholding or
> granting licenses *in every case,* such a possibility might occur. But
> as it is absolutely imperative that a license shall be granted to any
> or everyone exhibiting a diploma, license, commission or warrant,
> as described in the Act, and as every licentiate has it in his power
> to become a member at any time he may choose without the
> College having the discretionary power to refuse him, it is an
> absolute impossibility that any professional monopoly can arise
> out of this Act.
> But if by the word 'monopoly,' allusion is made to the power
> granted to the Fellows to augment their number by election from
> among their members, it remains to be shown how... this can
> produce the least 'inconvenience to the inhabitants of this
> Province.'
> Your Committee would ask, suppose that the Fellows be dis-
> posed to follow the example of the Council of the London College
> of Surgeons and make the College a close [*sic*] corporation, could
> that, under the existing Act, confine to their body the exercise of
> professional talent and information, so as to prejudice the health
> or interests of the community at large?
> The warm support which this Act received from the most re-
> spectable and influential portion of both branches of the Legisla-
> ture, shows that they did not apprehend that the community at
> large could suffer any serious inconvenience under it.[161]

The objections of the College were unavailing. On December 28, 1840,
the Lieutenant-Governor communicated to the College that a dispatch
from the Secretary of State for the Colonies informed him that the act
under which the College had been created had been disallowed.[162]

The provincial College's defense

On one point the provincial College's defense appears to have been correct. If the 1839 statute were to be disallowed on the grounds offered, why, then, had the medical acts previously enacted in the province not been struck down for the same reasons? Although the Colonial Office traditionally possessed veto power over colonial legislation, it had disallowed none of the earlier acts regulating the practice of medicine in British North America.[163] It is true that with the passage of the Colonial Laws Validity Act in 1865, the legal relationship between Britain and her colonies was altered and the broad authority hitherto accorded the Colonial Office to review colonial legislation was restricted. After 1865, only those provisions of colonial laws repugnant to an imperial statute extending "by express words or necessary intendment" to the particular colony or the colonies in general could be held void and inoperative.[164] But the medical act of 1839 could as easily have been disallowed under the Colonial Laws Validity Act as by action of the Colonial Office. In fact, it was under the terms of the Colonial Laws Validity Act that a British Columbia ordinance of 1867,[165] was held repugnant to an imperial statute[166] granting physicians and surgeons registered in Britain the right to practice anywhere within the Empire. (This law required a certain level of education of all physicians wishing to register as practitioners of medicine in the colony.) Yet, despite the authority of the government in London to disallow any medical act passed in Canada before 1931,[167] the Upper Canada medical act of 1839 and the British Columbia ordinance of 1867 were the only laws regulating the practice of medicine enacted in the British colonies of North America that were ever struck down by the Imperial government.

Chapter 2

The Period from 1840 to Confederation

THE PROFESSION IN CANADA WEST IN THE 1840s

With the disallowance of the 1839 statute, the provisions of the 1827 act once again came into force in Upper Canada, and its revived medical board continued in operation for another quarter of a century.

In the wake of the rebellions of 1837 and the report of Lord Durham, the act of union of Upper and Lower Canada passed the Imperial Parliament in July, 1840,[1] and the union of the two provinces was brought into force on February 10, 1841. Because of the joining of the two separate provinces, it was thought expedient to enact a statute at the first session of the united parliament permitting all practitioners of medicine licensed in either Upper or Lower Canada to practice in either area without penalty.[2] The previously distinct provinces, now commonly designated Canada East and Canada West, continued to operate their own licensing boards throughout the period of union, and the provincial parliament often enacted separate legislation for each area.[3] Certainly with respect to legislation regulating the practice of medicine — with but the one exception of the act of 1841, permitting licensed physicians to move freely from one section of Canada to the other — the unification of the two provinces might as well have never occurred.

The profession in both parts of the united province continued to agitate for stronger legislation. In Upper Canada — more properly, Canada West — numerous attempts were made to re-establish a College of Physicians and Surgeons and bills to that effect were presented in the legislature in 1845, 1846, 1849, 1851, and 1860. In addition, established physicians bombarded the government with a substantial number of petitions demanding more effective laws restricting entry into the profession. These petitions proved unavailing and the law under which the practice of medicine was regulated in Canada West remained unchanged until 1865.[4]

King's College Medical School

Established physicians were more successful in their demands for the creation of a medical faculty at King's College.[5] In September, 1843, a committee of the University was struck to establish a medical school, and in November of that year, six physicians were appointed professors in the various branches of medical study. The first session of the new medical faculty began on January 15, 1844.[6] It is instructive to quote from the report of the medical committee respecting the requirements to be instituted at the University for a degree in medicine:

> The following shall be the medical requirements for a student presenting himself at the final examination for his degree: A certificate that he has attained the age of twenty-one years, that he has passed five years in acquaintance of medical knowledge, three of which must have been occupied in attendance on medical lectures in schools recognized by the University, and one, at least, in the Medical School of this University. That he shall produce certificates of attendance on the following lectures and hospital practice: Chemistry, one course of six months; Anatomy and Physiology, two courses of six months; Medicine, two courses of six months; Surgery, two courses of six months; Materia Medica and Pharmacy, one course of six months; Midwifery and Diseases of Women and Children, one course of six months; that he has attended for, at least, eighteen months on the Medical and Surgical practice of an hospital, containing not less than eighty beds, twelve months of which shall be during winter sessions, when lectures on Clinical Medicine and Surgery will be delivered.[7]

In contrast, the requirements for a degree in most American medical schools at that time, including many of the better ones, specified attendance at two four-month terms (comprising a curriculum similar to that specified by King's College) and study under a preceptor for three years, these three years to *include* the eight months of formal instruction.[8] And even these requirements were commonly not strictly enforced; a survey of thirty medical schools undertaken by the American Medical Association in 1849 showed that only four schools required proof of a three-year apprenticeship, nineteen others required certification of at least *some* apprenticeship, without specifying the length of time required, and seven others did not require any proof of apprenticeship at all.[9] Additionally, most schools in the United States did not preclude a student from taking both four-month terms in the same calendar year.[10] It was thus theoretically possible to gain a medical degree from a few schools in one year, and even at the best of them, a degree in medicine took no more than three years.

Exacting standards

The requirements established at King's College—in 1850, the school was renamed the University of Toronto—for a degree in medicine were totally incongruous with those of American universities during the period. Yet the medical board of Canada West soon incorporated the faculty's curriculum requirements as part of its examination of all applicants wishing to practice in that portion of the province.[11] And, lest practitioners with lesser credentials attempt to evade the authority of the board by applying for a license in Canada East and then setting themselves up in practice in Canada West under the terms of the 1841 act, the board corresponded with the medical boards in Montreal and Quebec "on the subject of the institution of a uniform system of examination for candidates for certificates."[12]

Between the re-establishment of the medical board of Canada West in 1841 and the end of 1849, 137 candidates applied for licenses to practice. Of these, 40 percent of the applicants were rejected. The board's minutes during this period seldom provide the reasons why a candidate was refused a license, but an account of its meeting of July, 1845, might be indicative. It is there noted that only one of six candidates passed his examination, and of the five that failed, "four were rejected for ignorance of the classics. One of the rejected was an M.D. of Jefferson Medical College, and another, an M.R.C.S. of Edinburgh."[13] The board was equally severe in its attitude towards applicants at its next meeting in October. The minutes note that "the new broom continued to sweep clean, as all the candidates, five in number, were rejected. One was an M.D. of the Willoughby University, in the State of Ohio."[14] During the decade of the 1840s, the medical board of Canada West accepted only 84 candidates for licensure. During that same period, the population of the area increased by over 290,000,[15] providing a ratio of newly-licensed physicians to new residents of 1:3,450. Given these figures, it is little wonder that large numbers of unlicensed doctors continued to practice throughout the country.

CANADA EAST AND THE MEDICAL ACT OF 1847

The number of medical schools operating in Canada continued to multiply in the 1840s. In 1843, the same year as the inauguration of the medical faculty at King's College and the re-establishment of Dr. John Rolph's medical school in Toronto, the Ecole de Médecine et de Chirurgie was established at Montreal; the medical faculty of McGill had, since its founding, provided instruction exclusively in English

and the Ecole de Médecine was created to meet the needs of franco-
phones wishing to study medicine in Canada East. Five years later, in
1848, a second French-language medical school, the Incorporated
School of Medicine of the City of Quebec, began offering courses in
Quebec City, and in April, 1854, was reorganized as the medical faculty of the newly-created Laval University.[16] With the establishment
of the Upper Canada School of Medicine at Toronto in 1850 (soon to
become the faculty of medicine of Trinity College), no fewer than six
medical schools were operating in the united province by mid-century.

This proliferation of schools offering instruction in medicine was
viewed with some alarm by the profession. Physicians were especially
fearful that these new schools might be raised to the level of universities, either by Royal charter or by affiliation. Holders of medical
degrees from universities within the British Empire were, under the
provisions of the medical acts of both Canada West and Canada East,
exempt from examination by the licensing authorities; they were permitted to enter practice simply by having their educational credentials
endorsed by the appropriate medical board. In consequence, the established profession agitated for new legislation that would empower
the medical boards not only to regulate entry into medical practice via
examination but also to exercise control over the study of medicine.

Medical education

Thus, in commenting on the propriety of the provisions concerning
medical study contained in a proposed medical act to govern both
areas of the province, introduced in the legislature in 1845,[17] the
editor of the *British American Journal* gave voice to the feelings of the
established profession throughout Canada, albeit in somewhat sancti-
monious terms, when he observed:

> Should not the preparatory studies of those who propose devoting
> themselves to such important objects, be a matter of deep solic-
> itude? The laws of Canada provide for no such precautionary
> and prudential training; and it becomes the bounden duty of the
> Government, anxious for the welfare and happiness of its
> subjects, to enact laws to supply the desideratum. The existing
> Medical Boards of the Province have no *legal power* to regulate
> the *education* of candidates for license. The respective Acts of
> Canada East and Canada West, under which they are constituted,
> distinctly define their duties, which consist simply in the *examina-*

tion of candidates, and we maintain that they have nothing whatever to do with the *mode* in which the knowledge of the candidate has been obtained, nor even with his *age.* It is high time that this evil should be removed, and that these crude and imperfect Acts should be superseded by another, suitable to the exigency of the case, and more consonant with the progress of science. If young men desire to adopt the profession of medicine, and to engage in its practical duties, an intimate acquaintance with its principles should be enforced upon them. Medical education, then, will be found to constitute an important feature of the Bill.[18]

Not only must the applicant have successfully completed the examination set him by the medical board but, should he hold a degree in medicine or not, the mode of education and the age of the candidate are now offered as relevant criteria in determining whether a license should be granted! How these criteria are "consonant with the progress of science," we are not told.

The Ecole de Médecine

The 1845 bill having failed of passage, another measure, applying solely to Canada East, was introduced in the provincial legislature the following year. However, one of its clauses met with the strong opposition of the Ecole de Médecine in Montreal. Had the bill been enacted, the Ecole's diplomas would no longer have been recognized by the licensing authorities as exempting its graduates from examination. The bill provided that only diplomates or degree-holders from "some University, College, or School of Medicine incorporated by Royal Charter" were so exempt, and the Ecole de Médecine was incorporated not by royal charter but by an act of the provincial parliament. The Ecole sought to alter the language of the bill, but was bitterly attacked by a substantial segment of the profession in Canada East and particularly by its English-speaking members. Dr. Archibald Hall, the editor of the *British American Journal,* "whose caustic pen," we are told, "was never more fiery than when it was defending professional rights,"[19] devoted a lengthy editorial to denouncing the Ecole's modest request as destructive of the whole licensing system in Canada East and, in the process, supplied in clear and unambiguous language the true reasons behind the profession's ceaseless demands for restrictive legislation. "We lay it down in the first place, as an axiom," Dr. Hall observed at one point, that the more general and substantial the preliminary acquirements of a candidate, the more solid the professional education which he receives is rendered, the greater the impediments thrown in the way of acquiring degrees or diplomas, the more stable, elevated, and enlightened will become the general character of the profession of which he is to become a member. This we lay down as an axiom, upon which every step of legislation for medical education should be based, and which should be steadily kept in view. If young men are admitted to the study of medicine with improperly trained and educated minds, rendering them incapable of receiving, or profiting by, scientific truths, and if easy access be afforded to the acquisition of degrees or diplomas, the character of the profession *will surely deteriorate.* That the latter will become an inevitable and certain consequence of a multiplicity of interested licensing boards to a very limited population, and that the former is an equally legitimate consequence of an opposite state of affairs, facts based on the medical history of nations will abundantly testify.

....

What shall we say of the United States, where the free trade principle in medical teaching, has run riot; where the cry of "no monopoly" has ever been the order of the day, where Universities granting *ad practicandum* degrees have sprung up, and are daily springing up like mushrooms. What, we ask, has been the effect on the profession there? ... Are we asked whether similar consequences would follow here, if the Montreal School of Medicine obtained the power of granting *ad practicandum* diplomas? The question is a delicate one, but we will meet it. *We* would not say that similar abuses, and similar consequences to the character of the profession, would positively follow the delegation of the power sought for, but *who could say that they would not.* It is not too much to state, that we are men of like passions, sentiments, and feelings, with those of the United States, and that by similar actuating causes, we would not be dissimilarly influenced.

....

In thus exposing the dangers to the best interests of the profession, which will certainly follow the concession of the power demanded by the School of Medicine, our observations have been dictated by no special feelings of hostility to that body. As long as they did well we let them alone; indeed, we have not breathed their name in previous pages of the Journal; and this silence would have been still further prolonged until some cause for praise was found, or reason for censure, as in the present case;

but it could scarcely be expected that our silence would be longer
maintained, when they are endeavouring to sacrifice what we certainly consider the best and truest interests of the profession on
the altar of their own selfish and paltry ambition.[20]

The effect of the controversy was to postpone passage of any new
medical bill, for which the *British American Journal* took much of the
credit.[21]

Renewed attempts to gain stronger legislation

The established members of the profession in Canada East had meanwhile attempted to organize a medical association in 1845,[22] and the
area's leading practitioners met again at Quebec in September, 1846. It
was there recommended that the various district medical societies submit for the consideration of their membership a substitute medical
bill, incorporating the profession in Canada East into a College of
Physicians and Surgeons.[23] At a subsequent meeting at Trois Rivières,
held the following month, the established profession,

> while it deeply deplores the inadequacy of the existing laws, for
> regulating the Medical Profession in this section of the Province
> of Canada, both as regards the education of intending members,
> or the protection of those duly licensed to practise the same [felt
> confident that it could] devise ways and means by which such
> difficulties may be obviated, and the Profession of Medicine
> made to assume that position to which it is entitled among the
> other learned professions.[24]

It was there resolved to petition the legislature, that

> based on the inadequacy of the existing laws to regulate the prac-
> tice of Medicine, Surgery and Midwifery, in this section of the
> Province: to establish a certain and fixed course of study pre-
> viously to obtaining license to practice these branches.... It
> shall pray for the repeal of all the existing acts or portions of acts re-
> ferring to these subjects; and it shall further pray for an Act of
> Incorporation, by which the persons, whose names are appended
> to the said petition, shall be embodied and incorporated into a
> College, to be styled, "The College of Physicians and Surgeons of
> Canada East," and that the said persons constitute the original
> Corporation of the said College....

> That power be granted to the Corporation to legislate in all matters affecting the Medical Profession, whether in reference to education, practice, the protection of its members from inroads of unlicensed practitioners, the regulation of the practice of midwifery, the supervision of druggists' establishments, and the protection of the public health, in regard to Medical Police and Hygiene.[25]

Inadequacies of the existing law

The medical establishment in Canada East viewed the need for a stronger medical act as pressing. The area was still operating under the medical statute of 1788, which provided that all holders of university degrees in medicine — without regard to where the degree was obtained or what requirements had been met for its award — were entitled to a license.[26] Additionally, the penalty provisions of the act were so onerous — a £20 fine for the first offense, increasing to £100 and three months' imprisonment for a third offense — that conviction for illegal practice was virtually impossible. The result was that large numbers of practitioners trained in the United States — both licensed and unlicensed — operated in the province in competition with the area's established physicians, whose medical education was commonly undertaken in England or Scotland. In the spring of 1847, no doubt in order to achieve maximum effect on the forthcoming deliberations of the legislature, the *British American Journal* reprinted an editorial that had appeared two months earlier in the *Morning Courier,* bemoaning the prevalence of illegal practitioners in Canada East and calling for stricter legislation. "We presume," commented the *Courier,*

> that there is no occasion for us to state a fact which is sufficiently well known, that is, that this Province is inundated with Medical practitioners who are utterly unqualified to prescribe for the bodily ailments of the lieges, in fact, quacks, under whose diabolical "simples" and other nostrums hundreds of the population are annually murdered. Against this infliction we believe there is no "specific" remedy. At least we remember some time ago having occasion to notice the arrival among us of a Yankee, who pretended to be an oculist, aurist, or some thing of that class. We mentioned the circumstance to a Medical friend, and advised him, if there was any law by which it might be done, immediately to institute a prosecution against him. We were then told that there was no law which could be resorted to in order to put a stop to irregular practice. This we thought rather extraordinary, and

wondered at the existence of a Board of Medical Examiners and the formality of a license to practise, so solemnly promulgated in the Official Gazette. It is true that we were always aware that the examination before this Board was to a certain degree a farce, for to our own certain knowledge men have passed their examination there and been admitted to practice who knew nothing of anatomy but what they had learned from books; they had never in their lives dissected a subject, yet a good memory enabled them, by dint of severe cramming, to undergo the ordeal. But still to enforce an examination on Canadian students, while there are no means of preventing foreigners, not only really educated men from the American Colleges, but the most abominable quacks, from practising when and where they please, certainly does seem to us a little bit of a farce.

Medical men, who come to this Colony, and have obtained their diplomas from regular institutions in England, Ireland, and Scotland; medical men natives of Canada, who have gone home to study and there taken their degrees, and men who have studied and taken their degrees in Toronto, and Montreal, have obtained their skill and their standing in their profession at an immense expense and after years of hard study; is it either just or right, or expedient, that these men should not be protected from the intrusion even of educated foreigners? If so, is it not still more imperative that they be protected against quacks? We think this will be readily conceded. . . .

We believe this to be one of those questions of practical reform of an existing abuse, which is of much more importance than disquisitions on abstract questions of government.[27]

A new statute

The legislature was not remiss in heeding the requests of the profession. In July, 1847, it enacted a statute creating the College of Physicians and Surgeons of Lower Canada,[28] comprising the 181 physicians whose names had appeared on the petition earlier submitted to it. In conformity with the terms of the petition, the College was to be directed by a Board of Governors, to be chosen from the College by its membership, and which also constituted the Provincial Medical Board. The Board was empowered to certify applicants for a medical license, granted by the governor upon its recommendation. All applicants were required to sit an examination by the Board, excepting those holding "a Medical Degree or Diploma in any University or College in Her Majesty's Dominions."

Additionally, the Board was given authority to regulate the study of medicine within Canada East, including preliminary qualifications, duration of study, and the curriculum to be followed. The act stipulated that

> the qualifications to be required by the Board of Governors from a person about to commence the study of Medicine in this Province, shall be: A good moral character, and a competent knowledge of Latin, History, Geography, Mathematics and Natural Philosophy; and that from and after the end of the year one thousand eight hundred and fifty, a general knowledge of the French and English languages shall also be indispensable,[29]

and that

> the qualifications to be required from a candidate for examination to obtain a certificate for a license to practise shall consist in his not being less than twenty-one years of age; that he has followed his studies uninterruptedly during a period of not less than four years under the care of one or more general practitioners duly licensed; and that during the said four years he shall have attended at some University, College or Incorporated School of Medicine within Her Majesty's Dominions not less than two six months' Courses of General Anatomy and Physiology—of Practical Anatomy—of Surgery—of Practice of Medicine—of Midwifery—of Chemistry—and of *Materia Medica* and Pharmacy,—one six months' Course of Medical Jurisprudence,—and one three months' Course of Botany, if obtainable in Lower Canada; also that he shall have attended the general practice of an Hospital in which are contained not less than fifty beds under the charge of not less than two Physicians or Surgeons for a period not less than one year, or two periods of not less than six months each; and that he shall also have attended two three months' or one six months' Course of Clinical Medicine, and the same of Clinical Surgery, and to remove all doubts with regard to the number of Lectures which the Incorporated Schools of Medicine of Quebec and Montreal are bound to give yearly; Be it enacted that it is and shall be sufficient that the said Schools of Medicine, respectively, shall yearly cause to be delivered one hundred and twenty lectures on the subjects by law provided....

Female midwives were exempt from the provisions of the 1847 act, except for those practicing in Montreal, Quebec, and Three Rivers, who were required to receive a certificate of competency from the

Board. The penalty for practicing medicine, surgery, or midwifery in violation of the statute was set at £5 *per day* of illegal practice, the testimony of two witnesses being sufficient to convict.

Fears respecting implementation

The profession had high hopes for the new act[30] and was pleased with its penalty provisions which, regardless of their weaknesses, were viewed as a vast improvement over those contained in the 1788 statute. There were some reservations, however, concerning whether they would be effectively implemented. The *British American Journal* observed:

> The penal clause, we think, will give general satisfaction to the country physicians. The process against illicit practice is as summary as it can possibly be made; but, summary as it is, we are not disinclined to the opinion... that conviction will be by no means an easy task, because the private feelings of the Justices of the Peace are as likely to be elicited in favour of the quack, and against his punishment as they appear to have been....[31]

One physician, writing of the competitive conditions prevailing in the countryside on the eve of the new act's passage, was somewhat skeptical that the bill would significantly reduce the amount of unlicensed practice in the rural areas of Canada East, although he felt that it might partially ameliorate the circumstances under which licensed physicians operated. The author, who signed himself "Rusticus," complained bitterly about the competition he faced from unlicensed practitioners and, in passing, offers an interesting summary of orthodox medical practice at mid-century. "Allow me to say," he writes,

> that I consider the penalty clause the *best* that has ever been suggested to fulfill the wishes of the country surgeon.
> The interests of the country practitioner seem to be entirely lost sight of in all that has yet been done. Too much attention has been paid to the mere preliminary and collegiate courses of rival schools, to allow much time to be wasted on his interest; and yet where, in the whole profession, do you find any so grudgingly requited for his laborious exertions, or the daily and hourly annoyances he is forced to bear, or how his preserves are poached upon by a host of rapacious quacks....
> Under my very nose lives neighbour B., who bleeds and extracts

teeth at exactly half the professional charge. This to you may appear a trifling grievance, yet I assure you, the receipts before this infringement of my rights, has helped greatly to condition my horse for a hard midnight's ride. In the extirpation of tumours, &c., my scalpels have grown rusty for want of use, as Dr. B., so called, takes this branch under his care, and unblushingly promises a cure in all cases, malignant or benign, at a moderate cost!... In midwifery, not to mention a host of illiterate mid-wives — until late, there was a Dr. S. who used to *do the natives*.... Even the storekeepers have so far forgotten the sphere nature intended them for, as to encroach on my privileges, by dispensing such articles as strychnine, arsenic, tartar emetic, calomel, quinine, and, in fact, the whole contents of a well-ordered surgery.

These illegal pretenders make regular charges, ay, and get paid too, and what must surely surprise you, it has been decided in our Commissioners Court here, that it was of no consequence whether a person was licensed or not, *and that decision was acted upon.* Under circumstances such as these, is it surprising that many have abandoned the profession in disgust, and entered other pursuits where their exertions are better requited? How long are such practices to be tolerated, inflicting, as they do, incalculable injury both on the regularly qualified medical man, as well as the public? The existing remedy is *totally* inadequate to stop them. The proposed medical bill — however stringent the penal clauses — if the enforcing of them is to be left to the complaining party himself, will, I venture to say, never answer. Where is the medical man who will incur the *onus* of becoming the prosecutor? Where the willing witnesses to back him? Who would travel forty, or it may be one hundred and forty miles, or go before a country magistrate, merely to *stop for a time* the inroads of some quack, and thus enable him to insult you with greater impunity than ever? Constituted as society is in this country, such a plan will never do.

[Yet, as] I have already said the penal clause in the proposed bill for the College of Physicians and Surgeons is the best that has been suggested. I repeat this conviction.... For my part,... I would be content to... join the College of Physicians and Surgeons of C. E., with all its disadvantages, merely from the fact that half a loaf is better than no bread.[32]

In order to strengthen the position of the College in prosecuting offenders and to simplify the procedures whereby unlicensed physicians could be convicted, the act was amended in 1849,[33] to provide that fines for practicing without a license, plus reasonable costs, were recoverable by an ordinary civil suit, brought in the name of the College itself. But, despite the act and its amendment, unlicensed practice flourished throughout Lower Canada, as patients continued to frequent physicians whose fees for medical care undercut those of licensed doctors, and as courts remained reluctant to convict.

POLITICAL RESISTANCE TO STRONGER LEGISLATION IN CANADA WEST

Although the profession in Canada East was incorporated into a College in 1847, established physicians in Canada West, despite numerous attempts, were unsuccessful in gaining a similar governing body for another two decades. In 1846, the Toronto Medico-Chirurgical Society[34] initiated a petition to the legislature calling for passage of a new medical act, with provisions similar to the earlier-disallowed statute of 1839, creating a College of Physicians and Surgeons for the region.[35] The petition was novel in that it called not only for the enactment of stricter legislation to combat the large number of unlicensed practitioners in Canada West, but also for the creation of district and provincial medical societies, empowered to set and enforce fee schedules and, presumably, to discipline members whose professional behavior was unorthodox. The petition, in part, observes:

> That your Petitioners have found, that the law now established has proved ineffectual for the object apparently designed; as empiricism flourishes to an extraordinary extent—to the discouragement of your petitioners, and the serious detriment and danger of the community. Men of skill and eminence are deterred from settling in the province; and several, such now residing here, have been induced to relinquish their profession, to follow other vocations better calculated to ensure them a competence, and to advance the interests of their families; moreover, no sufficient inducement is held out to young men of talent, to adopt a profession, in which there is so slight a prospect of obtaining an adequate return for the necessary, laborious, and expensive study required.
>
> Your Petitioners are of opinion, that the act regulating the practice of physic, surgery, and midwifery (8th Geo. IV, c. iii,) is inoperative, from two causes—one of which is, that no prosecution can be commenced one year after the offense. Parties transgressing, can thus readily evade the penalties of the law, by refraining from claims for their illegal practice, until more than that period has elapsed. Another, and probably the principal rea-

son of the inadequacy of the law, is, that although the whole community suffer from infractions of it, they have been in the habit of looking to the regularly qualified practitioners to enforce its enactments; and it will not seem surprising that but few have been found willing to endanger their own prospects, by incurring the odium attached to the capacity of an informer.

Your Petitioners, therefore, deeply impressed with the uncertainty of individual action in promoting the interests both of the public and of the medical profession, beseech your Honourable House to take into favorable consideration, some measure, to unite into one body, the whole of the medical practitioners in Canada West. And as a preliminary step to establish *Medical Societies* in each district — to which it shall be imperative on all medical practitioners to attach themselves in their respective districts.

Your Petitioners pray, that these District Medical Associations shall be authorized to make By-laws for the management of all local matters connected with the profession — such as their tariff of fees, the suppression of illicit practice, and other objects calculated to advance the combined interests of themselves and the public.

Your Petitioners further consider it desirable, that, for the examination of candidates, granting licenses, the expulsion or suspension of unworthy members, and other purposes, there should be established a *General Provincial Medical Board or Council*, possessing the confidence of their brethren in the profession. They, therefore, humbly pray that each District Society shall be authorized to nominate to that honourable office, two of its members, subject to the approval of the Governor General, and to be annually re-elected.

A *Provincial Medical Society, or Board*, so constituted, would unite in one common centre, the views and wishes of the whole profession; and it is earnestly hoped, that it would confer upon the practitioners of medicine, the independence, respectability, and advantages, which the incorporation of the Law Society has obtained for its members, and thus ultimately raise the medical profession to that position in public regard to which it is, by its utility and importance, so justly entitled.[36]

The petition's self-serving nature

The petition evidences the same approach as has always been used by special-interest groups seeking protective legislation, the linking of the interests of the group with those of the public. Why it should be to the advantage of the consumers of physicians' services to reduce the number of persons supplying that service, we are not told. Nor is the reader informed of the reasons why the public would benefit from the enforcement of a tariff of fees, below which practitioners were reluctant to charge without jeopardizing their status within the profession. The petitioners contend that there are no inducements for men of talent to enter the profession given the "laborious and expensive study required." Yet these same men were in the vanguard of those demanding that these studies be, by law, made more laborious and expensive. We are not told why empiricism, as opposed to orthodox practice, flourished, that is, why those seeking medical care chose to seek the services of empirics. If, as the petition elsewhere states, "the majority of the public cannot reasonably be expected to justly estimate the qualifications of those who tender them Medical services," then why did these heterodox practitioners prosper relative to other physcians? If no distinction whatever was made on the basis of competence—which was extremely unlikely—it must have been at least partially made on the basis of price. Needless to say, the petitioners nowhere indicated that the passage of the proposed bill would increase the costs of physicians' services and thereby deprive at least some of the poorer residents of the province of medical care.

Strong support for a new medical act

Both the petition and the proposed medical bill were predictably lauded in the medical press. One Toronto practitioner called upon all licensed physicians to organize in support of the measure, which he recognized as having as its sole object the benefit of the established profession:

> It is not to the metropolitan portion of the profession that we are to look for the power by which this great object is to be attained, it is the force of numbers alone that can effect it. A system of organization must be adopted that will extend itself over the whole province, from Sandwich to Gaspe. From all the towns and villages invitations should go forth from societies and influential individuals, to every licensed practitioner within the limits of each district, to assist with his advice and influence in furthering the grand object, and let it be proclaimed that the object embraces *protection for ourselves, an elevated standard of education for the rising generation, and nothing more.*[37]

The author had in an earlier letter concluded that a stricter medical law was essential to the profession, and had contrasted what he regarded as the inferior status of physicians with that of attorneys in Canada West:

> "Help yourself, and the Lord will help you," is a time-honoured precept: it must have been one of the first lessons taught by experience. It is certainly one of those the breach or the observance of which is of the greatest importance in the business of life. Believing, as I do, that the degraded state of the medical man, may be traced to the breach, the prosperous condition of the lawyer, the divine, and others, in a great measure, to the observance of this maxim, and in the hope that this view of the case, if well sustained, either by direct or analogical evidence, may assist to arouse the slumbering energies of my brethren, I shall endeavour to furnish... a short but faithful description of the respective professional positions of the members of the bar, and the physicians, and surgeons in this part of Canada. It is scarcely necessary to go beyond the limits of this city for materials to fill up the picture; the family likeness is strongly marked everywhere. We learn from the statistics of Toronto, that there are within its boundaries at the present time, thirty regular practitioners of medicine and surgery, and about eighty barristers and attorneys at law. The whole population, according to the last census, amounts to 20,000 or thereabout, and if we add to this number the incidental practice of the rural districts in the neighbourhood, the number of medical men, though large, does not appear altogether out of proportion to the population; but alas! we have also twenty unauthorized practitioners, in the shape of druggists, apothecaries, venders of nostrums from the United States, and quack doctors par excellence: the consequences resulting from this state of things, are, of course, most injurious to the *privileged?* practitioner; shall we ascribe them to the ignorance and credulity of the public, or to the apathy of the victim?[38]

Eighty barristers and attorneys, and, at best, fifty druggists, apothecaries, and physicians, including "quacks," serving a population of over 20,000 and we are asked to believe that this is indicative of the degraded state of the medical profession, especially when compared to that of law!

The apathy of Parliament

Despite the absence of apathy on the part of the physician-as-victim, the profession's pleas for a stronger medical law appear to have fallen on deaf ears. The members of the provincial parliament were prepared to furnish a new medical act to Canada East in 1847 largely, it would seem, through the concerted vote of the representatives of that region. These representatives were likely impressed with the unanimity of sentiment for a new medical law among both the French-speaking and English-speaking physicians of Canada East.[39] Nevertheless, during the same period the legislature remained hopelessly divided on the question of a statute for Canada West.

The province's wandering capital had temporarily settled in Toronto in 1849 and in 1851 the established profession in the area, hoping to take advantage of the legislature's presence in Canada West, once again made a concerted effort to gain passage of a stronger medical statute. The *Upper Canada Journal* decried the state of the profession in western Canada in much the same language as had been employed five years earlier. It called upon the area's physicians both to petition the provincial parliament and to exercise any influence they might have with its members in order to gain passage of a new and more effective medical law. Respecting the condition of the profession in Canada West, it editorialized:

> Did we propose to examine the matter merely in a pecuniary point of view, we believe that we should have no great difficulty in bringing our enquiry to a speedy termination—it would be this: that medical men are the hardest worked, have the least leisure allowed them for domestic enjoyment, are the most grudgingly remunerated, have their services the least appreciated, and are the worst protected and least encouraged by the State of all other classes of men, let their profession or calling be what it may.... We want mutual and cordial co-operation to protect ourselves and our interests. And how is this to be [accomplished?]...
> It is obvious as it is simple: to obtain from the Legislature, by means of an Act of Incorporation, the power to regulate our own affairs—to manage our own concerns. Is the Medical Profession of Western Canada less capable of doing so than that of the Eastern section? Is it less qualified to decide upon the amount or nature of the acquirements, both preliminary and professional, to be possessed by its future members, before they be intrusted with the lives of Her Majesty's lieges in this portion of the British empire?...
> With such data before us, let us here sink, as politicians say, all minor differences; let us set shoulder to shoulder in the emancipation of ourselves and our brethren from the thraldom which now oppresses us; and while we are prepared to throw open our doors to educated practitioners of all countries, on the most reasonable

conditions, let us endeavour to secure protection against those
who would fain represent Medicine to be nothing but a trade, and
capable of being exercised by the veriest clodhopper or the most
ignorant artizen.[40]

A resolution

In May of that year, a meeting of the leading practitioners of York
County resolved, among other things, that

> the interests of the Medical Profession generally, as well as those
> of its members individually, can only be effectually secured and
> protected by the incorporation of the same into a body endowed
> with power to regulate its own affairs; [and]
>   that the members of the Medical Profession, considering them-
> selves the best, inasmuch as they are the only true judges of the
> requisite qualifications for the exercise of the Art of Medicine,
> claim the power of regulating the amount of those to be possessed
> by candidates for practice, and of granting licences accordingly.[41]

They thereupon drafted a medical bill for the consideration of the profession and for eventual submission to the legislature. The bill provided for the establishment of a College, to be directed by a Board of
Governors acting as a medical examining board. This board would be
empowered to make rules respecting the preliminary qualifications,
duration of study, and curriculum to be followed by all candidates
submitting themselves for a license to practice.[42]

   More controversial was a provision empowering the Board to make
its own determination respecting the universities and faculties whose
diplomas and degrees would exempt the holder from sitting the
examination. Some of the more prominent practitioners in western
Canada, who were themselves graduates or licentiates of British
schools and faculties, objected that the clause would almost certainly
be employed to exclude others like them from practicing without first
taking the Board's examination.[43] This agitation led to the offending
clause being amended before the bill was finally submitted to parliament.[44]

Parliamentary resistance

To the great annoyance of the profession, the bill met fierce resistance
from some members of the legislature, who opposed any restrictions
on the practice of medicine. Indeed, one M.P.P. went so far as to propose a substitute bill, amending the medical act of 1827 — under which

Canada West was still operating—to provide that "no person shall be liable to any criminal prosecution or to indictment for practising Physic, Surgery, or Midwifery, without license, except in cases of malpractice, or gross ignorance, or immoral conduct in such practice."[45] To this, the *Upper Canada Journal* retorted:

> That it is a Bill for legalizing quackery, and at the same time opening a very wide door for the vexatious persecution of the "benevolent, but well-qualified persons" whom the Honourable Member has taken under his especial protection, must be admitted by all; for who, in the cases supposed, can prove malpractice, or gross ignorance, on the part of the offender but regularly educated medical men? And we only trust, that on any occasion of the kind, the latter will lay aside all feelings of delicacy, and endeavour to support the law, should this Bill ever become such.[46]

The *Journal* was astonished and irritated that the act proposed by the profession should meet with opposition from otherwise sensible men. In June, 1851, it editorialized that the proposal

> as submitted to Parliament for its sanction, is a measure calculated to protect the interests of the public, as well as to advance the progress of medical science; these it is proposed to effect, by the organization of the profession into a body: unity of action and concentration of forces have at all times been considered indispensable to the successful operation of a large number of scattered or separate pieces of machinery; the same obtains with regard to communities of men. Acts of incorporation are daily sought for and granted by the Legislature to bodies of individuals, certainly for the most indistinct and even inconceivable purposes: for example, to Mechanics' Institutes, Sons of Temperance, &c., &c.; and yet we are astonished to learn, that when notice was given of intention to introduce a Bill for the incorporation of the Medical Profession of Upper Canada, the hon. member so moving was warned of strenuous opposition to be offered to the measure. . . . We are told, that the country desires free-trade in physic, and that people will employ whom they choose as their medical attendants. Then we say, that these men, if guilty of malpractice should be subject to criminal prosecution, and punished for felony or misdemeanour, according to the extent of the mischief done by them. It is said, that no jury will convict in civil process a quack prosecuted at the instance of another party. Then we answer, amend the law, and convict by summary process.[47]

Medicine still regarded as a trade

That the practice of medicine was a trade and, as such, deserved no greater protection than that afforded other trades in a free society, and that the criminal and civil law was sufficient protection against the consequences of incompetent and negligent practice, were clearly unfamiliar responses to physicians' demands for protective legislation. So outraged was the profession in western Canada by this attitude, that the *Upper Canada Journal* devoted no less than ten pages of its July, 1851, issue to ridiculing both the position and its adherents in the legislature.[48]

Notwithstanding the unflagging exertions of the profession in Canada West to gain a new and more restrictive law governing medical practice, the 1851 bill did not pass the provincial parliament. The *Upper Canada Journal* noted that

> nearly every body of men who sought for corporate rights from the Liberal Legislature have obtained them, except those whose welfare is so intimately associated with the personal interests of all classes of the community, and with the general well being of society. We approach the consideration of this subject with feelings of much disappointment, mingled with no small share of painful regret, for our convictions lead us to the belief that this failure to obtain what is so earnestly required by the large majority of the profession, has been brought about as much by the successful intrigue of enemies within the camp, as by the openly avowed hostility of a few who differed on minor points from the measure itself, and the want of a proper management on the part of the gentleman who had charge of it.... When we feel that the privileges sought for by us are those best calculated to ensure the common weal, we ought not to shrink from performing the great duty we owe to ourselves and to the country, and seek by every legitimate means in our power, to secure the return to Parliament of those men only who will see that justice is dealt to all with a fair and impartial hand.[49]

THE LEGAL RECOGNITION OF HOMEOPATHY AND ECLECTICISM

A powerful free-market faction in the Canadian legislature[50] emerged following the repeal of the Corn Laws and the election of an anti-protectionist Whig government under Lord John Russell in London in

1846. This made it extremely unlikely that the medical profession in Canada West would be successful in gaining passage of a more stringent medical act. Additionally, it had become increasingly clear that large segments of the Canadian public strongly opposed legislation to restrict competition and to curtail the activities of heterodox practitioners. In 1852, the *Upper Canada Journal,* in typical protectionist language, complained of the public's attitude towards the established physicians of the province and their lack of sympathy with the profession's attempts to institute tighter restrictions on medical practice:

> Look at the man who with all the advantages of a liberal education, embarks his capital and engages in some speculative undertaking of the true nature and risks of which he knows nothing—how certain and signal is his failure. But to him alone the consequences are serious and prejudicial, or if his rashness should have involved others, the loss is a pecuniary one, which experience and prudence may repair. Yet the world punishes him with ridicule and censure. If an artisan should undertake to construct some mechanism, being ignorant of its principles, and unacquainted with the use of the requisite tools—the law punishes him for the injury done to his employer by the waste of material, and breach of contract. But on him only falls the penalty of his wayward presumption;—and so through nearly all the ramifications of the social scale. But, if a man, who one day is a journeyman hatter or a stage coach driver, the next day dubs himself a doctor, a Homoeopath, Hydropath, or Mesmerist, the credulous world flock around him to be duped, irreparably injured, and *probably murdered*—aye, to be hastened on to a premature grave, by the administration of the most powerful and subtle agents, whose composition, whose relative affinities, whose *modus operandi* are all a dark and incomprehensible mystery; to this scelerate impostor. And what is the result of all this? If the properly qualified practitioner seeks to avail himself of the slender protection extended by the law for the punishment of the fraud committed on the public, and the injustice done to himself—straightway the public voice is raised against the proceeding and its justified instigator, whose motives are characterized as invidious, selfish and mercenary. But who shall restore the poor deluded victim to the comfort and enjoyment of his wonted vitality? What compensation will cheer the widowed hearth, give back again the joyous prattle of the cherished infant, heal the wound of

blighted love, or bring together the severed links of fraternal happiness! And yet it is desired to countenance and promote these evils, by removing all legislative restrictions against unqualified practice, by lowering the standard of education and the cost of its acquisition, and so encourage the adoption of medicine as a profession, by those who are unprepared for the study by lacking the most elementary knowledge—a proper acquaintance with their native language, and the ability to impart information by the art of writing. We hope for a better issue, and look for a renewed effort on the part of those who are striving after the wiser course.[51]

The editorial does not inform us how lowering the costs of medical education would encourage unqualified practice and do a disservice to the consumers of physicians' service. Nor does it explain the similarities between the person suffering a tort and the effect on licensed physicians of unlicensed practice.

Paternalism

Two years later, the *Medical Chronicle* echoed the views of the *Upper Canada Journal* and advocated that consumers of medical services, like children, must be kept from injurying themselves, through passage of restrictive legislation that they opposed:

Very few appreciate the real merits of the case, or have a sufficient sense of equity to comprehend why the profession requires the same protection, and is entitled to the same privileges in Upper as in Lower Canada, and why without these its condition must border on anarchy. Nor can they admit that the simple right of men sanctioned by law to practice a profession obtained at heavy personal cost, and after compliance with prescribed enactments, is to be defended, from the debasing aggressions of those whose knowledge is intuitive, and who, perhaps, are disabled from following their proper callings, and find in medicine a better business than in horse-shoeing or sow-gelding. But such things cannot continue long. Learned men must be encouraged in their undertakings, for if their art be without a premium, its worshippers will disappear, and its sphere become a chaos. We hold that the expression of a people in behalf of quackery is entitled to no regard, for if they be so simple minded and grossly ignorant as not to know the difference between an educated physician and a boasting empiric, they must be, like children, taught better, and like imbeciles, kept from injuring themselves.[52]

Among all the heterodox practitioners — contemptuously lumped together by the established profession as "empirics" — the groups that had made the most substantial inroads into orthodox practice were the eclectics and the homeopaths. Both were comparatively well-organized and had substantial followings,[53] especially in western Canada. As a result, they were singled out for the most scurrilous attacks in the medical press. In 1851, the *Upper Canada Journal* thought it worthwhile to carry a report of the Provincial Medical and Surgical Association of England, denouncing homeopathy, in which the association resolved that "homoeopathy, as propounded by Hahnemann and practiced by his followers, is so utterly opposed to science and common sense, as well as so completely at variance with the experience of the medical profession, that it ought to be in no way practiced or countenanced by any regularly educated practitioner," and that "it is derogatory to the honour of members of this association to hold any professional intercourse with homoeopathic practitioners."[54] And the *Canada Medical Journal,* during its first year of publication, printed an extensive review of a monograph denouncing homeopathy, in which a British medical journal is quoted as concluding of homeopathic physicians:

> They are not to us disinterested enquirers after truth, patient endurers of unmerited contumely, followers of a faith which the dictates of a deep conscientious conviction required them to adopt. They are rather men who follow their profession, and who suffer their pseudo-martyrdom for no higher or holier motive than the need to make money. Their motto is "REM." No sophistry, however elaborate, no manifestation [of] scientific research, however profound; no protestations of deep conviction, however loud, can blind the observer of their proceedings to the damning fact, that before they embraced homeopathy, they had no success, pecuniary or curative, in ordinary practice. Their failures in the former sense are patent to the world, in the latter are loudly proclaimed by themselves.[55]

Eclectics

Eclectic practitioners were treated no better. At the third annual meeting of the Canadian Eclectic Association, in 1851, it was resolved that the association support "the expunging from the statute books of all protecting and prohibitory enactments in relation to Medical practitioners." It was further resolved:

That we recommend, and urgently though most respectfully insist, that all friends of Medical Reform shall exert their influence in every manner proper to procure at the earliest day possible, a repeal of the offensive laws against which we complain; [and]

That the friends of the Reformed Practice have already strength sufficient to hold the balance of political power; and that we will employ our influence, one and all, to obtain liberal and enlightened enactments, and to effect all we can in this important particular.[56]

To these resolutions, the *Upper Canada Journal* responded:

When those who are opposed to us evince this spirit of combination, it is surely time to act on the defensive. Again we entreat the profession to be unanimous and energetic. The dearest interests of true science now call for our exertions. The community at large will view with a keen and jealous eye the proceedings of the two respective parties now existing in the Province — these spurious pretenders, and the regularly educated men. Let not public judgment be warped by the industrious efforts of the one, and the indifferent apathy of the other. It will not suffice to say that the educated and more enlightened portion of the community will be able to discriminate between us. It is with the same mass we have to deal. It is our high prerogative to protect them from presumptive ignorance on the one hand, and persevering imposture on the other.[57]

In the following issue of the *Journal,* the editors again turned to the same subject and, under the guise of speaking in the interests of a confused and gullible public, attacked the eclectic association as an illegal combination, seeking to subvert the laws of the province.

Now, it will not be denied, that a large proportion, if not all of the members of that association are not licensed to practice, have no legal authority to prescribe or administer medicines, and therefore do not possess any legitimate right to ask, sue for, or recover remuneration for their proffered services. Thus much said, and our duty to the public is discharged. But we *are* influenced by other, and to us more cogent motives in drawing the attention of our professional brethren to these proceedings. If an organization, apparently maturely devised in its character, can take place among these quacks, having for its ostensible purpose the subversion of the existing law for regulating the practice of Medicine, is it not time that we should exert ourselves in self-defence.... It would be wrong to conceal from ourselves the fact, that when a body of individuals act in concert to promulgate among the ill-informed masses doctrines, however injurious their tendency, and however unscrupulous the means employed, they will succeed to a great extent, if not counteracted by the dissemination of proper information, and the resolute opposition of those in whose keeping the welfare of the community has been justly and wisely placed by the acts of the Legislature. The records of every country contain many examples of the success of such illegal combinations, and the unhappy results arising from them. Nor is it the more self-interested desire to protect ourselves as a legally qualified profession from the assaults of this predatory faction, which should govern us, however natural and excusable such a motive may be; but we have a higher and more imperative influence to govern us. As the duly authorized guardians of the public health, we are bound to see that no infringement of our prerogative takes place.[58]

There is perhaps no clearer instance of the habit of mind of large numbers of established physicians than that they could contenance the vilification of a group that wished not for special favors nor restrictions on their competitors, but solely for the right to minister to those who, without compulsion, chose one of their number as their physician. We are asked to believe that it was not out of a "more self-interested desire" to protect themselves, that the established profession attacked eclectic practitioners who were winning away their patients and reducing their incomes. But it is difficult to believe that any reader of the medical journals of the day could have thought otherwise.

Antagonism to heterodox medicine

Even legally qualified physicians who opted to practice heterodox medicine were not spared from attack in the medical press. When a graduate of McGill and a licentiate of the College of Physicians and Surgeons, Lower Canada, announced his intention to set up practice as an eclectic physician in Hamilton, he was denounced by the *Medical Chronicle* as violating the terms of his license, which granted him the right solely to practice "such medicine and surgery as he had been taught at McGill College, and which, at his examination, he distinctly affirmed he would practice."[59]

Given the antagonism of the established profession towards heterodox medicine, it was with particular dismay that regular physicians witnessed both homeopathy and eclecticism receive legal recognition in Canada West. In 1859, despite the protests of regular practitioners, the provincial legislature passed a bill recognizing the existence of homeopathic physicians by providing them with their own board of examiners.[60] In language paralleling that of the 1827 statute respecting regular practitioners, the law provided that an applicant passing the examination set by the homeopathic board and having satisfied the authorities of his loyalty, integrity, and good morals, was entitled to a license to practice homeopathic medicine in Canada West. Additionally, candidates were required to have spent at least four uninterrupted years in the study of medicine, at least two years of which must have been spent at some medical school. (No such educational requirement had yet been instituted in Canada West for the certification of regular physicians.) In 1861, a second act was passed extending to eclectic physicians the same powers granted homeopathic physicians two years earlier.[61] The statute created a board of eclectic examiners with the power to set examinations for prospective eclectic practitioners. The provisions of this law were almost identical to those of the homeopathic act of 1859, with one variation; of the four years of medical study required of eclectic applicants, two years were to be spent at a medical school and one year was to have been devoted to training at a hospital.

No grandfather clause

The acts respecting homeopathy and eclecticism, unlike other medical acts passed in the province, contained no grandfather clause. All members of these irregular sects, regardless of how long they had been practicing, were required to sit the examinations and meet the other provisions of the law to receive licenses.[62] The 1859 and 1861 acts did not contain penal clauses but, inasmuch as the practice of homeopathy or eclecticism was still, in law, considered the practice of medicine, unlicensed physicians were subject to the penalties provided in the medical act of 1827.

In Canada East regular physicians were better organized, possessing as they did a stricter medical licensing law for some eighteen years. Even here, however, despite the fact that fewer heterodox physicians had set up practice, homeopaths were able to secure an act granting them legal recognition in 1865.[63] The statute created the Montreal Homeopathic Association, and empowered it to establish both a dispensary and a hospital, together with a medical school in Canada East. Such a medical school was authorized to teach "by regular courses of lectures, the principles and practice of medicine and *materia medica* according to the doctrines of homeopathy, to such persons as have received or are receiving instruction in all other requisite branches of the medical profession." In addition, the association was granted the right to appoint a homeopathic board of examiners, for the purpose of examining applicants wishing to practice in Lower Canada; its members were required to have been either medical graduates of a British or provincial university or medical licentiates of a British or provincial college or board. The educational requirements for licensure were almost identical to those provided in the 1847 act respecting regular physicians. As in the 1859 law governing homeopathic practice in Canada West, no grandfather clause was included in the act. All homeopathic practitioners were required to meet the provisions of the statute under penalty of violating the medical act of 1847.[64]

Reaction of orthodox practitioners

It is hardly surprising that the medical press was disappointed that the provincial legislature saw fit to sanction the practice of irregular medicine. The recognition of homeopathy was more easily comprehensible, since it was the creation of a physician possessed of a rigorous formal medical education and its adherents were, for the most part, well-trained and respectable doctors who had proved themselves not inflexible on therapeutic questions. But to legally recognize eclecticism, the invention of a self-educated American farmer, whose practitioners confined their therapeutic arsenal to herbs and other botanic substances, smacked too much of sanctioning quackery.[65] Indeed, the *British American Journal* went so far as to suggest that the representative in the legislative council who rescued the bill from defeat in that body, himself an M.D., was a quack, whose name did not appear on the list of licentiates of either Canada East or Canada West. "Supposing" it observed, "that he has been practising for years and years without a legal authority to do so, the fact sufficiently accounted for his proclivities towards charlatanism."[66] "Toiling as we have done during the best portion of our life," it editorialized, for the advancement and true recognition of a profession to which we are ardently attached, a profession whose annals are adorned by the names of the noblest and best of our race, and with no other ultimate object in view, than that of placing at the disposal of the inhabitants of these Provinces, a class of men whose medical attainments should pre-eminently qualify them, for the relief of the various illnesses to which the human body is incident, we feel it hard that all our labour should have been thus thrown away.[67]

REGISTRATION IN CANADA WEST: THE MEDICAL ACT OF 1865

Despite these setbacks, however, the regular profession was able to wring some concessions from the legislature. In the same year as the provincial parliament passed its bill creating the Montreal Homeopathic Association, it finally succumbed to the demands of the profession in Canada West by revising the medical act to provide for a medical board empowered to set the educational requirements necessary for licensure in the area. The medical act of 1865[68] created a General Council of Medical Education and Registration of Upper Canada. The Council's membership comprised one representative from each of the educational bodies in Canada West empowered to grant medical degrees, together with elected representatives of the regular profession from each of twelve designated districts. The Council was empowered to license and register physicians issued a certificate of qualification by one of the medical schools represented on the Council,[69] and to any practitioner (1) licensed under earlier medical statutes; (2) holding a medical degree from any university within the British Empire; (3) holding a license from the Royal College of Physicians or the Royal College of Surgeons, London; (4) duly licensed in Lower Canada; (5) holding a commission as a physician or surgeon in the military; or, (6) licensed to practice medicine under the Imperial Medical Act of 1858.[70] Although the Council was purely a registration body—it was denied the authority to examine candidates—it was authorized to establish the preliminary qualifications necessary for undertaking the study of medicine and to determine the curriculum to be followed in the medical schools of western Canada. Registration was henceforth to be the sole means by which a practitioner could be licensed. In addition, only registered physicians were entitled to employ any name or title indicating they were licensed practitioners (e.g., physician, doctor of medicine, licentiate in medicine and surgery, bachelor of medicine, surgeon, general practitioner, etc.), under penalty of a $50 fine.[71]

Educational requirements

The educational requirements instituted by the Council were similar to those operating in Canada East and consistent with the graduation requirements of the area's medical schools: four years' study, comprising terms of at least six months' duration.[72] The act might have proved a potent weapon for introducing stricter educational requirements, but initially it seems to have accomplished very little. There had been some complaint respecting the length of the academic term and the curriculum of study necessary for a medical degree at Queen's University soon after its establishment in 1854.[73] In response to the attacks of the medical fraternity that the University was cheapening the value of a medical degree in Canada West, however, the school soon made the necessary alterations. Inasmuch as the creation of a Council of Medical Education did not lead to greater educational requirements than those already in place and since the Council could not examine applicants, its authority being the purely mechanical one of registration, control over the number of entrants into the profession passed from the provincial medical board to the schools of medicine operating in western Canada.

Although female midwives were no longer exempt from the penal provisions of the medical law, it now became necessary to show that unlicensed practitioners "wilfully and falsely pretended" to be registered under the act in order to convict. This change in the penalty clause represented a radical departure from previous licensing laws in the province. No longer was it illegal in Upper Canada to practice medicine without a license,[74] but only to deliberately imply, by title or otherwise, that one were a registered physician under the act.[75] The statute permitted only registered practitioners to be appointed to any public institution or to sign official certificates, but, beyond this, and being prevented from suing for the recovery of fees, no penalty attached to engaging in medical practice without government license.

MEDICAL LEGISLATION IN THE REST OF BRITISH NORTH AMERICA

Nova Scotia

The medical profession in the Maritime colonies did not remain idle in the period immediately prior to Confederation. The population of the area had been growing substantially. Nova Scotia's increased from 82,000 in 1817 to 123,000 ten years later; by 1851, the colony had a population of almost 227,000.[76] The number of physicians had clearly increased apace. Heagerty notes that in 1845, fourteen established physicians, thirteen of whom held degrees from Edinburgh, were practicing in the town of Halifax.[77] Additionally, large numbers of "empirics," most from the United States, had set up practice in Nova Scotia to serve its growing population.[78] In response to the competition of these less qualified physicians "who were finding their way into the province in alarming numbers,"[79] the regular profession founded a medical society at Halifax in 1844. In 1854, a committee of the society was formed "for the purpose of studying the entire problem of medical practice in the province. After due consideration of the question the committee drew up a memorial advocating the union of the profession throughout the province and the extension of the Halifax Society to include the entire province."[80] In October of that year, a meeting of the society drew up a petition to the colonial legislature calling for the introduction of licensing legislation in Nova Scotia and submitted a draft of a bill to that effect.[81]

The result of this agitation was that the Nova Scotia government enacted the medical act of 1856.[82] The act established a licensing body for the colony, to be appointed by the Governor, with powers to examine prospective practitioners and to certify them as qualified to receive licenses to practice from the Governor. Holders of degrees in medicine were exempt from examination but, together with other applicants, were required to register their credentials with the provincial secretary. Professing to hold a medical degree or a license to practice while not registered under the act was punishable by a $20 fine for each such offense. No penalty attached to merely practicing without a license.

New Brunswick

An attempt to institute restrictive legislation in New Brunswick[83] proved less successful. The established profession there managed to secure the enactment of a registration law in 1859, probably by appealing to the example offered by Great Britain. But the proximity of the colony to the New England states and the mobility of the population[84] made enforcement impossible and the law was effectively repealed by a new statute in 1863. The 1859 act[85] established the Medical Council of Education, Health and Registration for New Brunswick, to register medical practitioners in the colony. The statute allowed registration of all physicians then practicing in New Brunswick who (1) were possessed of a diploma from any medical college in Great

Britain, Ireland, Canada, France, or the United States; (2) had been granted a license to practice by the Lieutenant-Governor of the province; or, (3) had been practicing in New Brunswick for at least seven years. Future registrants were either to have been graduated or licensed by a medical school or corporation approved by the Council, or to have been registered as medical practitioners in Great Britain or Ireland.[86] Military physicians and medical practitioners residing in the neighboring areas of Canada, Nova Scotia, or Maine who occasionally practiced in New Brunswick were exempt from registration. Penalties were provided for attempting to falsely secure registration (imprisonment for up to twelve months) or for using any title or designation suggesting the practitioner were registered (a fine of up to £20). There was no provision in the act making unlicensed practice itself illegal.

The law appears to have been almost impossible to enforce and in 1863 the registration provisions of the act were repealed.[87] The provisions of the 1863 statute were similar to those of New Brunswick's act of 1816. The Governor was once again empowered to grant licenses to practice medicine and surgery in the colony, with holders of diplomas from medical schools in Great Britain, Ireland, Canada, any other British colony, any European country, or the United States, qualified to receive a license without examination. All other applicants were required to undergo an examination by judges appointed for that purpose by the Governor. Military physicians were again exempt from the provisions of the law. As in the 1816 act, no penalty attached to practicing without a license. However, only licensed physicians could sue for the recovery of fees.

British Columbia

Lobbying for protective legislation was not limited to the profession on the Atlantic coast. On the opposite shore of British North America, a small but energetic group of physicians on Vancouver Island sought passage of a medical bill aimed at limiting the number of medical practitioners. Lobbying for restrictive legislation began even before the union of the separate colonies of Vancouver Island and British Columbia in 1866. Practitioners residing on the Island who possessed British and Canadian medical diplomas petitioned the colonial legislature for a law aimed at preventing supposedly less qualified American and continental physicians from practicing in the colony. The bill was hotly debated in the colonial assembly, but had no popular support and it failed to pass. The *British Colonist* commented on the measure, while it was under consideration in the legislature:

> After doctoring bills for three months without curing any of the diseases of the body politic, the assembly has hit on the bright expedient of considering a doctors' bill. And such a bill it is, that the sooner it becomes waste paper, the better for the community. Nothing but the anxiety of some obliging members to have their constituents killed scientifically, could ever have induced any one to father it. As ali nice schemes to benefit a particular class are usually surrounded by a show of parental anxiety to protect the dear people from injury, so this doctors' bill is not a whit behind that to regulate the legal fraternity, and benefit the community by an invidious monopoly to benefit themselves. The preamble to the bill says, 'Whereas it is necessary to distinguish qualified from unqualified practitioners, Be it therefore enacted,' etc. Our opportunities to learn whether any such want has been expressed by the public, are rather extensive, and we have failed to discover any evil demanding such an enactment. We have discovered, however, that the doctors' bill is another selfish contrivance to throw the practice of medicine entirely into the hands of British Surgeons and Physicians. Were we to require the services of a physician, it would be but natural to employ one of that illustrious faculty. But we cannot see why the Americans, Germans, or French, who form a very considerable portion of our population, should be prohibited from employing those who graduated in their own country, as well as ourselves. A natural inference from the bill would be that foreign practitioners are not as good as British. Such a proposition is too absurd to be listened to; for some of the most eminently scientific doctors in the world are Americans, Germans and French, and some of the more profound works on medicine are from their pens. But a consequence of such an enactment would be to drive foreign practitioners from the colony. That is amply sufficient to order it to be laid under the table for six months, to purge itself of public contempt.
>
> The last clause of the bill prohibits apothecaries from prescribing medicine for the commonest ills that flesh is heir to, under penalty of fine and three months' imprisonment. If a person is attacked by the toothache, he must first fee [*sic*] Doctor Sangrado for a prescription, and pay the apothecary for compounding it besides. Such good Samaritans as the medical authors of this bill, are models in their way. Their antiquated notions indicate a mind diseased, and the sooner the rooted idea of their

own sorrow at the want of patients is extracted, by liberalizing the profession through leaving it as it is, the better. Such an exploded idea as imprisoning for three months an apothecary, or an old woman, for prescribing nostrums, is a fitting finale to a narrow-contracted bill designed for individual benefit; and the public money spent in examining it ought to be charged to their account. Society will protect itself sufficiently without any enactment; and in fact no enactment can suppress quack medicines or quack doctors, or ever make good surgeons and physicians out of medical students with merely parchment diplomas. So the whole thing deserves a severe letting alone.[88]

Despite this blistering attack on special-interest laws, the profession proved somewhat more successful seven years later. In 1867, an ordinance with provisions resembling those of the imperial statute of 1858 and the New Brunswick law of 1859 was enacted at the first session of the colonial assembly following the union of British Columbia and Vancouver Island.[89] The 1867 ordinance[90] created an office of Registrar for the colony, whose function it was to keep a medical register. Only physicians possessing a medical diploma already in practice in British Columbia or prospective practitioners holding a medical degree from some school or body requiring a compulsory course of at least three years' duration could be registered. Under the act, it was illegal to attempt to falsely procure registration or to employ any title or designation implying that one were registered. The ordinance was soon held in violation of the provisions of the Imperial Medical Act of 1858, which had granted to all physicians and surgeons registered under the imperial act the right to practice anywhere within the British Empire.[91] As a result, British Columbia amended its ordinance in 1870[92] to allow all physicians registered under the British statute to enroll with the Registrar of the colony upon payment of the requisite fee.

THE LEGAL CONDITION OF THE MEDICAL PROFESSION ON THE EVE OF CONFEDERATION

Although Canada had an uninterrupted history of medical licensing legislation going back to the period before the British conquest, the condition of the profession in British North America on the eve of Confederation was, in many particulars, not dissimilar to that which prevailed in the United States at the same time. The major exception was in the area of medical education. In 1867, Upper and Lower Canada possessed seven medical colleges, all of which had their origin as proprietary schools, and five of which remained as such. The medical laws governing each part of the province had established both the preliminary qualifications necessary to embark on the study of medicine, and the curriculum and duration of courses to be exacted by the province's medical colleges.

These requirements, more demanding than those exacted by the majority of schools in the United States, were incorporated into the curriculum of the Canadian schools. They included four years of study, comprising two sets of lectures of six months' duration and clinical experience in a hospital. It was in the area of education that the regular profession in Canada had achieved its greatest success prior to Confederation. It had effectively agitated for laws requiring of all prospective medical graduates a level of education offered only in the British universities and at the best American schools.

The effect of such laws, no doubt, was to open the profession only to those students possessed of the financial resources needed to acquire the training necessary to pass the provincial boards' preliminary examinations and to devote four years to the study of medicine. In the United States, on the other hand, the large number of medical schools[93] permitted a good deal of differentiation. Only the leading colleges, appealing to wealthier students, required extensive preliminary education and offered a longer and more rigorous course of studies. Poorer students were still able to embark on a medical career by attending the less demanding colleges. These had few, if any, preliminary requirements, and exacted two or three years of study, comprising two terms of eighteen weeks each, and a minimal amount of clinical and hospital instruction.[94]

Unlicensed practice common

It was the lack of effectiveness of the licensing provisions of the various statutes then in place in British North America that led to a situation closely resembling the unfettered competition that characterized the American profession at the close of the Civil War. The law in Lower Canada alone seems to have been in any way effective in curtailing unlicensed practice, and even there it appears that such practice was not uncommon. Indeed, the *Medical Chronicle* at one point complained that, while the educational requirements for licensure were strictly enforced in that area of the province, the College of

Physicians and Surgeons of Lower Canada became "completely dulled, amaurotic in fact, whenever the doings of an unlicensed practitioner is brought before them."[95] It continued:

> The College is much to be blamed for not protecting more carefully the rights of their licentiates; and for not preserving the people from the designs of any ignorant, unprincipled, rapacious fellow, who may choose to dub himself Doctor.[96]

Nor does it appear uncommon for licensed physicians in Lower Canada, among them members of the Board of Governors of the College, to employ unlicensed practitioners as assistants or to consult with them when it was profitable.[97]

However common unlicensed practice was in Canada East, it was far more prevalent in Canada West. Even under the 1827 statute, which provided for a fine of £25 and six months' imprisonment for practicing in violation of the act, there were "such impediments in the way of the execution of this law, that quacks of every kind run riot throughout the land."[98]

Canada West's registration law

The situation could not but have deteriorated after passage of the 1865 statute, regulating the educational requirements and requiring the registration of qualified practitioners. The 1865 law was modelled in almost every particular, including its preamble, after the Imperial Medical Act of 1858. And like the imperial act, it contains no provision for the punishment of unregistered physicians. The imperial statute was deliberately designed solely for the purpose stated in its preamble, to make it "expedient that Persons requiring Medical Aid should be enabled to distinguish qualified from unqualified Practitioners."[99] It was not intended to either discourage or prevent unregistered practitioners from offering their services to the public.

The chief sponsor of the bill at Westminster, Francis Cowper, explicitly disavowed this goal and was "disposed jealously to guard the right of private individuals to consult whomever they pleased."[100] The 1865 statute, like the imperial act, provided solely for the punishment of unregistered practitioners who attempted to register under the act in defiance of the requisite qualifications, or who led patients, by assuming a title or otherwise, to infer that they were registered. Even here very little seems to have been done to enforce the law in Upper

Canada. One physician, a graduate of Victoria College, boasted in a letter to the Toronto *Globe* that, although convicted of using his titles though unregistered under the statute, and fined twenty-five cents, he refused to pay the fine. Two months later, the writer was served with a warrant for committal but it was quickly withdrawn and the physician continued in practice without harassment.[101]

The condition of the medical profession in the other colonies was, if anything, more competitive than in Upper Canada. Neither Newfoundland nor Prince Edward Island had any medical statute whatever, and there were no penalties of any consequence attached to violating the New Brunswick law. The statutes of Nova Scotia and British Columbia, like Upper Canada's, were modeled on the Imperial Medical Act and did not provide any penalty for unregistered practice *per se*. Even when unregistered physicians advertised their services, a not uncommon practice, these laws were apparently unenforced.

Osler's views

In his presidential address before the Canadian Medical Association in 1885, Sir William Osler advanced the view that Canadian legislation had traditionally imposed strict limits on entry into the medical profession. He further maintained that the medical statutes of British North America were modelled on the legislative treatment consistently accorded the profession in Great Britain. But the history of medical licensing in England — including the complex and sometimes conflicting system of rights and privileges accorded the guilds of physicians, surgeons, and apothecaries incorporated in the sixteenth and seventeenth centuries — belies this view. More importantly, a careful reading of the Imperial Medical Act of 1858 and of the Upper Canada statute of 1865 disproves Osler's contention that the medical statutes of Canada and Great Britain were habitually of the most restrictive kind. In the face of what must have been clear evidence to the contrary, Osler declared:

> In a well-arranged community a citizen should feel that he can at any time command the services of a man who has received a fair training in the science and art of medicine, into whose hands he may commit with safety the lives of those near and dear to him. For the State to regulate and determine the individuals to whom the citizen may apply, is not by most persons thought unreasonable. There are those, however, who would have no

restrictions, but allow the utmost freedom and permit assumption and assurance to have full sway, and give to any man without education the right to practice medicine. This has never been the case in Canada. The men who came here in the early days to practise medicine were chiefly English and Scotch licentiates, who brought with them the traditions and customs of the profession in Great Britain.[102]

Indeed, Osler's comments constitute the traditional rationale for government regulation of the profession. But his argument neglects the less obvious but substantial costs to the public incident to restricting entry into the medical profession: that the licensing of physicians reduces the number of medical practitioners, that it increases the costs of medical services, that it permits the enforcement of anti-competitive practices among licensed doctors, that it discourages innovation in the field, and it adds considerably to the costs of entry into the profession, and, more significantly, that it increases the incomes of medical practitioners from what they would have been in the absence of licensing statutes. Most importantly, there is no hard evidence that licensing, as opposed to certification,[103] improves the quality of physician care available to the public; indeed, there is a good deal of evidence that suggests the contrary is true.[104] And doubtless these effects account for why medical licensing laws have originally been enacted at the urging of the profession itself, and have seldom been promoted by the consumers of medical care, their supposed beneficiaries.

Public antipathy to restrictive legislation

Certainly these factors in part determined the bitterness of the editors of the *British Colonist* in 1860, when it appeared that the profession on Vancouver Island might prove successful in gaining legislation to restrict competition. Indeed, by the 1850s, the sympathies of the public throughout British North America were strongly against restrictive legislation. Nor were the attitudes of a significant segment of the Canadian parliament any different. The legislature had recognized homeopathy in both Upper and Lower Canada and, more distressing to the profession, had sanctioned the practice of eclecticism in Upper Canada. It had removed criminal sanctions for unregistered practice in the western part of the province and had abolished the professional faculties at the publicly-supported University of Toronto, leaving the education of physicians in the hands of private universities and proprietary schools.

Even where unlicensed practice was illegal and subject to fines, as in Lower Canada, no effective enforcement existed and unlicensed practitioners abounded. There are, of course, no hard data on the number of unregistered or unlicensed doctors practicing in British North America; indeed, no reliable data exist even for the number of legally qualified practitioners during this period. But the figures offered by the Medical Council of Ontario in 1870 are perhaps indicative of the situation prevailing throughout the various colonies three years earlier. It was then estimated that approximately one-third of all physicians practicing in the province were unlicensed.[105] It would be legitimate to regard this as a base figure for British North America as a whole in 1867.

The profession at mid-century

In response to a letter complaining that some physicians had recently taken to "drunkenness and other vices," the *Upper Canada Journal* summed up the state of the profession at mid-century:

> The causes of this deep degradation are, we believe, dependent upon the want of that just and proper position which the science of medicine should occupy in the social condition of this province: it is a matter that requires from the legislature a searching inquiry as to its causes, and the national interest demands that a sufficient remedy should be found for its effect.... Placed in juxtaposition with the quack, who charges for his services whatsoever he can get — payment not being compulsory — he is generally preferred to the licensed practitioner on that very score. The consequence is that the professional medical man gets disappointed, disgusted, and quite out of heart; takes to the bottle to drown his cares — a fashionable remedy with all parties in this country.... [Canadians] cannot understand the distinction between the physician and the quack, save it be in the license, which they are too apt to look upon as a monopoly; so that they are more inclined to pity the impostor and spite the physician, than to encourage his exertions....
>
> In the vast strides of material improvement now making in Canada, almost every individual, save those connected with the professions of physic and divinity, are advancing at no tardy

rates. The professions alone appear to be deteriorating in public estimation. Many will instance the facts of our correspondent as pointing to the cause. We maintain they are only the effect — an effect produced by the unjust and insane treatment which the profession has long experienced at the hands of the legislature and of the public. We fear that this degradation of the professions is an evidence of the downward tendency of the Anglo-Saxon race, — this condition evincing itself most powerfully at the circumference of the empire, in the colonies. Such was the case with the ancient Roman Empire when it tottered to its fall. The Roman Empire was a kingdom established by military prowess and successful war; the Empire of Britain has been the fruit of the successful cultivation of science and the judicious application of knowledge. The first mark of weakness in the Roman power was the necessity for the withdrawal of her troops from the distant colonies, and the successful irruption of barbarian and undisciplined hordes. And we take it that one of the first marks of Britain's decline is a want of appreciation of the sciences, and a due estimate and encouragement of knowledge, which has ever been the source of her wealth and power. As far as Physic is concerned, take Canada for an example. Hence we confess we have our fears that the great mass of the public and the legislature will fail to see their error — will still endeavour to perpetuate a condition that only leads to public disadvantage and political degradation, while it stays the onward progress of science that might lead to more powerful and permanent results.[106]

Such, then, were the consequences of weak and poorly enforced laws restricting entry into the medical profession: the decay of a great civilization, its science enfeebled, its professionals degraded, its empire on the verge of collapse. It was indeed fortunate that physicians in Canada were successful in turning the tide over the course of the next half-century, else Britain was sure to suffer the fate of Rome.

TABLE 2.1

CANADIAN MEDICAL SCHOOLS, TO 1920, WITH DATES OF OPERATION

St. Thomas Dispensatory, Toronto[1]
1824 = 1826

Medical Faculty, McGill University, Montreal[2]
1824 = present

Toronto School of Medicine[3]
1832 = = :   = : 1887

Medical Faculty, University of Toronto[4]
1843 : = = = = :   : = present

l'Ecole de Médecine et de Chirgurie, Montreal[5]
1843 : = present

Medical Faculty, Laval University, Quebec[6]
1848 = present

Faculty of Medicine, University of Trinity College, Toronto[7]
1850 = = =   : = = = = = = = = = = = = = = = = = = : 1903

St. Lawrence School of Medicine, Montreal[8]
1851 = 1852

Medical Faculty, Queen's University, Kingston[9]
1854 = present

Medical Department, University of Victoria College, Toronto[10]
1856 = = = = = = = 1874

Halifax Medical College[11]

1867 = present

Medical Faculty, University of Bishop's College, Montreal[12]

1871 = = = = = = = = = = = = = = = = = = 1905

Medical Faculty, Laval University, Montreal[13]

1879 = = = = = 1890

Medical Faculty, Western University, London[14]

1881 = present

Women's Medical College, Kingston[15]

1883 = = = = = 1894

Ontario Medical College for Women, Toronto[16]

1883 = = = = = = = 1906

Manitoba Medical College, Winnipeg[17]

1883 = = = = = = = = = = = = = = = = = = present

= = = = = 10 years

Sources: Maude E. Abbott, *History of Medicine in the Province of Quebec* (Montreal: McGill University, 1931): 58–61, 63–67; Murray L. Barr, *A Century of Medicine at Western* (London, Ont.: University of Western Ontario, 1977): *passim*; Charles-Marie Boissonnault, *Histoire de la Faculté de Médecine de Laval* (Quebec: Les Presses Universitaires Laval, 1953): *passim*; William Canniff, *The Medical Profession in Upper Canada, 1783–1850* (Toronto: William Briggs, 1894): *passim*; Charles M. Godfrey, *Medicine for Ontario: A History* (Belleville, Ont.: Mika Publishing Co., 1979): *passim*; John J. Heagerty, *Four Centuries of Medical History in Canada* (2 vols.; Toronto: The Macmillan Company of Canada, Ltd., 1928), II:55–141; H. E. MacDermot, *One Hundred Years of Medicine in Canada* (Toronto: McClelland and Stewart Ltd., 1967): 95–109; Ross Mitchell, *Medicine in Manitoba: The Story of Its Beginnings* ([Winnipeg]: Manitoba Medical Association, [1954]): 84–91; Hilda Neatby, *Queen's University*, Vol. I: *1841–1917* (Montreal: McGill-Queen's University Press, 1978): *passim*.

Notes to Table 2.1

[1] In 1824, Drs. Charles Dunscombe and John Rolph set up a medical school in the Talbot settlement of Toronto and advertised its opening in the *Colonial Advocate*. It appears that the school operated for only two years and there is record of only one student having attended.

[2] The Montreal Medical Institution opened in 1824 with twenty-five students. Five years later, the Institution became the medical faculty of the newly-created McGill University.

[3] In 1832 Dr. John Rolph established a school of medicine in Toronto, which continued to hold classes until the rebellion of 1837, when Rolph was forced to flee to Rochester. In 1843, he returned to Canada and re-established his school, which was incorporated as the Toronto School of Medicine in 1853. The following year, Rolph affiliated his school with the University of Victoria College at Cobourg, where he was made Dean of its medical faculty. His teaching staff, however, resigned and carried on its functions as the Toronto School of Medicine. In 1874, the Medical Department of the University of Victoria College united with the Toronto School of Medicine and, in 1887, the united medical school was engrafted onto the University of Toronto as its medical faculty.

[4] In 1843 a medical faculty was created as part of the newly established King's College, later the University of Toronto. The faculty continued as a teaching department until passage of the Hincks Act in 1853, whereby the University of Toronto was reduced solely to an examining body. In 1887, the University was once again permitted a teaching faculty in medicine and the medical staff of the University of Victoria College—at that time united with the Toronto School of Medicine—became the faculty of medicine of the University of Toronto.

[5] The Ecole de Médecine et de Chirgurie was founded in 1843 and possessed degree-granting powers until passage of the Medical Bill of 1847, which created the College of Physicians and Surgeons of Lower Canada and which restricted medical licenses to those holding university degrees. As a result, the School affiliated itself with McGill University in 1847 for degree-granting purposes, students being required to spend their final year of medical study at McGill. This arrangement lasted only until 1850. In 1866, the School arranged affiliation with the University of Victoria College at Cobourg and this situation prevailed until 1890, when the Montreal School of Medicine absorbed its rival Francophone medical school, the Medical Faculty of Laval University at Montreal, on condition that Laval University, Quebec, would award its graduates the required university degrees. Finally, in 1920, the School was engrafted onto the newly-created University of Montreal as its medical faculty.

6 The Incorporated School of Medicine of the City of Quebec, inaugurated in 1848 by Dr. Joseph Morrin, was, in 1852, constituted as the medical department of Laval University.

7 The Upper Canada School of Medicine, at Toronto, was organized in 1850 by Drs. Edward Hodder and James Bovell. Two years later, the School was reconstituted as the faculty of medicine of the University of Trinity College. As a result of internal difficulties, the faculty was disbanded in 1856 and was not re-established until 1871. In 1903, Trinity's medical faculty was amalgamated with that of the University of Toronto.

8 The St. Lawrence School of Medicine was incorporated in 1851 by Dr. Robert L. MacDonnell and was awarded degree-granting powers by the College of Physicians and Surgeons of the province in that year. It appears to have originally been successful in competing for students with McGill University's medical school, having been located in downtown Montreal, but McGill's move to its downtown quarters near the Montreal General Hospital in 1852 deprived the St. Lawrence School of its primary attraction and it closed its doors after only one academic year.

9 The Medical Faculty of Queen's University was established in 1854; in 1865, it reorganized itself as the Royal College of Physicians and Surgeons, in affiliation with the University. Finally, in 1891, the medical faculty reverted to its original status as an integral part of Queen's University.

10 The Medical Department of the University of Victoria College, Toronto, was created in 1856, when the University's attempt to affiliate with the Toronto School of Medicine proved unsuccessful. The merger finally occurred in 1874 and, three years later, the united medical school became the faculty of medicine of the University of Toronto.

11 The medical school at Halifax was originally established as the medical faculty of Dalhousie University, which inaugurated a partial medical course in 1867 and a full course three years later. Because of financial difficulties, the medical school was detached from the University in 1875 and separately incorporated as the Halifax Medical College. At this point, the Medical College affiliated with the newly-organized University of Halifax for degree-granting purposes. When the University of Halifax became defunct in 1885, Dalhousie University replaced it as the degree-granting institution. In 1911, partly as a result of criticism aimed at the College by the Flexner Report, the Medical Faculty of Dalhousie University was re-established, absorbing the Halifax Medical College.

12 Established in 1871, the Medical Faculty of the University of Bishop's College continued in operation until 1905, when it was fused with the Medical Faculty of McGill University.

Notes to Table 2.1 — Continued

[13] In 1879, after a series of abortive negotiations to affiliate with the Ecole de Médecine et de Chirgurie, Laval University of Quebec opened a branch, or *Succursale*, of its medical faculty in Montreal. In 1889, the Montreal branch became virtually independent of the parent institution in Quebec, except for the granting of degrees. Finally, in 1890, the Montreal branch of the Laval medical faculty and the Ecole de Médecine were united; affiliation continued with Laval, Quebec, for the purpose of granting the requisite university degrees upon certification of the Ecole de Médecine.

[14] The Medical Faculty of Western University was founded in 1881, coincident with the establishment of the University at London. The London Medical School was virtually independent of the University during its early years and was owned and governed by its faculty, its connection with the University being primarily for degree-granting purposes. A reorganization in 1913 made the medical school an integral part of the University.

[15] In 1883, Queen's University opened a separate medical college for women, affiliated with the University for instructional and degree-granting purposes. The College was closed in 1894, however, ostensibly on the grounds that similar facilities for the education of female doctors existed in Toronto.

[16] In the same year as the establishment of a women's medical college at Kingston, a similar school was started in Toronto. The College did not possess specific university affiliation, but most of those completing its course were graduated through the University of Trinity College and the University of Toronto. The College remained in existence until 1906, when, for the first time, the University of Toronto admitted women to its medical school.

[17] The Manitoba Medical College, established in Winnipeg in 1883, was affiliated with the University of Manitoba for degree-granting purposes. In 1918, the Manitoba Medical College ceased to exist as a separate institution and became the Faculty of Medicine of the University of Manitoba.

Appendix to Chapter 2

Medical Politics

The following comments, under the title "Medical Politics," appeared in the editorial section of the *Upper Canada Journal of Medical, Surgical and Physical Science,* I (July, 1851): 158–168, and were occasioned by opposition in the provincial legislature to new legislative restrictions on the practice of medicine in Canada West, and the suggestion that, in place of a stricter law, all existing restrictions be repealed.

We can conceive a man being so completely blinded to his own interests, by a variety of causes combining to influence and overshadow his reason and judgment, as to consent to sacrifice social position, personal comfort, nay even life itself, in exchange for the accomplishment of one desire, the gratification of one passion.

Such a man, it will be said, would be a fit inmate of the Provincial Asylum, where, under the admirable management of our friend, Dr. Scott, and the wholesome restraint and discipline of the institution, he would be restored to the enjoyment of a rational exercise of his faculties.

In such a condition we regret to find, not only one, but several members of the Provincial Legislature. This epidemic mania, for we can regard it in no other light, reveals itself most conspicuously on the subject of the Medical Profession. It would appear that this body is considered by those unfortunates as a superfluous and noxious part of the community, whose extermination is to be accomplished at any hazard. What other explanation can be given of the desire evinced by those who seek to throw the practice of medicine open to every uneducated impostor? Who would de facto *legalize murder*, by rendering its detection impracticable. If we examine the bearing of the arguments put forth by these champions of charlatanism, we shall find them resolvable into the following general axioms:

1st — That the practice of medicine is as much a *trade* as any of the other mechanical pursuits of life or speculative occupations of commerce, and therefore ought to be as free and unfettered in its exercise as these are.

2nd — That the criminal law of the land is a sufficient protection against the evil consequences of ignorance and malice, and therefore it is unnecessary to restrict by statutory regulations either the

education or the conduct of those who profess to treat disease.
3rd—That every person ought to be as much at liberty to employ their own *doctor!* (save the mark), as they are to select their
own parson or lawyer; and that no one will give the preference to
an ignorant quack, when he can obtain the services of an educated
practitioner.

We propose to review these preposterously absurd conclusions
for the especial benefit of Messrs. Richards, Flint & Co. [oppo-
nents of the proposed medical bill in the provincial legislature].

What, let us ask, is it that brings the study and practice of medicine to the level of a trade? Is it the necessity of acquiring an intimate knowledge by long-continued and intense study, of one of
the most intricate pieces of mechanism which has ever, at least in
human belief, been framed by Almighty wisdom? Mechanism endowed with a spiritual vitality—which raises it far beyond the
other works of His creative hand—the mysterious connection of
which is apparently so intimate, yet really so frail, that the
slightest violence will sever the tie for ever! Is it because, successfully to acquire even a limited knowledge of this comprehensive
subject, an intellect of no ordinary capacity, tutored by preparatory education for the task, must be kept serene by abstinence
from all other pursuits, and be directed towards that object, and
that object alone; aye, even through a long life of toil, anxiety,
and disappointment. Is it because, in the prosecution of our
calling, we are brought to view the weakness of our common nature, to watch its changeful character under the trials of physical
suffering, to have our humanity wrought upon by the agonies of
pain, the contemplation of mental anguish, the appeals of helpless poverty, and the heartless forgetfulness of ingratitude? Is it
the consciousness of the fearful responsibility which attaches to
our vocation, when we see the life of a fellow-being depending
upon our still finite knowledge—however successfully acquired—a being in whose existence is wrapped up the hopes and
affections of a dependent family, the love and devotion of a
parent, or the interests and welfare of a community? Is it because
the peculiar nature of our intercourse with our patients makes us
frequently the depository of their fullest confidence, reveals to us
their most private concerns, which nought but the highest sense of
honour, and a just appreciation of moral obligation, can enable
us to preserve inviolable and protect with discretion? Is it
because, at all hours, in all places—under the meridian sun or
through the midnight storm, from the warmth and comfort of a
home to the dark and dismal cell of houseless outcasts, from the
happy communion of the domestic circle to the wailing abode of

sin and sorrow, from the social enjoyment of the festive board to the bed of death, the dwelling-place of grief, — we must pass and repass at the bidding voice of need, regardless of personal comfort, of mental anxiety, the rack of feeling, or the wants of a languishing frame. Yet these are the materials we have to barter, these the glorious instruments of our trade; it is with these chattels we enter the great mart of the world, the workshop of life.

The mason, the carpenter, the cobler, are all obliged to serve a probationary period of time, in order to obtain a practical knowledge of their handicraft; and no one will employ a tradesman who has not been regularly initiated in his occupation; but it would appear that any one can practice medicine, that such preparation is unnecessary for him who is to deal with human existence! The greater the ignorance, the grosser the imposture, the bolder the quack, the more successful he is in obtaining the encouragement and favour of those with whose lives he tampers, whose credulity and whose pockets are *his* stock in trade. We defy our enemies to say that this picture is overdrawn. Let every one, in the full enjoyment of his reflective powers, ponder over the duties which a medical man is called upon to fulfil in the instance of his own household, and he will soon discover, that the relationship existing between them is one of a most peculiar character; the requirements for a faithful and conscientious discharge of its obligations such, as he can hope to find only in one who has been educated with a full sense of their magnitude and importance, with every precaution as to his acquisition of knowledge; and who has obtained by examination the approval and sanction of properly constituted authorities among — those who only are competent to decide upon his qualifications — the seniors of his profession. And yet it is required by these legislative quidnuncs to permit any man, no matter what his principles, his education, or his other qualifications may be, or whether he be deficient in all, to undertake the treatment of the diseases of a body of which, unless so educated, he can know nothing.

We say it is wise, it is right, it is necessary, that the Legislature *should interfere* to protect the lives, the interests, and the physical happiness of the people, by placing such restrictions upon the study and practice of medicine, that those who enter upon the one, and commence the other, shall be duly and sufficiently qualified; and that no one unless so legally recognized, should be permitted to attempt the cure of the sick or the administration of drugs, as a profession or calling.

That the criminal law is equally applicable to the educated and licensed practitioner and to the ignorant and presumptuous quack, in the cases of injury to person or of loss of life, is true. True it is, that both must answer at the same tribunal, and before a jury of their country, for their delinquences and misdeeds. But the means of proof in both cases is not the same; the evidence for conviction or exculpation not equally ascertainable. The educated and licensed practitioner, when danger threatens his patient, is required by a sense of moral obligation, by custom and the rules of his profession, to call in the aid and seek for the advice of one or several equally or more experienced than himself, to counsel him in the difficulty which exists, to corroborate his opinion, correct his errors of judgment, and sustain him in his treatment; thus dividing the responsibility of his position, and providing at once a means of proof, either that his proceedings have been founded on the principles of science universally established and inculcated; that his attention to the sufferings of his patient and the exigencies of the case, have been sufficient; or, that he has displayed a want of knowledge and been guilty of neglect. It may sometimes occur that the precaution of consultation has not been resorted to, either from some circumstances, such as pressing emergency and want of sufficient time, the great distance from which additional assistance could alone be obtained, the repugnance of the patient, and physical obstructions of various kinds, or from a wilful disregard of common usage and obstinate opposition to such a course when suggested to him by those interested in the welfare of the sick; the practitioner, thus assuming to himself the entire responsibility of his acts, is bound to state in self-defence, the views he entertained of the nature of the illness under which his patient laboured, the plan of treatment he pursued, and the medicines he administered. This information obtained by his own declaration, and by cross-examination, is then submitted to the ordeal of comparison with the opinions of other medical men, celebrated for their skill and learning, who are required by the administration of justice to sanction or condemn the course pursued, and by their judgment and opinion so expressed, to enable the jury and the Court to acquit or convict the accused party.

But in the case of the ignorant pretender, how is this evidence to be obtained, how is the conclusion to be arrived at? If he calls to his assistance, in the time of need, a properly qualified person, his ignorance and presumption must necessarily be exposed; and should injury follow his charlatanry, he ought to be punished. And simply because such result does not ensue, is he to be permitted to go at large unrestrained, and place again the life of another human being in jeopardy? If he is brought into court, and submitted to the same investigation and the same ordeal as the educated and licensed practitioner, which justice would demand, how can his ignorance there escape the scrutiny of knowledge and experience? To whom can he appeal? Surely not to one as ignorant as himself; certainly not to the court or the jury, who in all that appertains to the body and its ailments are not presumed to be one whit better informed. On whose judgment then, can and must the people rely for the detection of the violence which has been perpetrated – the evil which has been consummated, in order that the ends of justice may be met? On that of those who are the duly recognized emissaries of the educational establishments of the country. Those who, from a life devoted to the zealous and careful discharge of their professional duties, have earned for themselves a reputation for skill and knowledge. Those who, from the promptings of a good conscience, and the dictates of sound reason, have first sought to learn how fearfully and wonderfully we are made, before they have *dared* to deal with the handiwork of God. Here, then, a similar result must ensue. Imposture will be laid bare, and held up to the contumely of the good, and ignorance will be punished for its presumption.

By permitting, therefore, all who feel so disposed, to engage in a pursuit for which they possess none of the requirements, would be to multiply the objects of criminal jurisdiction, to load the calendars of crime with victims scarcely less unfortunate than the poor sufferers on whose account they are punished. By such a law you would encourage the idle and dissolute to plunge into the vortex of danger which would momentarily surround them; for it is not to be supposed that they would voluntarily undergo the discipline, labour, and expense of a proper education, when they might at once dub themselves doctors, and commence the work of carnage and pillage. By holding out a premium to 'untutored genius,' this law would entice from other avocations more fitted to their capacity and wants men, who ready to cast character and even life on the hazard of a die, would seek by what they erroneously conceive to be a ready access to wealth, for the means of livelihood they find it irksome to gain by the plough, the anvil, or the hatchet.

Again, we say, it is wise, it is right, it is necessary that the Legislature should interfere to prevent such a calamitous state of things, by placing restrictions on the study and practice of medicine. We require a preventive, not a remedial law; a law which would guard and protect the community, not entrap and punish the individual.

We may as well answer at once, a very frequent but fallacious argument employed against a statutory provision of the nature for which we contend. It is asserted that such a restriction would prevent a man from giving a dose of medicine to his household, and might debar him from acting the part of the good Samaritan. Now the law always looks to the motive or intent as that which constitutes the offence; and it must, we think, be admitted, that it is not against the occasional exercise of individual judgment in cases of emergency that the spirit of such an enactment would apply, but against the wholesale imposture, the wicked assumption of a character to which they have no just claim, by those who openly undertake *as a means of livelihood, as a profession,* to practice medicine, of which they are entirely ignorant. No sophistry whatever can make it appear that — however unfortunate — the consequences of an act done under the influence of parental anxiety or charitable feelings, could reasonably be brought under the operation of a law framed expressly to prevent deliberate and wilful malfeasance. No jury of rational and conscientious men could fail to recognize the difference which exists between such cases, and to give their verdict accordingly, supposing a vexatious prosecution to be brought before them, founded on the provisions of this Act [the bill regulating the practice of medicine in Canada West then before the provincial parliament].

We pass now to the consideration of those arguments, by which it is maintained that such a law would interfere with the exercise of private personal rights, as far as liberty of choice is concerned, in the selection of those who shall minister to the spiritual wants of an unquiet conscience; who shall counsel in the mysteries of litigation; or who shall prescribe for the pain and threatened decay of the frail body. We distinctly assert, that there could be no interference with the right of selection among the *individuals of a properly qualified and educated body* of medical men; the superiority of the acquirements of some, the peculiar manner of others, would be certain to attract the good opinion and confidence of different sets of people, and to limit the exercise of private opinion and judgment in such a matter and to such a degree, would indeed be to trample on the liberties of the subject. But are the cases parallel? Is there any analogy between the duties of these respective professions or the consequences of an ignorant assumption of their functions? We trow not. Our convictions lead us to believe that the evil consequences of misdirected faith manifest themselves in every relation of life; and that we are bound to be most careful in the formation of our religious principles and the selection of our pastoral counsellors. Still the office of the clergyman consists principally in promoting the spiritual welfare of mankind, — they have to deal with the mysterious agencies of thought and conscience, to direct the efforts of repentance, and point the way to salvation. Any abuse of their functions involves the eternal welfare of individuals, but brings no temporal or, apparently at least, no physical evils on those connected with them. They are responsible alone to the God whose majesty they offend, — who, looking into their hearts, knows the hypocrisy and counterfeit hidden from the finite sense and imperfect knowledge of mortal and erring man. With such an awful accountability, from which there is no escape, no human contrivance could possibly interfere.

In the regulation of commercial pursuits, of monetary transactions of every description, and in the maintenance and protection of the social rights, either of communities or individuals, where the exercise of legal knowledge is called forth, men have a safeguard in the general information which is acquired by the daily intercourse of differing interests. If in the higher and more abstruse departments of legal science, where professional knowledge of principles and familiarity with technical detail is essential, an ignorant pretender should intrude, the consequences of his act are confined to the loss of money or of property, — a loss by no means comparable to that of life, or of that which makes life desirable — health, corporeal integrity, and functional vigour! Moreover, the errors of the ignorant, the evil deeds of the designing, may still be remedied. The means which brought about the casualty, if properly employed by competent persons, will restore to the unjustly suffering victim, his precious and accustomed liberty, his jeopardized property. But who shall replace the amputated limb — who soothe and quiet the troubled brain, unhinged by ignorant error or wilful malice — who can bring again, from the cold and silent grave, the body animated by the life prematurely cut short, to tell its tale of suffering unrelieved or disorder aggravated, to reveal the cause of its destruction? No! the tomb swallows up the best evidence of ignorance and crime, — in the smouldering clay lie buried alike, the records of deluded hope, of blind and helpless credulity; the secrets of unprincipled and murderous fraud.

Nor will it avail any thing to say that quackery is an evil which will cure itself, — that no one will countenance or employ the impostor, when they can obtain the assistance of an educated man. Daily experience teaches the reverse. We see even among intelligent and enlightened communities some instances of weak and perverted judgment, who are easily caught with the glitter of pretentious ostentation, which invariably characterizes the professional quack. With many, the very novelty of a new man has its peculiar attractions:

> Some praise at morning what they blam'd at night,
> But always think *the last opinion right;*
> While their weak heads, like towns unfortified,
> 'Twixt sense and nonsense daily change their sides.

But by far the largest proportion who give employment and support to the quack are those who are really ignorant of the risk they run, the danger they incur, in so doing, — they are unable, from a want of it themselves, to appreciate the advantages of education; and influenced and guided by the example of the really better informed though unthinking class, who set them so pernicious an example, they readily fall prey to the cunning and avarice of the unscrupulous pretender. It is for the protection of these, the very largest portion of the population of a new country like this, that the Legislature ought to evince a jealous desire to pass such laws, as will not only secure the careful and efficient education of every one who wishes to embrace medicine as a profession, but laws also which will prevent any but men educated under such legally established regulations from presuming to engage in its practice.

It may appear to be almost superfluous to adduce any instances of the evils of empirical imposture, to substantiate the assertion that such evils really do exist, of a nature and to an extent of which probably few dream. But as these remarks are intended for the benefit of our senatorial readers we will favour them with one of the most recent, kindly sent to us by our esteemed contributor, Dr. Rolls of Wardsville. He states that the case was related to him by Dr. S. of London. The practitioner was a homoeopathist, one who has lately taken up his quarters in that part of the country. The patient, a poor woman, was delivered of a child, by a midwife residing in the neighbourhood, but she could not succeed in bringing away the afterbirth, which it would appear was retained by hour-glass contraction of the womb. She sent for the globulist, who it may readily be conceived was somewhat staggered by the urgency of the symptoms. He had heard or read that the ergot of rye was a good thing to promote action of the womb; and therefore he presumed that as there was something to be brought away *by some means* from the womb, the best course to pursue would be to give some of the ergot, which was accordingly done, and in *very large doses.* The result of this drugging was such as to endanger the poor woman's life, and to whose assistance Dr. S. was most fortunately though tardily called in. The issue of this case will be made equally public with this account of its progress. [It is worth observing that, in fact, the alkaloids contained in ergot of rye (e.g., ergonovine, ergotamine) have a contractile effect on smooth muscle.]

We shall in a subsequent number enter into the consideration of
another most important division of the abuses which exist in one
department of medicine, namely, — the universal and unrestricted
custom of retailing drugs, now so prevalent, by persons entirely
unacquainted with their nature and properties. In this it will
perhaps be somewhat more readily admitted that much danger to
the community exists, and that it is an evil which ought to be
checked by legislative interference.

The balance of the editorial, which continues for another three pages,
is addressed "to our professional readers more particularly." The
editors of the *Upper Canada Journal* remind the profession of its
traditions of selflessness and devotion to duty, chide those physicians
who have engaged in the "too eager pursuit of individual benefit, at
the expense of the body to which we belong," and call upon every
established doctor to use all his influence, political and moral, to
"secure the attention and support of Government" for passage of an
effective law restricting entry into the profession.

Chapter 3

First Steps Towards the Professionalization of Medicine, 1867–1887

CREATION OF THE CANADIAN MEDICAL ASSOCIATION AND AGITATION FOR DOMINION RECIPROCITY

The confederation of the provinces of Quebec and Ontario with the Maritime colonies as the Dominion of Canada in 1867 coincided with renewed efforts on the part of the medical profession to create a Canada-wide association to represent their interests.[1] According to MacDermot's history of the Canadian Medical Association, the original impetus for the founding of a national medical organization following Confederation came from Dr. William Marsden of the Quebec Medical Society. Marsden had attended the 1867 convention of the American Medical Association at Cincinnati. He was particularly impressed by the nature of the suggestions put forward by the American profession for stricter educational requirements in medicine and for the establishment of but one licensing board for all physicians throughout the United States.[2] His report encouraged the Quebec Medical Society to pass a series of resolutions in June of that year, advocating a uniform system of granting medical licenses throughout Canada and the creation of a central licensure board to examine all prospective practitioners, irrespective of whether or from whence they held a medical degree. Additionally, the Society called upon all regular physicians throughout the Dominion to assemble in Quebec City on October 9, 1867, for the purpose of creating a Canadian medical association.[3]

The first resolution to be submitted for the consideration of the physicians attending the Quebec meeting was the following: "That in the interest of the public, and the Medical Profession, it is desirable to adopt such means as will insure an uniform system of granting license to practise Medicine, Surgery, and Midwifery, throughout the Dominion of Canada."[4] The great majority of practitioners favored such a move. It would provide mobility to licensed physicians who otherwise would be legally entitled to practice only in that province from which their license issued. At the same time, it was thought that a nation-wide law would provide a more effective method of curtailing the large number of unlicensed physicians operating throughout the country. The *Canada Medical Journal*'s views on the question were not atypical:

> The law under which the profession in Canada is governed is very defective, and is no terror to wrong doers. It is indefinite and inoperative; a conviction under the law as it stands for practising Medicine, Surgery or Midwifery without a license, is next to an impossibility; as a result we have throughout our country, but more especially in the larger cities, all sorts of quacks: Thompsonians, [*sic*], Steam Doctors, Bone Setters, Eclectics, Homoeopaths, Tumbleties, Electricians, Vacuo Vacuas (a novel genus), Phrenological itinerant lecturers, and every shade and degree of wonder monger all clamoring for public favour and public support. It is with a view of remedying this condition of things that the proposal has been made to endeavour, if possible, to secure an uniform system of granting license to practise in the Dominion.[5]

A national organization

The prospect of a national association comprising all regular licensed physicians throughout Canada was welcomed by many members of the profession. Such a national organization was thought to offer an effective mechanism for the punishment of practitioners who offended against the profession's rules respecting fee schedules, consorting with irregular practitioners, advertising, and so on. As early as 1851, one of the major medical journals had suggested the formation of some society for this very purpose:

> It is undoubtedly a source of reproach to the Medical Profession in Upper Canada, that there exists no means of regulating its internal economy, no tribunal of Professional opinion, before which offenders against etiquette and morality—which in other countries and from a remote period of time, have been respected and unheld—can be arraigned and punished. There are offences and delinquencies of a grave nature, involving important results to the honour of the Profession of Medicine and the welfare of the community, which do not strictly come within the pale of ordinary jurisprudence. Moral crimes, which can be, and often are perpetrated, under the cloak of the professional character, cognizable principally by those engaged in similar pursuits, and susceptible of restraint only by those against whose interests and

reputation they so materially militate.... Every attempt which
has hitherto been made to engage the co-operation of the Legislature in securing the right of self-government, has proved a
failure. A question naturally arises as to the practicability of
establishing a jurisdiction such as would be efficient for the end
desired, independent of Legislative authority by association
among ourselves.[6]

In light of this, the response to the Quebec Medical Society's invita-
tion for a convention of all licensed physicians to form an association
was, as one historian put it, "most encouraging."[7] Some 164 delegates
attended the meeting, held at Laval University in October, and the
Canadian Medical Association was duly formed by unanimous vote of
the assembled body.[8] Charles Tupper of Nova Scotia, later Prime
Minister of Canada, was elected as the Association's first president by
acclamation.[9] Dr. Tupper's brief comments on assuming the chair give
some indication of the purposes to which the Association was to be
put. He remarked that

I trust our deliberations will show to the world that our leading
objects are to protect the health and lives of the poeple of this
Dominion from the unskilled treatment of incompetent men, and
to provide in the most effectual manner for the due qualification
of the members of a profession so important as our own.[10]

The convention proceeded to establish a series of committees on the
following subjects: (1) framing of constitution and by-laws; (2) preliminary education; (3) medical education; (4) granting of licenses; (5)
statistics and hygiene; (6) medical registration; and (7) code of medical
ethics.[11] No committee was created for the advancement or dissemination of scientific or medical knowledge.

The Quebec Medical Society

Although the recommendations of the Quebec Medical Society respecting medical education and a central licensing board were not formally endorsed by the Association at its Quebec meeting, they were
taken under consideration by its various committees and discussed at
the succeeding meeting held in Montreal in 1868. The Association
apparently endorsed the principle of licensing legislation similar to
that proposed by the Quebec Society,[12] but the reports of the various
conventions of the CMA do not indicate that any clear recommenda-

tions emerged concerning preliminary and professional educational requirements until the annual meeting of the organization in 1869. The Montreal meeting did, however, frame the internal structure of the Association on the basis of the report of its committee on the organization's constitution and by-laws. More importantly, the convention accepted the report of its committee on medical ethics by adopting a code of ethics identical to that earlier drafted by the American Medical Association.[13] The code provided, among other things, that all physicians adhere to any fee schedule established in their area, that they refrain from advertising, and that they avoid dealing in any professional capacity with heterodox practitioners.[14]

The provision against consorting with irregular physicians was of singular importance to orthodox practitioners, whose ultimate goal was to eliminate all heterodox sects entirely. The immediate effect, however, was sometimes ludicrous. For example, at the CMA's meeting in Toronto in 1869, a number of physicians present, including the president of the Ontario Medical Council, were charged with associating with homeopaths and eclectics. The debates over whether these physicians should be admitted to membership in the Association appear to have occupied most of the time and attention of the delegates.[15]

Medical education

Despite this divisiveness, the question of medical education was not neglected at the Toronto meeting. The committee on preliminary education submitted a series of recommendations calling for a preliminary examination of all prospective medical students in the following subjects:

> Compulsory English or French language, including grammar and composition; arithmetic, including vulgar and decimal fractions; Algebra, including simple equations; Geometry, first two books on Euclid; Latin, translation and grammar; natural history and logic, and one of the following optional subjects: Greek, French or English (according to the nationality of students); German — and the Committee are of the opinion that mental and moral philosophy should be made compulsory at as early a period as possible.[16]

One delegate from Quebec objected that the examination was not sufficiently broad and should also include mineralogy, astronomy, geology, and rhetoric, subjects "taught in even the little girls' schools at Quebec," but the report was unanimously adopted in its original form.[17]

The recommendations of the committee on professional education were equally unrealistic, comprising four years' study, consisting of three courses of lectures of nine months' duration each, at some college or school of medicine approved by the Association. Graduates of recognized schools in the United States were required to have passed their preliminary examination before commencing the study of medicine, complied with the duration of study and curriculum specified by the CMA, and, additionally, to have completed one full course of lectures at some medical school in Canada.[18]

Finally, the CMA, after having expressed its dissatisfaction with the Imperial Medical Act of 1858 as a model for Canadian legislation, unanimously adopted a resolution appointing a committee to draft a medical bill for the Dominion, "providing for a uniform system of Medical education and examination in conformity with the views of this Association and the registration and licensing of Medical practitioners by a central board of examiners."[19]

Slow progress

The CMA's progress towards achieving a dominion-wide medical act was slow and uneven. Discussion of the provisions of such a bill occupied the Association for the next few years.[20] However, it soon became apparent to most physicians that more stringent legislation concerning medical education and licensure would have to come from the provinces, which were constitutionally empowered to legislate on these issues, rather than from the federal government.[21] The goal of a national licensing law was never abandoned however, although it was not until 1912 that the profession finally proved successful in obtaining the concurrence of both the federal and provincial authorities to such a measure. In 1874, in his presidential address before the CMA, William Marsden summed up the feelings of the profession at the time when he remarked:

> Doubts have been expressed by lawyers, as well as legislators (and by no less an authority than Dr. Tupper) of the legislative powers of the Parliament of the Dominion to pass any Medical Act for the whole Dominion, unless or until previous concerted action has been taken by the Local Legislatures; and to this opinion I strongly incline. In the American Medical Association progress is being steadily made in that direction by state legislation, and I

think the best thing we can do is to agitate the subject in each Province of the Dominion, and separately and gradually lead them up to the highest standard required.

Thus only can we hope to succeed in Dominion legislation. I would, therefore, respectfully suggest that, when this matter comes up, some member will move that its consideration be indefinitely postponed and thus put an end to a fertile source of discord.[22]

THE ONTARIO MEDICAL ACT OF 1869 AND ITS EFFECT ON HETERODOX PRACTICE

Attempts to gain passage of stricter licensing legislation on the provincial level following Confederation had, of course, never ceased. The profession in Ontario had been most dissatisfied with its 1865 act and particularly with the continued operation of the province's homeopathic and eclectic medical boards.[23] It soon became clear, however, that no improvement in the legislative condition of the profession would be possible unless regular physicians were to temporarily compromise with irregular practitioners regarding the enactment of a more restrictive statute. Many physicians thus found themselves in a moral quandary. To cooperate with heterodox practitioners violated the code of ethics established by the profession; on the other hand, not to act in concert with homeopaths and eclectics would likely deny regular physicians in Ontario a licensing law of greater severity and would perpetuate the existence of competing licensing boards in the province. The Ontario Medical Council early opted for compromise. At its Ottawa meeting in May, 1867, it was moved by Dr. Horatio Yates and resolved by the Council

that in the next amendments to the Medical Act, the committee [of the Council charged with proposing changes in the law] be instructed to endeavour to obtain a clause to the following effect: "That hereafter all Homoeopaths and Eclectics, before obtaining a license to practice, shall conform in all respects, save examination in treatment in practice of physic, and then, that all licensed be admitted to registration and representation under the Act."[24]

In 1868, the *Dominion Medical Journal* editorialized on the need for some check on prospective homeopathic and eclectic licentiates:

We believe it to be the duty of the legislature to place all the sects of medicine upon a somewhat equal footing. At the present time the public has *no guarantee* for the competency of Homoeopathic and Eclectic practitioners. Their respective "Boards" are to all intents and purposes closed corporations. They may abuse their privileges to an unlimited extent (and we have good reason to believe that the latter does do so) for they are beyond the restraining influence of public, or even professional opinion.

We are not going to discuss the relative merits of these rival systems of medicine.... Nor do we intend to discuss the wisdom displayed by the Legislature in granting charters to the Homoeopathic and Eclectic bodies. It is our duty... to recognize the fact that they have received the authority of the Legislature to grant licenses. Such being the fact, it is the duty of the Legislature to make such further enactment as may be deemed necessary to ensure the competency of their licentiates before they are allowed to engage in the responsible duties of their profession.

Certain "regulations" of the Medical Council (which have the force of Legislative enactments by virtue of their having received the sanction of the Executive) require that all persons who study medicine shall spend four years in studying *before being allowed to present himself for examination*; not only is the period of study fixed, but it commences at the time when an examination in preliminary education has been passed.... Here is a very complete guarantee of competency, but to make the matter surer, the Legislature has given the Medical Council power to enforce these regulations. This system of "checks and guarantees" complete as it is, remains practically useless, because it cannot be applied to the Homoeopathic and Eclectic Schools of Medicine.[25]

A new bill

In late 1868, the Ontario Medical Council unanimously agreed that certain amendments to the 1865 act were imperative and thereupon drafted a new medical bill, which it then submitted to the provincial legislature. The bill in its original form did not contain any provision for abolishing the homeopathic and eclectic boards nor did it provide that these sects be represented on a unified Medical Council. The most important provision contained in the draft proposal, and the only principal change from the previous act, was the requirement that all prospective practitioners applying for a license to the Medical Council not only satisfy the educational requirements stipulated by the Council, but also undergo a qualifying examination before being licensed to practice.[26]

The addition of a clause requiring candidates for licensure to sit an examination was thought essential inasmuch as the medical schools in Ontario, despite their having complied with the General Medical Council's educational requirements, were still turning out large numbers of physicians. The University of Victoria College alone had graduated 195 medical students between 1867 and 1869.[27] The *Dominion Medical Journal,* in supporting this provision, noted that "the competition between the rival schools of medicine in this Province for the last five years at least has been so great that it has become a public scandal."[28] The bill was introduced into the provincial legislature by Dr. William McGill. McGill's remarks in the assembly during second reading indicate that the practice of homeopathy and eclecticism were omitted from the original draft only because it was feared that irregular practitioners would object to being included under the act. However, he explained that the profession would be happy to incorporate both these sects within the Medical Council. The *Globe* reported his comments on this occasion:

> He would explain why the representation of Homeopaths and eclectics on the Board was not provided for. The promoters of the Bill did not seek to interfere with those gentlemen, but they would be more than happy to allow them to enter the Council and to be registered along with themselves after an examination on all the subjects with which all who presumed to practise medicine should be familiar . . . . If this had been proposed in the Bill, however, it might have been represented as a cause of severe persecution. But if these gentlemen could be induced to come in, those whom he represented would, as he had said, be more than happy to meet them.[29]

It was largely due to McGill's remarks that the legislature agreed to a new medical bill at all.[30] A completely amended bill, incorporating both homeopathic and eclectic representation on the Medical Council was enacted in Ontario in 1869.[31] The General Council of Medical Education and Registration, established in 1865, was transmuted by the act into a General Medical Council of the College of Physicians and Surgeons of Ontario. The College comprised all registered physicians in the province, including all practitioners registered under the 1865 and earlier acts. The composition of the College's governing

Council was similar to that of the old General Council, with the addition of five homeopathic and five eclectic representatives. The Council was empowered to set the preliminary education requirements necessary to pursue the study of medicine in the province; it was to appoint examiners to conduct its preliminary examinations, to determine the duration of study and curriculum of Ontario's medical schools, and to appoint a board of examiners to test all applicants seeking a license to practice.

The provincial register

All practitioners were obliged to register their names with the Registrar of the Council. Physicians who had been registered under the province's previous acts, including its homeopathic and eclectic licensing statutes, together with all applicants who had complied with the Council's educational requirements and passed its examinations, were entitled to be entered on the register. As was the case with the 1865 law, penalties were provided for fraudulently procuring or attempting to falsely procure registration or for employing any title or designation, such as physician, doctor of medicine, etc., implying that one were registered, unless one's name actually appeared on the medical register. Additionally, the law contained a provision permitting the Council to enter into reciprocal registration agreements with other jurisdictions whose licentiates met the requirements of the act.

To placate previously unregistered physicians who had been operating in the province, the act contained a clause allowing all orthodox practitioners who had been in practice in Ontario continuously since before 1850 to register, provided they had attended at least one course of medical lectures. Homeopaths and eclectics operating since 1850 were required to have practiced in Ontario for the last six years. They faced no educational requirement, but had to be recommended for registration by the representatives of their sect on the Council.

The new law's detractors

Despite the potential provided by the 1869 act for curtailing the number of physicians entering the profession in Ontario, the law had its share of detractors. The medical schools objected to it on the ground that its degrees were no longer, in themselves, sufficient to qualify candidates for a license. The *Canada Medical Journal,* long a devoted supporter of McGill's medical faculty, carried on a bitter debate with the *Dominion Medical Journal* on the proposed law and attacked the examination provisions of the bill. In December, 1868, it wrote:

> By the provisions of the act powers are sought by some of the members of the profession in Ontario, to restore the old Medical Board under a new name. They seek to establish a central board of examiners before whom all persons desirous of practising Physic, Surgery or Midwifery in the Province of Ontario, shall appear and submit to examination before they shall be entitled to registration. All persons no matter from whence they come, or from whatsoever college or university they hail, must as at present appear and pay fees to entitle them to registration. The promoters of this bill, however, regard the examinations of the colleges and universities in Canada as insufficient, and with pompous self-conceit deem themselves alone capable of administering the required test. . . .
>
> We regard this measure as narrow minded and highly injudicious, and fully hope that the promoters will be removed from their present position as members of the General Council of Medical Education and Registration for Ontario. All good and true members of the profession should see to it that these men, whoever they may be, have abused their high position, having endeavoured surreptitiously to introduce into the Laws of the Province of Ontario an enactment which will disgrace their statute book.[32]

In voicing such sentiments, the *Canada Medical Journal* was doubtless speaking for all the medical schools in Canada, whose authority stood to be diminished by passage of the bill. This was especially true of McGill, whose graduates, having taken their degrees from a university outside Ontario, were subject to whatever by-laws the new Council wished to establish respecting their matriculation and other certificates of medical education. This was exacerbated by the fact that the medical colleges of Ontario alone had representation on the new Council. It is hardly surprising, as Dr. McGill reported to the old Medical Council at its final meeting, that

> special representatives had been sent from Montreal to do all in their power to oppose the bill in its passage through the House, and indeed I understand that they paid a special visit to each member of the House, and stated their objections to it.[33]

It was solely to comply with the requirements of the Ontario Medical Council that the McGill medical faculty adjusted its 1869–1870 term so that its conclusion would coincide with the period fixed by the Council for its licensing examinations. In addition, and for the same reason, the University found itself compelled to add practical chemistry to its medical curriculum.[34]

Unpopularity of a mixed board

Certainly the most contentious aspect of the new law, however, was that it created a new Medical Council comprising representatives of the heterodox schools of medicine. At the final meeting of the old Ontario Medical Council in April, 1869, even before the 1869 act had come into force, Dr. James Richardson of Toronto moved that the sections of the statute providing for special treatment of homeopathic and eclectic applicants for registration, either by examination or via the law's grandfather clause, be condemned. The resolution was defeated, but only by a vote of 9 to 6.[35] At the same meeting, a resolution of the medical section of the Canadian Institute was presented, protesting the inclusion of irregular practitioners in the new law as repugnant to orthodox medicine and insulting to regular physicians. The communication was read but, by vote of the Council, was immediately tabled.[36]

No sooner had the new Council met, on July 14, 1869, than another resolution was introduced by one of its members calling for the repeal of those sections of the new act that had reference to homeopathy and eclecticism. The resolution condemned

> the Coalition, in a Council forced upon the Medical Profession, with two other bodies, known as Homoeopathists and Eclectics, for the purpose of legislating in regard to questions involving the most vital principles of medical science, [which] is viewed by nearly all the leading and thoughtful members of the profession as fraught with great danger, and likely to lead to the most pernicious consequences, alike subversive of the cause of science and of professional morality; for if the views held by all the great schools of the world are honestly embraced by the medical profession of this Province, and, if the so-called theories of the other bodies are honestly held by them, they cannot be compromised by either for any mere expediency, without dishonour;

and

> the incorporation of the medical profession with the Homoeo-
> pathic and Eclectic bodies in "the College of Physicians and
> Surgeons for Ontario," without distinction of any kind whatever,
> [which] is viewed by the profession as highly objectionable and
> calculated to compromise their status as recognised members of
> the great body of scientific practitioners of medicine throughout
> the world.[37]

There followed a lengthy discussion of the merits of the resolution,
which became somewhat acrimonious.[38] But, once again, supporters
of the act outnumbered its opponents, and the resolution was defeated. In its place another motion was passed by a vote of 20 to 7,
stating that

> inasmuch as three licensing bodies existed in medicine in the Prov-
> ince of Ontario, whose privilege was to send forth practitioners of
> an inferior medical education, and whereas it is highly desirable to
> protect the public by allowing only thoroughly educated men to
> receive a license to practice medicine, notwithstanding the objec-
> tions many of this Council may have and do now entertain to-
> wards some clauses of the new Bill, we are prepared to use our
> best efforts to make it acceptable to the profession, and beneficial
> to the community at large, by raising the standard of medical edu-
> cation throughout the country.[39]

Disappointment with the act

Opposition to the act was also voiced at the 1869 meeting of the CMA,
held in Toronto. Dr. Benjamin Workman, in his welcoming address,
expressed the disappointment of many physicians in the province with
the new law and remarked that the regular profession was now "as low
as the most modest and humble amongst us could for the sake of spiritual mortification, desire to go." But he regarded it as useless to petition an unsympathetic legislature for a better medical statute, since
"we are, I think, sure to come out worse than we went in."[40] Even the
president of the Association, Charles Tupper, took the occasion to
assault the Ontario law as a blot on the profession.[41]

But despite these attacks it was clear that the new act was supported
by the great majority of the profession in Ontario. Dr. Horatio Yates,
who sat on the Medical Council under the 1865 act as the represen-

tative of Queen's University's medical faculty, wrote in the *Dominion Medical Journal* that the existence of independent homeopathic and eclectic boards, abolished by the new act, had resulted in large numbers of ignorant "knaves and fools" becoming licensed. A mixed board with standardized educational requirements, he contended, would reduce the number of irregular practitioners receiving licenses in the future. "I have been censured by some medical friends," Dr. Yates commented,

> whose good opinion I value, for having originated the scheme for admitting *Homoeopaths and Eclectics* to registration, and representation in the Medical Council. This is, upon condition of their first undergoing the same curriculum of studies, and submitting to the same examinations, save in the practice of physic, &c, as students of orthodox medicine. And it is upon *these examinations* that the whole efficacy of the new act depends. It is true that the respective "Homoeopathic" and "Eclectic" acts also require of their students for admission a certain curriculum of studies, but it is also true that these requirements have not been carried out *bona fide*. I know of licentiates, under the Eclectic Act at least, who never attended a lecture or a hospital in their lives. . . . I felt convinced that every conscientious and intelligent student who had at first contemplated entering either of the two bastard branches of medicine, would, long e'er his curriculum was finished, be purged of his heresy, and would become a faithful disciple of genuine medical science and practice. That the ranks of Homoeopathy, Eclecticism so called, would be replenished exclusively by knaves or fools. That as in every profession, *some* knaves and fools will ever succeed in crawling in, so in our profession, the same misfortune must, though I trusted very rarely, happen; and it would be a great gain to have them hereafter sifted — the chaff from the wheat — and the knaves and fools left among the base coins of the profession. . . . The registration, &c., of the Homoeopaths and Eclectics, does not in the least involve the necessity of our meeting them in professional intercourse, any more than we are now called upon to meet every rascal who may chance to disgrace our own profession.[42]

Eliminating irregular practitioners

In spite of any initial fears that it might implicitly sanction heterodox practice, it did not take long before most of the regular profession in Ontario shared Dr. Yates' views. Indeed, it soon became apparent that

TABLE 3.1

ONTARIO LICENTIATES, BY LICENSING AUTHORITY, 1867-1870

School or Licensing Board	1867	1868	1869	1870
University of Toronto	15	14	20	
University of Victoria College	78	49	68	
Royal College of Physicians and Surgeons, Kingston (Queen's University)	17	16	18	
Toronto School of Medicine	6	3	5	
Homeopathic Board	7	4	21	
Eclectic Board	19	17	25	
Medical Council (1869 Act)				42
Total	142	103	157	42

Source: "Medical Legislation," *Dominion Medical Journal*, II (July, 1870): 193.

the new act would result not only in a sharp reduction in the number of newly licensed physicians, but also in the virtual elimination of licensed irregular practitioners. Under the terms of the 1865 act, the medical colleges in the province were entrusted with the authority to issue certificates of qualification to those students who had successfully completed the schools' examinations. Additionally, both the homeopathic and eclectic boards remained empowered to issue licenses to practice in the province. Table 3.1 gives some indication of just how successful the Medical Council created by the 1869 act was in reducing the number of new licentiates in its first year of operation.

Reduction in the number of medical graduates

These figures so impressed the *Dominion Medical Journal* that in 1870 it editorialized:

> The passage of the bill is a matter of history, but its influence on the profession is yet an experiment. We confess... that we feel strongly disposed to tolerate the combination in view of its influence on the numbers and qualifications of those entering the profession. For, while we were prepared to find *some* reduction in the numbers licensed, owing to the greater uniformity of the examination, and the usual dread which students feel at being examined by others than their own teachers, we were *not at all* prepared for the immense falling off, exhibited by a comparison of the numbers graduated during the last four of five years.[43]

It had been earlier pointed out by one anonymous correspondent that the educational requirements promulgated by the new Council were as demanding as those in operation in any country in the world and were bound to reduce the number of graduates from the province's universities:

> Remembering how many have graduated during the last fifteen years, we should not be surprised that censorious persons accuse the schools of sending out men unprepared either by preliminary education, or professional training, to discharge safely, satisfactorily, or creditably, the onerous and important duties devolving upon them, either as professional men, or private citizens, nor shall we forget that the establishment and enforcement of such a curriculum, as that promulgated by the Ontario Medical Council, while it removes all possible ground for such censure and accusation, will likewise enable our future licentiates to compare favourably with those of any other country, and command that respect in any position in life, to which, as members of a liberal profession, they are entitled.[44]

The 1869 statute even won the support of William Marsden, one-time president of the College of Physicians and Surgeons of Lower Canada, and later president of the Canadian Medical Association, who concluded that the Ontario act would lead not only to the destruction of homeopathy and eclecticism in the province but to the more expeditious suppression of unlicensed practice. In these respects, he wrote, it compared favorably with the medical act then in effect in Quebec. "I now participate," he noted in late 1869, "in the common opinion of most of my Quebec confreres, that the Act is not only the best that could have been obtained at the time, but superior in some respects to the Lower Canada Act."[45] Marsden appears to be one of the very few physicians to remark on the penalty clauses of the new statute, which provided, among other things, that registration alone entitled a person to practice medicine, surgery, or midwifery "for hire, gain, or hope of reward," under penalty of a fine of $25 to $100 per offense. No longer were unregistered healers permitted to offer their services to the public. Ontario's experiment with a hobbled free market in medical services had lasted a scant four years. Addressing the penalty provisions of the Ontario act, Dr. Marsden observed:

> The "Ontario Medical Act," which we were lately so ready to condemn and repudiate, is in fact, rather a boon to Ontario, than

otherwise. It is in my opinion, in some respects, superior to the Act of the College of Physicians and Surgeons of Lower Canada, (which regulates the practice of medicine in the Province of Quebec;) and especially in its penal clauses. In Quebec, we can, and occasionally do succeed in convicting unlicensed practitioners, and did so for the first time under my adminstration as President of the College of Physicians and Surgeons, after repeated failures during the preceeding ten years. Under... the "Ontario Medical Act," however, it is scarcely possible to fail, if the action be properly brought; as, (like the English Act,) you have a wider field of action, than the Lower Canada Act gives. The Ontario Medical Act proceeds against three separate and distinct offenses: Firstly, "wilfully and falsely pretending" to be something he is not; secondly, practising "for hire, gain or hope of reward;" [no such provision appeared in the British act] and thirdly, "falsely taking or using any name, title, addition or description" calculated to mislead. Whereas, the Lower Canada Act... names only one offense, "practising without license" under a penalty; "and such penalty shall be recoverable on the oath of any two creditable witnesses, &c;" but, it is very difficult if not impossible to obtain *two witnesses to every fact*, as the quack is very careful to avoid committing himself in the presence of third persons.[46]

Treatment of heterodox candidates

The treatment of heterodox applicants by the Medical Council was so biased at the first meeting of the Council that Dr. Duncan Campbell, earlier president of the homeopathic board and spokesman for its homeopathic and eclectic representatives, petitioned the provincial legislature in late 1869 for amendments to the act. The proposed amendments provided that all applicants be examined by a mixed board of examiners, comprising homeopaths and eclectics as opposed to a board consisting entirely of regular physicians, as was then the case. (Under the provisions of the 1869 act, sectarian representatives were granted the right to examine prospective homeopathic and eclectic practitioners only, and solely in the areas of "Materia Medica, or Therapeutics, [and] in the Theory or Practice of Physic, or in Surgery or Midwifery, except in the operative parts thereof.") Additionally, the amended bill, as proposed by Dr. Campbell, would have required that at least one homeopath and one eclectic sit on all committees of the Council. These amendments were fiercely opposed by the established profession and after passing through second reading in the provincial parliament in December, 1869, were referred to a committee of the legislature comprising several regular physicians. With passage of the amended bill thus doomed to defeat, it was withdrawn by its sponsors.[47]

Dr. Campbell reprimanded

When the Council next met, in Hamilton in April, 1870, Dr. Campbell was chastised by the representatives of the regular profession for "unbecoming" conduct in claiming to speak for the Council's heterodox representatives and in daring to suggest that the Council's orthodox members were in any way "unfair." To this, one of the other homeopathic members responded that

> if this Council was—as it was reasonable to suppose it to be—a reflex of the feeling and spirit that animated the medical profession in Canada, it would be sheer madness not to doubt [that the majority of the Council was unfair]. They [homeopaths and eclectics] had been studiously and assiduously treated with contempt. The regular profession affected to look down upon their qualifications with disdain, and to treat their claim to honor and respectability with derision. This feeling was unmistakably evinced at the last meeting of the Medical Association, by refusing to admit to membership a Homoeopathist or Eclectic. Their own members were expelled from the Association for consulting with the Homoeopathists, and could only be reinstated by humbly confessing their sins, and promising, like obedient though erring children, never to do the like again. If [the president of the Council's] own words were to be taken, they had a right to distrust; for he remarked that "in ten years the Act would snuff them out of existence." He assisted in preparing and carrying through a Bill that he believed would wipe out the Eclectics and Homoeopathists in ten years.[48]

At the same meeting, a motion was put to elect, by majority vote, an executive committee of six members of the Council "to prepare all items of business to be brought before the Council." The motion was carried, but an amendment by Duncan Campbell requiring that at least one homeopathic and one eclectic representative be included on the committee lost when all of the Council's members representing the regular profession voted against it.[49] As a consequence of this action, a formal protest, signed by the sectarian members of the Council, was included in the minutes of the meeting.[50]

Graduates of American schools

Perhaps the greatest blow to heterodox applicants came with the decision of the Council to pass the following regulation respecting graduates of American medical schools seeking licenses in Ontario:

> All graduates from recognized colleges in the Unites States shall be allowed to proceed to the examinations of the council after having matriculated and passed two full courses of lectures in some medical school in Ontario.[51]

Since no homeopathic or eclectic college existed in Canada, the requirement, which amounted to adding an extra two years to the educational requirements demanded of graduates of American medical schools, would have had a lethal impact on heterodox medicine in the province.

At the final session of the succeeding meeting of the Council, held at Toronto in June, 1871, Duncan Campbell, in attempting to undo the damage to homeopathic and eclectic applicants caused by this onerous requirement, introduced a resolution, with the full support of the Council's sectarian representatives:

> That graduates in Medicine from the homoeopathic colleges in the United States, known as the Cleveland Hospital College, the New York Homoeopathic Medical College, the Chicago Hahnemann Medical College, and from the eclectic colleges known as the Bennett College of Chicago, Eclectic Medical College of New York City, and the Eclectic Medical Institute of Cincinnati, after attending one full course of lectures in one of the medical schools of Ontario, shall be admitted for final and primary examinations, upon giving proof that they have been engaged in the study of medicine for not less than four continuous years under the direction of one or more of the homoeopathic or eclectic members of the College of Physicians and Surgeons of Ontario; that they have passed the matriculation examination of this council previous to the commencement of their studies, and that the degree has been conferred after having attended not less than two full winter sessions in separate years.[52]

Objections by the Council's heterodox members

Despite the innocuous nature of the motion, it was dismissed as out of order by the chair, having been made without prior notice. Campbell's insistence that the question was one of life and death to the irregular practitioners of the province did no good, and the Council was adjourned *sine die.* At that point, Campbell announced that the Council "would never meet again as presently constituted."[53] That October, Campbell wrote to the Registrar of the College in the following terms:

> The action of the majority of the Council of the College of Physicians and Surgeons of Ontario, on the last evening of the meeting in Toronto in June, has led to the very general belief in our section of the profession, that our continuing to act in concert with the members of the "General" School will not lead to beneficial results; and that it would be better for our body and for the Eclectic School also, that the connexion should cease. I am instructed to take immediate measures to apply to the Parliament of Ontario for the repeal of the "Medical Act," and to ask either for the re-establishing of the Homoeopathic and Eclectic Medical Boards, or for the entire removal of all restrictions upon the practice of Medicine, putting it on the same footing as in the adjacent State of New York. . . . I cannot resist the appeal made to me to take action in this matter, admitting as I do the justice of the complaint made both by the Homoeopathic and Eclectic Schools, that their students are compelled to pay exactly double for their education than the students of the "General" School do. Two years' attendance upon lectures in any Medical Institution gives a right to all subsequent sessions free; when three sessions are exacted from students at the *same* College, it adds only the board to the expense; but when Homoeopathic and Eclectic students, having as yet no College in Canada of their special Schools of Medicine, go to the United States for their education, they are compelled, no matter how complete that education may have been, or how well qualified they might be to pass any ordeal however searching, they are, I say, compelled by the Council to pay in full for another medical education in Ontario, before they are admitted to examination. This is no mere imaginary or fanciful grievance; it has begun to tell very seriously upon the number of students applying to enter with practitioners of our School, and several young men have distinctly stated that they cannot afford to become Homoeopathists, when they can enter the Old School for half the money. This may be a matter of exultation to those who have looked upon the Medical Act as the means of extirpating Homoeopathy from Canada; but it is scarcely a creditable mode of proceeding when arguments have failed to have recourse to fining students to coerce them into the "General" School.[54]

A compromise clause accepted

Nothing was accomplished with respect to this contentious issue at a special meeting of the Council held in December, 1871,[55] except to temporarily placate the heterodox representatives, but the matter was reintroduced at the 1872 Council meeting. In an attempt to preserve unanimity, Dr. Campbell was elected vice-president of the Council and the following clause respecting American medical graduates was substituted for the earlier provision in the Council's 1872 Announcement:

> All candidates from recognized colleges outside the Province of Ontario and Quebec, shall pass the Matriculation Examination and attend thereafter one full winter course of lectures in some one of the Ontario Medical Schools and such other course or courses as may be necessary to complete the curriculum and pass the primary and final examinations before the Board of Examiners of the College of Physicians and Surgeons of Ontario.[56]

The profession, for the most part, was pleased that the Medical Council had been preserved in its existing form. Since the creation of the joint council in July, 1869, not one homeopathic or eclectic candidate had presented himself for examination,[57] and regular physicians had good reason to believe that a unified College — with independent homeopathic and eclectic licensing boards eliminated — would soon lead to the extinction of heterodox medicine in the province. The following table gives some indication of the progress of these sects under the new law and those that preceded it.

During the period the homeopathic and eclectic boards were in operation, 79 homeopathic and 139 eclectic physicians were licensed in Ontario.[58] Not one irregular practitioner was licensed in the province during the succeeding four years by the College of Physicians and Surgeons!

In light of this, it is understandable that two eclectic representatives on the Council concluded that eclecticism as a distinct sect was doomed to disappear in Canada "as the facilities afforded students in Canada for preparing for the allopathic examination were more favorable than for Eclectics, [and] it would be better to merge into the general body, as there was not enough difference to warrant the perpetuation of a sect."[59]

TABLE 3.2

HOMEOPATHIC LICENTIATES, 1859-1873, AND ECLECTIC
LICENTIATES, 1861-1873, ONTARIO

Year	Homeopathic Practitioners	Eclectic Practitioners
1859	10*	
1860	5	
1861	4	7**
1862	9	10
1863	4	5
1864	2	13
1865	5	7
1866	8	36
1867	7	19
1868	4	17
1869	21	25
1870	.	.
1871	.	.
1872	.	.
1873	.	.

* Of which 5 were licensed by the act of parliament creating the homeopathic board.
** Licensed by the act of parliament establishing the eclectic board.

Sources: *Canada Medical Journal*, VI (November, 1869): 196, and *Canada Medical Record*, II (August, 1873): 25.

Disappearance of eclecticism

With the virtual surrender of eclecticism to orthodox medicine, the homeopathic representatives on the Council found themselves standing alone against its regular members, whose explicit goal was the elimination of heterodox practice in Ontario. Surprisingly, the homeopathic members appear to have had no objection to the Council's policy of instituting more rigorous requirements for licensure and of reducing the number of entrants into the profession. Indeed, their votes on the Council were consistently cast with the majority on any motion touching on these subjects. It is clear that they were unaware of the grave implications these policies would have on the future course of sectarian medicine in the province.

An example of the homeopathic position on the question of limiting the number of new licentiates is found in Duncan Campbell's response to a deputation of Toronto medical students in November, 1872. The students had passed a series of resolutions condemning the high examination fees exacted by the Council and the fact that candidates were denied copies of previous examination questions. In dismissing these complaints, Campbell, speaking on behalf of the Council, expressed his hope that "in the future, the students would not take up any stand of antagonism to the Council,"[60] noting that "the effect of the Act [of 1869] ... was that the prospects of students had been very materially raised since the standard was made higher, the number entering the profession diminished, and the competition consequently decreased."[61] In supporting such measures, homeopathic practitioners in Ontario were acting contrary to their own interests. Any move to restrict competition would obviously fall most heavily on the heterodox sects, whose minority status would, at best, become rigidified. Since effective licensing laws, by their nature, discourage innovation and change in favor of the contemporary orthodoxy, homeopaths were inviting their own eventual destruction as a distinct school of medicine. The elimination of eclecticism was the strongest testimony to this rule.

A rift between orthodox and homeopathic members

It is somewhat ironic that when the short-lived harmony between the regular members of the Council and its homeopathic representatives did break down, it was not over the introduction of more restrictive regulations governing the admission of new physicians into the profession, but because Dr. Campbell, who had been made vice-president of the Council in 1872, was not elected president in the following year, in accordance with custom.[62] As a result of this slight, the homeopathic representatives resigned from the Council in December, 1873,[63] and in May of the following year met separately and resolved

> to abstain from presenting themselves at any meeting of the said Council until full justice is done by said Council to Homoeopathy both in the matter of the examination of students and of an equality of rights of the representatives in the Council satisfactory to the general body of Licentiates in Homoeopathy in Ontario.[64]

The homeopathic representatives thereupon had a new bill introduced into the provincial legislature seeking the incorporation of a Homeopathic College of Physicians and Surgeons of Ontario, with powers similar to those of the existing College.[65]

Meanwhile, at the instigation of the Council, a new medical bill, amending the 1869 act, was passed by the provincial legislature. The 1874 act[66] contained several provisions that appear to have dealt adequately with homeopathic objections, inasmuch as they did not proceed to press their own bill and returned to the Council in 1875.[67] The new act's provisions dealing with homeopathy included clauses permitting homeopathic applicants to fulfill the educational requirements of the Council at any homeopathic medical school in the United States or Europe recognized by the majority of homeopathic representatives. Additionally, for a period of four years following passage of the act, homeopathic candidates were permitted to take their preliminary examination at any time prior to their professional examinations. As was to be expected, the act further provided for the elimination of eclectic representation on the Council upon the expiry of its current members' terms in 1875, and for the immediate abrogation of any special status for eclectic applicants.

Other changes in the act included a provision allowing the Council to levy an annual fee on all members of the College of not more than two dollars. Additionally, any association of practitioners in the province was permitted to submit to the Council a tariff of fees for its approval, such tariff to be held a "scale of reasonable charges" by the courts of the area in which it was declared to take effect. Finally, the penal clauses of the act were altered.

Ambiguous definition of illegal practice

The Council had sought broader and harsher penalty provisions in the province's medical law ever since passage of the 1869 act. The language of section 41 of that statute, referring to illegal practice, was drafted in language too ambiguous for some, and had left a number of questions unanswered. It read:

> Any person who shall wilfully and falsely pretend to be a physician, doctor of medicine, licentiate in medicine or surgery, master of surgery, bachelor of medicine, surgeon or general practitioner, or shall practice medicine, surgery or midwifery for hire, gain or hope of reward, or shall falsely take or use any name, title, addi-

tion or description, implying, or calculated to lead people to infer that he is registered under this Act, or that he is recognised by law as a physician, surgeon or accoucheur, or a licentiate in medicine, surgery or midwifery, or a practitioner in medicine, shall, upon summary conviction before any Justice of the Peace, of any such offence, pay a sum not exceeding one hundred dollars, nor less than twenty-five dollars.[68]

This section was interpreted by some members of the Council as prohibiting all medical practice unless the physician were registered, while other members saw its provisions as applying only to those practitioners falsely claiming to be registered.[69] The issue was further complicated with respect to practitioners who had been licensed under earlier acts and who had failed to register under the 1869 law. Large numbers of physicians in the province appear to have done exactly that. One member of the Council complained at the 1870 meeting that

many practitioners of the very highest standing utterly refused to comply with the Act. He had heard two strong reasons given for this course. One was that the law should not have been made retroactive in its operation; old practitioners claimed that their former Provincial Licenses could not be abrogated, and that they were entitled to free registration. The other reason was one with which he could heartily sympathize, namely, contempt for the motley College of Physicians and Surgeons the Act had created. In the meantime the law was set at defiance, and in the absence of any other means of enforcing it than resorting to prosecutions, the Act might be pronounced a failure, and we had virtually arrived at "free trade" in medicine.[70]

Further, it appears that some unregistered physicians had evaded the law by not charging for either medical services or medical advice, but solely for the medications that they had recommended.[71]

A call for stronger penal provisions

Because of these confusions, the president of the Council, at its 1871 meeting, called for "an amendment to the present Bill embracing a penal clause that would be unmistakably operative against ignorant and unlicensed pretenders, whether local or foreign peripatetic, including also power to prevent druggists prescribing."[72] As a result, a motion was put and carried at that year's session that after several years of practical working of our present Medical Bill, this Council is of the unanimous opinion that more stringent penal clauses should be obtained, whereby uneducated and unlicensed men may be prevented from practising as physicians, or dispensing medicines in the Province of Ontario. That this Council regrets that the penal clause of our Bill, as originally drafted, was struck out. Therefore each member pledges himself to use all his influence among his confreres throughout the Province, to have the necessary penal clauses incorporated in our Medical Bill, for the better security of all parties interested.[73]

Agitation for a clear and far-reaching provision against unregistered practice was even taken up by the medical students of Toronto in November, 1872. Among the resolutions presented by their deputation to the Council was the following:

Whereas the medical students of Ontario, while recognizing the benefits conferred on the medical profession generally through the establishment of a Central Examining Board for the examination of students in medicine, feel that the Act has signally failed in its main object, viz., in securing protection to regularly licensed practitioners, inasmuch as the country is literally flooded with quacks, druggists and others, with questionable qualifications, who, in open defiance of the presumed intention of the said Medical Act, are openly practising medicine, surgery, and midwifery, to the detriment of legally qualified practitioners. It is therefore resolved that the Medical Council of Ontario be requested to take action during the ensuing session of the Ontario Legislature, with a view to secure for the profession the protection so much desired.[74]

It was largely in consequence of these efforts to clarify the ambiguous language of the 1869 act and to put a stop to unregistered practice that the penalty clauses of the 1874 law were enacted. Under the new law, the burden of proof respecting registration was placed on the person charged as being in violation of the act. It was made unlawful for any person not registered to practice, profess to practice, or give advice in medicine, surgery, or midwifery. Further, in instances where fines for illegal practice were not paid, the court was empowered to commit the offender to jail for up to thirty days. Any person convicted under the act who intended to appeal was required to turn over as security the full amount of any penalty, costs of conviction, and appeal. Finally, all penalties recovered were to be handed over to the Registrar of the College. The Council was authorized to appoint a prosecutor or prosecutors for the purpose of dealing with unregistered practitioners. The only limitation with respect to prosecutions was that they were to be commenced within one year of the alleged offense.

The new statute

The new act was well-received by the profession, who now had the advantage of some five years under a mixed board to reassure themselves that regular physicians would not become contaminated by working in concert with heterodox practitioners.[75] In a lengthy letter to the *Canada Lancet,* Dr. Walter Geikie, one of the leading physicians in the province, observed that the law "may be said to embody the wants and wishes of the vast majority of our medical men,"[76] and underscored the value of a central examining board in reducing the number of applicants for licensure in Ontario. "Prior to the passing of the previous Medical Bill," he noted,

> we had a very sad state of things—eight or nine different licensing bodies—each having a more or less pecuniary interest in the number of its outgoing licentiates. They were in many cases rival bodies competing with one another, and what was the result? The rushing into the profession of vast numbers of persons with very imperfect preliminary education in many cases, and very imperfect professional education in many more. Greatly reduced numbers, it is true, attend all our schools since the adoption of this *Central Board system*, but how great already has been the gain to the public, and how great will it ultimately be to the Medical Schools themselves by their willing adoption of a high and uniform standard of medical education. The present Bill continues the Central Board system, and the profession with rare unanimity accord it a very hearty support.[77]

Appointment of a public prosecutor

An early order of business at the first session of the Council held under the new act was the appointment of a public prosecutor to suppress unlicensed practice in the province. Much of the discussion surrounded the question of how great a role registered practitioners should play in initiating prosecutions, some members contending that "few medical men would like to lay themselves open to the risk of being called informants," while others regarded licensed physicians as the obvious candidates for originating prosecutions and providing the necessary testimony.[78] One representative even went so far as to present a resolution that, if carried, would have charged practically every provincial official with the task of prosecuting offenders. Dr. William Allison proposed:

That in order to make the Medical Act effective against persons violating any of its provisions, in so far as any of the penal clauses are concerned, it is due to the public at large that in all cases where any infringement of the law has been proved the most stringent measures should be adopted with the view of suppressing quackery in all its forms, either by druggists or other pretenders, and the following persons shall be deemed public prosecutors under the Act: — The chief constable of every town and city, the bailiffs of every Court, all inspectors of tavern licenses, and all other constables throughout the Province, and further, that when a case is proved and a fine is inflicted, that one-half of said fine be given to the informant, and the other half shall be handed over to the treasurer of the Medical Council to be applied as said Council shall direct.[79]

The motion was defeated and, for lack of any further agreement, the Council finally decided to accept the following resolution:

That the Executive Committee of this Council be instructed to appoint one or more persons in each county of Ontario to prosecute unregistered practitioners, and to give in each case the whole of the fine to the person securing the conviction.[80]

Attacks on the Council by the *Globe*

The actions of the Council and the Executive Committee appear to have proven at least minimally effective since the *Canada Lancet* found it necessary to defend the prosecution of unlicensed practitioners against the Toronto *Globe,* which had remained a staunch opponent of the monopoly privileges the profession had obtained for itself in the name of protecting the public. In its issue of September, 1875, the journal editorialized:

There have been several prosecutions under the Medical Act in this city, within the past month. Three most noted quacks have been brought up, charged with practising medicine without license. One was fined $50 and costs; the second was dismissed because Dr. Miller, the public prosecutor, could not prove that the accused had taken a fee for the services rendered, and in the third case, judgment was reserved....

It is quite time... to weed out from our midst all who are unlicensed and unqualified to practice medicine, and those who have been actively concerned in doing so deserve the thanks of the community, although it is very doubtful if after all they will receive any. It is very much to be regretted that an influential journal like the *Globe* should be found on the side of the illiterate quack, ready to throw dirt at any member of the regular profession who has the boldness to come forward at a most opportune season, to rid the community of men who are not known to possess any of the qualifications necessary to deal with human life.[81]

The *Lancet*'s defense of the Council, however, was short-lived for eight months later it bemoaned the lack of a vigorous and coherent policy respecting the prosecution of unauthorized practitioners.

No one can move freely in medical circles, without noting the feeling of dissatisfaction which prevails against the Medical Council, on account of its want of action in suppressing quackery. The failure of the council to prosecute unqualified practitioners (after the promises that have been held out) is leading to the expression of a want of confidence in its utility, and to a very special feeling of disappointment....

Either by the Medical Council, by local associations, or by individuals, the machinery of prosecution will have to be set in operation. A great point has been gained in obtaining a stringent enactment; but it is useless to allow the law to become a dead letter. A few exemplary prosecutions throughout the province would have a wholesome effect in deterring illegitimate practice. Medical quackery continues to be a great evil, and it ought to be suppressed. We advise medical men to avail themselves of opportunities of collecting evidence, and to summon all offenders against whom evidence can be obtained sufficient to ensure conviction.[82]

Successful prosecutions unusual

Apparently during the first year under the new act successful prosecutions were rare, especially since the Council had adopted a policy of staying proceedings against unregistered physicians during this period in order to provide them an opportunity to register. In addition, the prosecutors originally chosen by the Executive Committee seem to have lacked sufficient initiative. At its 1876 meeting, the president of the Council complained that

> these gentlemen took but very little interest in the duties of their position, and would not undertake prosecutions unless a medical man would enter the complaint and take the whole odium of the case. . . . The Council should take some steps to rid the country of unlicensed practitioners who were swarming in the western part of the Province.[83]

As a result, the Council voted to appoint one public prosecutor for the entire province, with the task of instituting proceedings against all unlicensed practitioners and to collect the annual fees levied by the College on registered physicians.[84] It is clear that the two issues were linked in the minds of many practitioners in Ontario, who had periodically objected to paying a yearly tax while still suffering the consequences of having to compete with unauthorized physicians. One representative on the Council, in explaining the poor performance of local prosecutors, noted that

> many parties were not prosecuted owing to local prosecutors refusing to act against illegal practitioners in their immediate neighbourhood, and consequently many physicians refused to pay the annual fee. What [the Council] required was to satisfy the profession that they were doing something for those who were registered practitioners.[85]

And, in a long editorial denouncing the prevalence of "charlatans" in the province and decrying the fact that a large segment of the public was unsympathetic to their being prosecuted, the *Canadian Journal of Medical Science* linked the College's annual fee with the need to eliminate the competition coming from unlicensed practitioners.

> The successful working of the Act is confessedly expensive. We have a Medical Council that requires a large sum of money annually to keep it in successful operation. To meet this pecuniary demand students are heavily taxed from year to year, until the period of their probation has expired. When they engage in the practice of their profession they must submit to an additional annual tax so long as they remain within the limits of the requirements of the law. Against all this professional men have certain penal clauses supposed to protect them against illegitimates or irregu-

lars. But what benefit has thus far been secured from these penal clauses? Why, the very first attempt that is made to enforce them is met by the most violent opposition from almost every leading journal in the country, with the hearty concurrence of a large, and often very respectable, portion of the general public. The cry of prosecution is raised if we even try to bring to justice a *Corn Doctor.* We are told that our system must certainly rest upon a very questionable basis if it is unwilling to stand upon its own individual merits, and that, if the public are willing to give their countenance to such characters, we should not object. We are also told by persons totally incompetent to be the judges, but holding a commanding position in society, that these montebanks are very useful members of the community, and that much damage would result from their banishment from our midst. . . .

Such a state of things, it must be granted, is very disheartening to the honest medical man. After years of diligent application, in the course of preparation for his great life-work and the expenditure of a large amount of substance, he must settle down to work; and, despite the most conscientious devotion to his profession, the fact is ever present to him that a miserable charlatan is working side by side with him and deriving *much more substantial* support from the public in many instances.[86]

Increase in prosecutions

The decision to appoint a single prosecutor for the province appears to have proved successful in changing the conditions under which the licensed practitioner, "the honest medical man," was forced to practice. The number of prosecutions increased dramatically over the following ten years.[87] In order to encourage legal action against unregistered physicians, the College devoted a section of its 1877 Annual Announcement to instructing the profession on how to take advantage of the penal clauses of the statute;[88] soon thereafter, it began including the same information in the provincial Medical Register.[89] The public prosecutor, who received the amount of all fines collected less costs, was thus encouraged to be particularly zealous in the exercise of his authority. Indeed, it was reported that the College's first prosecutor, who resigned in 1881, had gone so far as to prosecute some nurses who had occasionally acted as midwives.[90] The number of unlicensed practitioners in Ontario had been reduced sufficiently by the middle of the next decade that the *Canada Lancet* enthused in 1885:

> Graduates are no longer turned out in hundreds, and none but competent persons find their way into the profession. To be sure,

we still have the quack with us, but "he is not numerous." Pressed
as he now is, and will be, according to natural law, a few years
more and he will all but have disappeared. A "look at this picture, and then at that," is surely enough to convince any reasonable mind that the Medical Act has most fully met the ends for
which it was created. All who remember the utter chaos, under
the old order, cannot but wonder how successful the law has been
and how much good has been accomplished, both in the interest
of the profession and the public at large.

The Medical Act does suppress quackery, and besides, does
many other good things, of which we should feel proud. It has
brought order out of chaos, harmonized discordant elements, advanced education, and given a standing and dignity to the profession not enjoyed in any other country.[91]

Public opposition

Despite the actions of the College to suppress unregistered physicians,
the public continued to firmly oppose prosecution of these practitioners throughout the nineteenth century. Nor did they believe the College and the medical journals when they insisted that their campaign
against "quacks" was designed to separate out educated from unqualified physicians. In fact, regardless of the number of educational requirements that the Council might impose on applicants for licensure,
the state of medical therapy during the course of the century had improved very little. The major advances were in the area of surgery,
where the use of effective anesthetics became common in the late
1850s and in which antisepsis became accepted procedure by the
1880s.[92] But the scientific advances in bacteriology of the late nineteenth century, although they were to revolutionize medical science,
had only limited impact on medical therapeutics until the chemothera-
peutic revolution of the 1920s.[93] Indeed, until the beginning of the
twentieth century, the therapeutic arsenal of clinical medicine
remained comparatively primitive and the distinction between professionally trained and less well-educated practitioners was small.

In consequence, many, especially poorer, Canadians persisted in
consulting unlicensed physicians, whose fees were lower and who appeared no less competent in prescribing medications than did their registered brethren. The profession's attempt to suppress these doctors
was not motivated out of a selfless interest in improving the quality of
medical care offered the public, but out of a desire to lessen competition, which would in turn increase their incomes.

British credentials

Besides providing for the more expeditious prosecution of unregistered physicians, the 1874 act had allowed the Council the option of registering British physicians upon terms it "may deem expedient." Under the 1869 act, practitioners listed in the British medical register were not exempt from any of the educational or examination requirements imposed on all other candidates. Indeed, when in 1871 the London *Lancet* had mentioned that Canada was an excellent field for medical men wishing to emigrate and that "an English diploma suffices," some members of the Ontario Medical Council were alarmed. "If medical men come from England, we want to know if they have to pass an examination or not before the Council, before receiving license to practice. If we are to have an immigration from England into the profession, how are we to protect ourselves?" one representative asked. These fears were put to rest, however, since the act provided no dispensation for British registrants, as other members were quick to point out. "There can be no doubt," commented one prominent physician on the Council, "about our ability to legislate for ourselves. The lawyers have the right to exclude English lawyers from practising here, and why should we not have the same power?"[94]

When the subject was introduced at the Council's meeting in 1878, the president proposed that an arrangement be entered into with the medical council in Great Britain. Under the proposed agreement, British registrants would receive Ontario registration on payment of the usual fee provided that Ontario registrants be treated similarly in Great Britain. This reciprocity, however, was not to extend to Ontario residents first certified in Britain, who would continue to be required to sit the Council's examinations. It was moved that:

> The Council of the College of Physicians and Surgeons of Ontario consider it inadmissible that Ontario students, intending to practice in Ontario, should have the option of undergoing in any other country than their own the examinations which are to test their fitness for practice, and that the recognition of registration in the British Medical Register, shall not be held to exempt from the examinations established by the Council of the College of Physicians and Surgeons of Ontario any one who had begun his medical studies at any of the medical schools in Ontario, or who could have been properly considered as a resident in Ontario before the commencement of his medical studies.[95]

Reciprocity

The resolution was introduced partly in response to a bill earlier presented to the provincial legislature that would have allowed any graduate of a Canadian medical school registered in Great Britain to receive registration in Ontario upon application.[96] The proposed measure, however, was withdrawn from the Ontario parliament after fierce opposition from the profession; doubtless the resolution moved at the Council's 1878 sitting underscored the antagonism of organized physicians to licensing any Ontario physician who had not completed all the formal requirements set down by the Council, regardless of the applicant's abilities. Although the Council expressed support for the resolutions permitting a limited form of reciprocity with Great Britain, it was thought expedient to set the matter aside until passage of a new British medical act, then under consideration in the Imperial Parliament. Notwithstanding the fact that no changes were enacted in the British law in 1878 or 1879,[97] a new bill was being considered during this period. This, among other things, would have provided that any British registrant be automatically registered as a physician in any British possession, whether or not the territory possessed its own medical legislation.[98] This provision of the proposed British act infuriated the profession in Ontario. The province's physicians immediately petitioned the provincial legislature to amend the Ontario act so as to empower the Council to levy a special registration fee of $400 on registrants applying under the proposed provision.[99] During the course of the debate on the Ontario bill, however, it was decided to make representations to the Imperial Parliament instead, and the bill was withdrawn. In order to gain the cooperation of the Dominion authorities, Dr. William Clarke led a deputation of Ontario physicians to Ottawa. He there won the support of both the Prime Minister and the Governor-General in seeking to prevent passage of any such clause in the new imperial medical act, Dr. Clarke noting that "the medical profession of this Dominion would be endangered thereby."[100]

Educational requirements

During the decade following passage of the 1874 act, the Council did not neglect the question of the preliminary and professional educational requirements of its own graduates. At its 1878 meeting, it approved the recommendations of its education committee to extend the period of formal study in a medical school from three to four years, effective April, 1879.[101] And in 1880, it was moved that the Council no longer hold its own matriculation examinations. In its place, it was decided to accept the provincial intermediate high school examination, "with Latin as a compulsory subject," which "would make the approach to the profession if anything a little more difficult."[102] In proposing the high school standard, the following argument was put forward by Dr. James Burns and is indicative of the habits of mind of the Council:

> It is . . . an elevation of the standard as a comparison with the present examination would show, and it has the effect of grafting the system of elementary medical education upon the governmental system. By accepting the High School Standard it would prove a mutual assistance, as it is but reasonable to expect that if the Council endorses the Government in this matter we would be benefited in return. No one would deny that we have a perfect right to receive assistance from the Government, and we would have a better claim to it if we endorsed the Government standard of teaching.[103]

Graduates of U.S. medical schools

The rule regarding graduates from American medical schools, established in 1872, was to remain unchanged for decades. Candidates were required not only to comply with all the preliminary and professional requirements of the Council respecting their medical curriculum and length of study, and to undergo all the necessary examinations, but also had to complete an additional year of study at some Ontario medical school. In 1881, the *Canada Lancet* noted that the United States consul at Simcoe had complained in an American medical journal that "great injustice has been done to the medical institutions of the United States" by the Ontario Council, which discriminated in favor of Great Britain. (The Council had passed its reciprocity provisions with Great Britain in 1879.) The American consul contended that the provincial law "should not require any other evidence of qualification than a diploma from a reputable college in the United States, and the identity of the person presenting it, in order to make him eligible to practice in Ontario, especially as no other evidence of qualification is required from a Canadian graduate in the United States."[104] To this, the *Lancet* responded:

It would be a great injustice to Canadian students and Canadian schools, to admit to practice American graduates of three years' study, and exact a four years' course from our own students. There may be instances where an American graduate may have spent four winters' sessions, and passed a matriculation examination equivalent to that required by the Ontario Medical Council; but such cases are exceptional, and as all laws are made for the benefit of the many and not the few, it would be impossible to discriminate.[105]

Why it would be impossible for the Ontario Council to discriminate among American medical schools or their graduates, since this was one of the functions within the Council's purview under the medical act, we are not told. It was clear, however, that the Council viewed its central purpose not as one of seeing to it that only "qualified" candidates were permitted to enter practice, but to restrict entry into the profession as severely as possible using every device at its disposal, whether the applicant were qualified or not. As early as 1869, one of the Council's representatives had remarked, to the delight of its other members, that "it would be a great boon to the country if not another student passed for ten years to come."[106]

Hostility towards Canada's medical colleges

The profession's animus towards the country's medical schools, though often veiled, never ceased, nor was it likely to as long as the medical schools viewed their function as one of supplying the Dominion with trained practitioners, while the profession's goal was to reduce the supply of physicians. In his presidential address to the Canadian Medical Association in 1884, Dr. Michael Sullivan, in speaking of the eight medical schools then operating in Canada, was candid enough to remark that "we think, in fact we are sure, we have four times too many schools."[107] And Sir William Osler, addressing the Canadian Medical Association at its 1885 meeting, observed that "unrestricted competition between numerous schools means free trade in diplomas, and free trade in this sense is synonymous with manslaughter."[108] Osler continued:

The universities and chartered colleges have contested, inch by inch, the rights of the profession... and the struggle has not everywhere concluded. The possession of a degree in medicine from a university, no matter how reputable, cannot on any reasonable ground carry with it the right to registration and practice. The schools are independent bodies, outside, in a large measure, of State, and altogether of professional, control; they are numerous, and the competition between them is close; the requirements for graduation are variable, and the standard of examination unequal. They are close corporations, and neither the public nor the profession ever know what transpires in their councils. In the majority the teachers are also the examiners. Such a state of things can only lead to relaxation, and is fraught with danger to the best interests of all concerned.[109]

Certainly by 1885, the profession in Ontario had won the struggle to which Dr. Osler refers. After the establishment of the medical school at Western University in 1881, no new degree-granting institution was established in the province until the organization of the medical faculty at the University of Ottawa in 1945.

THE PROFESSION IN QUEBEC

When in 1869 Ontario established a provincial medical board with the power to examine all prospective practitioners — in addition to being able to exact a set of preliminary and professional educational qualifications deemed necessary for practice in the province — Quebec was still operating under its medical act of 1847. The situation remained unchanged in Quebec even after the penalty provisions of Ontario's law were strengthened in 1874. It soon became evident to Quebec's physicians that a new, up-dated statute was needed if the standards for medical practice in that province were to remain equal to those of Ontario. Quebec had historically enjoyed a smaller ratio of licensed practitioners to its population than had Ontario, and this differential became more difficult to maintain after 1869. Not only did the Quebec board not have the power to independently examine all applicants for licensure, but the educational qualifications imposed on medical candidates were somewhat less stringent than those obtaining in Ontario. The College of Physicians and Surgeons of Lower Canada had, through a by-law, established a course of study extending over four years, consisting of at least three six-month sessions at an approved medical school devoted to a curriculum similar to that set by the Ontario Medical Council. However, the 1847 law did not mandate that every student of medicine undergo a preliminary examination immediately preceding his entering upon the study of medicine, nor did it explicitly disallow students to take two consecutive sessions at a medical school in the same year. Finally, and perhaps more importantly, the penal provisions of the 1847 act were significantly weaker than those established in Ontario, and successful prosecutions for unauthorized practice in the province were rare.

Agitation for a new act

Given the general discontent with the prevailing law, the Governors of the College of Physicians and Surgeons of Lower Canada appointed a committee in July, 1874, for the purpose of drafting amendments to the medical act to make it more consistent with the demands of the profession. The report of the committee, consisting of an entirely new bill, was prepared in time for submission to a meeting of the whole College in May, 1875, but does not appear to have been taken up for discussion at that time. The bill called for enlarging the curriculum of study. Although it did not provide for mandatory examinations of all prospective licentiates, it did empower the provincial medical board to examine those candidates whose diplomas were not from Canadian medical schools meeting certain standards. In cases where these standards were met, the board was entitled to audit the universities' examinations to insure that they were sufficiently exacting. The penalty clauses contained in the proposed act were substantially broadened and, in part, modelled on those of the Ontario act of 1874. Assuming any title implying that one were registered, practicing without being registered, and "offering through the public prints to sell medicines for the purpose of promoting abortion, or against morality" were all punishable through summary conviction before any justice of the peace by a fine of at least $25 and not more than $100 plus costs.[110]

Criticism of the bill

The proposed new law was discussed at the meeting of the Governors of the College in October, 1875, and every effort was made to present it to the provincial legislature at its 1875 sitting. But because so little time was allowed the profession to consider the merits of the bill, it was found inexpedient to formally present it to the Quebec parliament that year.[111] Indeed, over the course of the next twelve months, the bill came in for a good deal of criticism. The most common complaint appears to have been that it was not severe enough; the views of the *Canada Lancet* were typical. It noted:

> By the provisions of the present [1847] act, the College of Physicians and Surgeons are given entire control of medical matters in the Province. Under this regime the profession has prospered for almost thirty years and the new Bill sets out with the statement that it is "highly desirable that the medical profession of the Province of Quebec be placed in a more respectable and efficient footing." This fair opening would seem to promise something good to follow as a means of elevating the profession, but instead, on perusal, we find it void of any feature, at all calculated to effect this desideratum. Unlike the Province of Ontario, the regular profession alone governs in Quebec. Unlike the present law, we think foreigners or all-comers, rather, should not be entitled to enregistration and admission to practice without examination, because, unfortunately, the possession of a diploma does not always warrant the possession of the needful amount of knowledge. The portals to the profession should not be too numerous or too easily entered; in fact, there should be but one licensing body, and one examining body, in each Province independent of all Schools and Universities. The power of expulsion of unworthy members should be provided for in any new Bill, which is not done in the one proposed.[112]

On the other hand, the medical schools of Quebec strongly objected to the provision permitting a committee of the College to audit the schools' examinations and to either re-examine or withhold licensure from those graduates whose examinations were found deficient. McGill University particularly was opposed to this clause in the proposed measure and used its not inconsiderable influence in the legislature to delay consideration of the bill.[113]

A more radical bill

Meanwhile, weary of the provincial College's overly-conservative approach, the Medical Society of Montreal had a second bill drafted in 1875, and immediately introduced it into the Quebec legislature, where it was sponsored by Mr. J. A. Chapleau. The bill was far more radical than that proposed by the College; not only did it empower a newly-created Council of the College to set both the preliminary and professional educational qualifications of all applicants, but it provided that all candidates undergo a mandatory examination, to be administered by the Council. The proposal empowered the College of Physicians and Surgeons to make the rules and regulations which it shall judge necessary for the interior discipline, and the honor of the members of the College, – to regulate the admission of aspirants to study or practice of medicine, – for the administration of its property, – to regulate a uniform tariff of fees for prescriptions, visits and professional attendance, – for all that relates to the general register and its publication, and to demand a fee from every member who shall ask the insertion of his name on the register after its publication, – to regulate the procedure in the case of suspension of a member of a section, in order that the General Council may have power to carry into effect the said judgment of suspension, and generally all the rules and regulations of a general interest for the Corporation and its members to assure their execution, which rules and regulations, it shall have to change, alter, modify and repeal whenever it shall deem expedient.

These rules and regulations . . . shall have the force of law. . . .[114]

In addition, the definition of illegal practice was broadened to encompass the writing of any prescription, or the sale of "poisons or other injurious liquids or substances," and the receipt of payment for any and all "attendance, visits, treatment or prescriptions." Indeed, the bill was so broadly phrased that, had it been interpreted literally, it would have placed almost any service whatever, including the visit of a cleric to an ailing parishioner, under the definition of medical practice.

The proposed act's complexity

The language of the act was so complex that even the *Canada Medical and Surgical Journal* was forced to observe that "this bill appears to lack conciseness and simplicity – but then, it was drawn up by an advocate! The gentlemen of the long robe are so accustomed to quibbling and being bothered in wordy argument by an antagonist, that in framing a law they endeavour to stop all gaps, so as to prevent, if possible, the proverbial coach and six being driven through their act unannounced."[115] And the *Canada Medical Record* noted:

In general terms we may . . . say it is by far too complex, requiring to be read at least half-a-dozen times by a man of ordinary intelligence, before it can be understood, and that many of its details are of such a character as to be utterly impossible of accomplishment.[116]

Support for Mr. Chapleau's bill appears to have divided along linguistic lines; the French-speaking profession and its journal, *l'Union Médicale du Canada,* favored the measure, while English-speaking physicians and the two English-language medical journals of the province opposed it.[117] In any case, the bill did not succeed in passing through the legislature in 1875 and it was dropped at its second reading.

A provincial examining board

Both the College bill and that proposed by the Medical Society of Montreal continued to be actively considered by the profession into the following year. After extensive discussion at the October, 1876, meeting of the College of Physicians and Surgeons of Lower Canada, the College decided to amend its proposal to provide for a provincial examining board, as existed in Ontario, and the following clause was added to the bill:

> Every person wishing to obtain a license to practice medicine, surgery and midwifery in this Province... shall, before being entitled to such license and to registration in this province, possess a degree or diploma from a Canadian university or college, or incorporated medical school, approved by the Provincial Board, and pass an examination as to his knowledge and skill for the efficient practice of medicine, surgery and midwifery, before the examiners appointed by this Board; and upon passing the examination required, and proving to the satisfaction of the examiners that he has complied with the rules and regulations made by the Provincial Board, and on payment of such fees as the Board may by general by-law establish, such person shall be entitled to a license to practice medicine, surgery and midwifery in this province, and to be registered, and, in virtue of such registration, to practice medicine, surgery and midwifery in the Province of Quebec.[118]

The College bill, as amended, was widely circulated among the profession and won the approval of a large proportion of Quebec physicians, including almost all the members of the Medico-Chirurgical Society of Montreal, embracing the English-speaking profession of the city. Although the various universities in the province held the right by nature of their charters to license their medical graduates without further examination, it appears that the medical departments of McGill University and Bishop's University, and the University of Victoria College, to which the Ecole de Médecine was affiliated for degree-granting purposes, assented to a central examining board.[119] In addition, a petition containing the signatures of more than 200 physicians, both French and English-speaking, was presented to the legislature in support of the measure.

The Quebec legislature, confronted with the College bill and the bill introduced by Mr. Chapleau at its last session, referred the matter of new medical legislation to a special committee of its membership, comprising all physicians in the House. At that point, matters were further complicated by the introduction of yet a third bill, drafted by the Sorel Medical Society. When it became clear that Laval University would refuse to consent to any law requiring its graduates to be reexamined by a licensing board, the concept of a central examining board for the province was dropped and the committee deputed the drafting of a totally new act to a delegation representing the major factions of the profession in the province.[120] The result of their labors was the Quebec medical act of 1876.[121]

The Quebec Act of 1876

The act created a College of Physicians and Surgeons of Quebec, comprising all registered physicians in the province. The College was to be directed by a Board of Governors numbering forty members, two of which were to be elected by each of the province's four medical schools and the remainder by the physicians of the various districts specified in the act. The Board of Governors was further constituted the Provincial Medical Board for the purpose of setting the requirements necessary for licensure and registration in Quebec. All students of medicine in the province were required to pass a matriculation examination before the Board immediately before embarking upon their medical studies. Candidates for licensure were to be at least twenty-one years old and to have followed their studies uninterruptedly for at least four years, of which no less than three years were to be in attendance at a medical school approved by the Board. The minimum curriculum of study was set forth in the act, rather than, as formally, determined by a by-law of the College. Only graduates of Quebec medical schools were exempt from examination by the Board; all others were required to pass an examination respecting the applicant's knowledge and skill before receiving a license to practice. In addition, the Board was empowered to appoint assessors to monitor the examinations of the various medical schools in Quebec, and to refuse registration to those graduates whose university examinations were not sufficiently exacting.

The penal clauses of the act were far more severe than those contained in the 1847 law. Practicing "for hire, gain or hope of reward," assuming any title or description implying that one were registered, or offering or giving any medical service, were punishable by a fine of not less than $25 nor more than $100, plus costs, with the oath of one witness sufficient to convict. Proof of registration was placed on the defendant. Prosecutions could take place before any sheriff, district magistrate or recorder, or judge of special sessions of the peace having jurisdiction in the locality where the offense was alleged to have been committed. Should the fine and costs not be paid, the act permitted imprisonment for up to thirty days. All penalties recoverable under the act were to be paid over to the Medical Board, which was authorized to appoint any person to act as prosecutor in its name. No member of the College could be deemed an incompetent witness by reason of his being a registered physician.

Finally, the College was empowered to assess an annual fee of $2.00 on each member and to frame tariffs for the different areas of the province.

Prosecuting unlicensed practitioners

Once the new act was in place, the profession's highest priority was the prosecution of unlicensed practitioners. Even before the new law formally came into effect, the Governors of the College, at their final session under the 1847 act, resolved in June, 1877,

> that the President be requested to appoint the High Constable in each district, or some other persons as he may deem expedient, to act on behalf of the College for the purpose of prosecuting all unlicensed persons who may be practising the profession of Medicine and Surgery;

and, "that the prosecuting officers appointed by the College shall have allowed to them the whole of the penalties recovered from unlicensed practitioners."[122] The 1876 law, like its predecessor, had authorized the Medical Board to establish rules respecting the admission of females to the practice of midwifery.[123] The policy of the College respecting midwives had traditionally been that none should be certified in any district in which a licensed physician was operating. It was therefore decided at the first meeting of the Board of Governors under the new statute that the president of the College also proceed against all unlicensed midwives in parishes containing at least one practitioner registered under the law.[124]

In their attempts to eradicate unauthorized physicians and midwives, the Quebec Board confronted the same difficulties as had earlier faced the profession in Ontario in like circumstances. Physicians themselves were reluctant to bear the onus of initiating prosecutions. And the general population was unsympathetic to any scheme aimed at reducing the number of practitioners, licensed or otherwise, operating in the province. As a result, during the first years under the 1876 act, few prosecutions were initiated.[125]

It soon became evident that if the College were to achieve any success in stamping out unauthorized competition, it would have to follow the example of Ontario and appoint a single prosecutor for the province, whose sole function would be to initiate proceedings and effect convictions. The medical act, however, had made no provision for the appointment of a public prosecutor who could act in the name and with the authority of the College, nor did it permit the College to assign fines collected to such a prosecutor. Consequently, when the law was amended in 1879,[126] the re-enacted statute contained a clause authorizing the College to "appoint any person or persons other than any of the officers of the said College . . . to initiate any proceeding against any person who may be supposed to have infringed any of the provisions of this act, and to collect any and all sums of money payable to the said College." This apparently minor alteration in the medical law proved to have far-reaching consequences.

Protection against unregistered practitioners

At the triennial meeting of the full College held in Montreal in July, 1880, the secretary of the College is reported to have remarked that "if the College expected the support of the profession, it must, without delay, take means to protect its members from the unlicensed practitioners throughout the country."[127] The College thereupon struck a committee to report to the next session of the Medical Board on "the best means to be adopted to protect the profession against unregistered practitioners."[128] As a result of the committee's recommendations, the Board appointed a Mr. Lamirande as official prosecutor for the province, who was assigned any fines collected in consequence of his activities. The *Canada Medical and Surgical Journal,* in writing of the urgent need to vigorously prosecute unlicensed physicians operating in Quebec, expressed great hope in the new prosecutor and in the Board that appointed him. "It is quite certain," it observed,

> that the profession look, and we hope with confidence, to the present Board under its energetic president for better things. There is a provision in our existing law for the appointment of a prosecutor for the purpose of indicting any one who shall be found to have contravened the said law.... Such an official has actually been appointed and may be expected to enter at once upon his duties. He will not have far to seek in order to find quacks and irregulars, and it is to be hoped that he will not waste his energies at first upon the smaller fry, but will boldly attack those notorious individuals who, in the cities, with brazen-faced impudence, flaunt themselves before the public. Their names can readily be obtained and no doubt, on inquiry, ample evidence can be secured to convict them of being law-breakers. With the majority of these cases there ought to be no difficulty at all, for they are unregistered, and therefore, from that very fact alone, are deserving of the punishment inflicted for this misdemeanour by the law.[129]

The prosecuting officer seems to have thrown himself into his work with alacrity, especially in collecting fines from practitioners delinquent in paying their yearly fees. Less than three months after his appointment, the *Canada Medical Record* was delighted to report:

> Mr. Lamirande...has been making things quite lively among those who have neglected to comply with the new law. We understand that many feel annoyed at having to pay the fine imposed by the Act. They can, however, only blame themselves, for ample and sufficient notice was given of the requirements of the law. When Mr. Lamirande has brought the regular profession into line, we hope he will pursue the irregulars with unabated zeal. At last the Profession is commencing to realize that the College of Physicians and Surgeons of Quebec is a live institution.[130]

And in August, 1881, the *Record* noted that five unlicensed practitioners had already been convicted under the law and that actions against an additional seven were still pending in the courts. By the time of the forthcoming meeting of the Medical Board in September, it observed,

> it will then be just a year since Mr. Lamirande was appointed prosecuting officer for the College. During that time he has not been idle. A large number of Medical men who were not registered have been compelled to do [so]. Several who had never taken out their license, although entitled to it, have been brought to see the error of their way. A very large number in arrears for their annual contribution have been taught that punctuality in its payment is the cheapest way in the end. In the matter of prosecuting charlatans, at least good progress has been made.[131]

Penalties increased

In 1882, the penalty provisions of the act were further strengthened. The Medical Board had been concerned about the light penalty attached to unregistered practice in instances where the physician were qualified to be registered. The 1876 act had provided that such practitioners were subject to a modest fine of five dollars for each year they were delinquent in registering. In order to encourage the prosecution of these physicians and to rectify an anomalous aspect of the law, the College managed to secure a further amendment to the act in 1882,[132] whereby all unregistered practitioners, regardless of their qualifications, were subject to the same penalties.

The new policy of suppressing all unlicensed practice was energetically pursued by the College and all indications are that it was highly successful. By 1883, few, if any, unauthorized physicians were likely to have been operating in the cities and larger towns of the province. At the 1883 meeting of the full College of Physicians and Surgeons, the president, Dr. R. P. Howard, offered a retrospect of the activities of the College's Board of Governors during the previous three years. Respecting the prosecution of unlicensed practitioners, he noted:

> One of the first acts of the Board at its first semi-annual meeting was to appoint an officer whose special duty it is to institute legal proceedings against persons infringing the provisions of the Medical Act, and ... a *systematic* effort has been maintained during the past three years, for the first time in the history of the College, to prosecute persons practicing the medical art without legal qualifications in the Province of Quebec. ... I may here state

that 49 suits were instituted by the agent of the College; 35 of which were successful, and 9 were lost through want of evidence; 2 through exception to the form; 1 through the plaintiff's lawyer failing to appear in court; and 2 because the defendant *possessed the Governor's* license, and the court was of the opinion that that was a Royal privilege and exempted him from the operation of the Medical Act.

When the many difficulties which attend the establishing of criminality in courts of justice — I was going to say in a legal way, when these many difficulties, some of them legal, some of them social, and, I regret to say, some of them of our own making — are borne in mind, it will be admitted that something has been done; at least a good beginning has been made to protect the members of the College in the enjoyment of their professional rights.[133]

Hence, despite public opposition to the prosecution of unregistered physicians, the College had succeeded in convicting thirty-five practitioners in slightly less than three years. As these efforts to deter unlicensed practice continued, the competition to supply medical services in Quebec was undoubtedly reduced, thus raising the incomes of registered physicians — insuring "the enjoyment of their professional rights" — at the cost of denying the public the option of lower-priced medical services.

Raising educational prerequisites

In addition to their efforts to eradicate unlicensed practice in the province, the members of the Medical Board were concerned with raising the educational prerequisites of prospective licensees. The 1876 act had added several requirements to the medical curriculum and the medical colleges in Quebec duly made the necessary changes in their programs. In keeping with the provisions of the new law, McGill University's medical faculty announced in 1877 that henceforth no degree in medicine would be awarded to any student who had not first attended a series of lectures in hygiene and had compounded medicines for at least six months. In addition, the period of compulsory hospital attendance necessary for a degree was extended from twelve to eighteen months.[134]

The College of Physicians and Surgeons had also given serious consideration to lengthening the academic term from its then current six months to nine months. In 1877, only Laval University's medical faculty exacted an academic year of nine months' duration. However, late in that year, the possibility was first raised that Laval might open a branch, or *Succursale,* of its medical school in Montreal. The profession, predictably, was strongly opposed to the prospect of yet another medical school in the province. This was especially so since the Medical Board lacked a central examining system and the degrees awarded by the proposed branch at Montreal would, in effect, carry the right to registration with the College. The *Canada Medical and Surgical Journal* spoke for the great majority of the profession when it wrote:

> The establishment of another medical school, because this is virtually what this movement means, must be regarded as an element of weakness in our educational system, and one which if carried out will tend to lower the standard of medical education in this Province. There are already in full operation in the Province of Quebec four medical Schools, all possessing University privileges, and should a fifth be established it will be more than is required by the country, and will tend to laxity in teaching, as also in examination of candidates.[135]

In response, the Medical Board considered petitioning the provincial legislature to amend the medical act so as to require attendance at four nine-month terms at a medical school, instead of the four six-month sessions specified in the act. Since no medical school in the Dominion other than Laval had as yet extended its academic year beyond six months, the change would have been drastic and far-reaching, both on the costs of medical education and the number of graduates presenting themselves for licensure. The rationale for increasing the academic year by 50 percent at one blow was offered by the *Canada Medical and Surgical Journal:*

> It would appear that if the Laval University establishes a branch medical school in this city it would be on the condition that sessions of lectures will be of the same duration, and on the same terms as those delivered by the parent institution, and that unless the medical lectures of McGill University, Bishop's College, and Victoria College [l'Ecole de Médecine] are of the same length and duration an unfair advantage would be held by those schools.[136]

Inconsistent arguments

It is hard to imagine how such specious and self-serving arguments could have been presented as serious reasons for so substantially lengthening the required period of study. Physicians first complained that a fifth medical school in the province was "unnecessary" and would lower the standard of medical education in Quebec—an argument without the least merit, inasmuch as the Medical Board already had control over the duration of study, curriculum, and preliminary qualifications of all medical students, in addition to being empowered to audit examinations. The profession then adopted the position that the new school would be placed at a disadvantage unless its competitors offered an academic term no shorter than that of the proposed college. In fact, the primary motivation of the province's physicians was neither to maintain the quality of medical education nor to insure Laval's proposed Montreal branch against the loss of students to the other medical schools of the city. Rather, their concern centered on the number of physicians that would be entering the profession in the near future to compete with those already in practice. That many laymen thought the profession's motives were selfless speaks to the success organized medicine had in convincing the public to regard physicians, not as lobbyists for their private economic interests, but as spokesmen for the health of the nation's population.

Because of the radical nature of the proposed change and the strong opposition of the province's medical schools, the College eventually decided not to pursue the matter of a mandatory nine-month academic session. The Montreal branch of Laval's medical faculty was established in 1878, exacting the same requirements and offering the same course of instruction as did the parent institution in Quebec. Its academic year extended over nine months, but Laval's continued to remain the only medical faculty in Canada whose academic year was of such duration.

Degree-holders from American medical colleges

Soon after the enactment of the 1876 law, the Quebec Medical Board was confronted with the problem of how to deal with graduates of American medical schools. Under the term of the act, so assiduously fought for by the profession, the College was prevented from issuing a license to any medical diplomate who had not passed a preliminary examination acceptable to the Board "before an authorized college or licensing board in Her Majesty's Dominions." All candidates not holding degrees from Quebec medical schools were further required to pass a professional examination. The law respecting preliminary examinations was conveniently interpreted by the Medical Board in September, 1877, as legally preventing it from examining candidates who had taken their medical degrees in the United States. To "solve" this problem, a committee on the by-laws of the College included a clause providing that graduates from any recognized medical school outside the British Empire must first attend a six-months' course (i.e., one academic year) at a medical school in Quebec, at which point the candidate would be in a position to sit both the preliminary and professional examinations of the Board, should he elect not to graduate from the Quebec school.[137] Why candidates could not satisfy the requirements of the law by submitting to both examinations without first having to spend an additional year at a Quebec school was never explained. Lest there be any question about the policy of the Quebec Board respecting American graduates, the 1879 act[138] contained the following provision:

> All persons coming from any recognized college outside of Her Majesty's possessions, and who are desirous of obtaining a license from the College, must previously pass the preliminary examination, before the examiners appointed by the Provincial Medical Board, or establish, to the satisfaction of the Board, that they have already passed an equivalent examination; they must, more-over, follow, in one of the Schools of Medicine in this Province, a complete course (for six months) of lectures, and such other course or courses as shall be necessary to complete the curriculum required by the board; they shall also pass a professional exami-nation before the Provincial Medical Board. Such persons may pass their professional examination immediately after their pre-liminary examination.

The penalties attached to graduating from an American medical school appear to have been decisive. In his summary of the 1880–1883 term of the College's Board of Governors, the president reported that of the 153 licenses issued during the period, 144 were awarded to Quebec graduates. Only four licenses were granted to candidates pre-senting themselves for examination.[139]

Successes of the 1876 Act

All in all, the 1876 act and its amendments appear to have succeeded in accomplishing what they were designed to do. Unlicensed practice in Quebec was substantially reduced, if not yet eliminated entirely, and the educational requirements for licensure were sufficiently tightened to have a noticeable effect on the number of new physicians

TABLE 3.3

STUDENTS AND GRADUATES OF QUEBEC MEDICAL SCHOOLS,
BY SCHOOL, 1878 TO 1890

Year	McGill University (S)	(G)	Laval University* (S)	(G)	Bishop's University (S)	(G)	Total (S)	(G)
1878	161	27	70	15	43	10	274	52
1879	166	37	65	9	30	9	261	55
1880	166	30	56	16	28	6	250	52
1881	168	38	97	13	31	5	296	56
1882	154	27	104	12	55	6	313	45
1883	188	30	117	26	34	3	339	59
1884	212	34	109	25	39	10	360	69
1885	234	36	85	22	23	4	342	62
1886	237	46	97	36	23	4	357	86
1887	231	45	136	27	31	5	398	77
1888	239	54	132	34	28	5	399	93
1889	233	38	149	35	39	5	421	78
1890	260	56	169	72	35	7	464	135

(S) = Students;   (G) = Graduates

* Laval University figures include both Quebec and Montreal faculties.

Sources: Figures are taken from the tabulations made by Dr. John Rauch, secretary of the Illinois State Board of Health, on medical education in the United States and Canada. See, *Medical Education and Medical Colleges in the United States and Canada, 1876-1886* (Springfield, Ill.: Illinois State Board of Health, 1886): 44-47; and, *Medical Education, Medical Colleges and the Regulation of the Practice of Medicine in the United States and Canada, 1765-1891* (Springfield, Ill.: Illinois State Board of Health, 1891): 15-17.

entering practice. If the profession had any complaint with the act, it was that it did not provide for the establishment of a central examining board. As early as 1877, Dr. William Hingston, in his presidential address before the Canadian Medical Association, observed that "the Province of Quebec has, as yet, no central board, yet nothing short of it will satisfy the wishes of those who look only to the well-being of the profession, and of the community."[140]

The profession renewed its efforts to empower the Medical Board to examine all prospective practitioners in 1886. The number of medical students and graduates in the province had shown a slow but steady increase since 1882 — McGill, which had graduated twenty-seven medical students in 1882, awarded forty-six medical degrees in 1886 — and physicians were keenly aware that if this trend continued, the increase in the number of practitioners would soon wipe out the gains achieved through passage of the 1876 act. Table 3.3 gives some indication of the increase in numbers of students and graduates at the province's medical schools between 1878 and 1890.[141]

Agitation for an examining board

These figures convinced most physicians that some check on entry into the profession independent of the medical schools themselves was essential. The *Canada Medical and Surgical Journal,* in calling for the creation of a central board of examiners, observed:

> There can be no doubt of the existence amongst the profession of this province of a sincere desire to promote a high standard of general excellence. Although, perhaps, the attainments of the average practitioner here may compare favourably with those of the same class, *e.g.,* many of the neighbouring states, yet it is distinctly felt, and fully admitted, that the time has come when a move towards reaching a higher plane may well be taken — is indeed demanded — if we are to hold our own. The only means by which such an advance can be made is by increasing the severity of the tests for admission to practice.[142]

In July, 1886, the Medical Board struck a committee to suggest changes in the medical act and to report back to the triennnial meeting of the full College later that year. The committee's recommendations not surprisingly contained a provision that all candidates for licensure should henceforth be compelled to undergo a professional examination by the Board. The recommendations were strongly endorsed by both the Board of Governors and the membership of the College.[143]

In addition, lest a professional examination not act as a sufficient deterrent, the College voted to increase the stringency of the preliminary examination by adding to the list of compulsory subjects upon which all prospective medical students would be tested, physics, elementary chemistry, and intellectual and moral philosophy. The decision to raise the preliminary requirements was made in face of the fact that, as the *Canada Medical and Surgical Journal* reported, "a very large percentage of those presenting themselves for the first time are rejected and obliged to appear for examination at the end of another year," and "the proportion of failures under the existing requirements is very great."[144] The draft amendments finally recommended to the Quebec legislature also provided that the Board be given disciplinary powers over members of the College who engage in unprofessional conduct and strengthened the penal clauses of the act.[145]

Opposition of the McGill Medical School

The draft was eventually introduced into the provincial legislature and considerable pressure was brought to bear to attain its enactment. But opposition to a central board of examiners by the province's medical schools was formidable. McGill University, especially, was unyielding in defending its traditional right to issue licenses to practice medicine in the form of its medical diplomas, a right secured to it by its Royal Charter. McGill's petition also took exception to the proposed changes in the preliminary qualifications required of medical students, arguing that the subjects to be added were "not in harmony with the system of education approved of, and in use in, the English Schools and Universities of this Country." Instead, the University suggested that

> the Degree of B.A., as given by the Universities of this Province, should be received as the best guarantee for adequate preparation for professional study, and that this is especially important as tending to induce students to take a regular University course, instead of merely cramming for arbitrary examinations.[146]

In the end, the legislative committee delegated to consider the new amendments, impressed by the vigorous opposition to certain provisions contained in the College's proposal, decided unanimously to report against the bill, which consequently died.[147]

Continued lobbying

In 1892, the College once again attempted to amend the medical act to establish a central examining board.[148] Like its 1886 predecessor, the new bill proposed that all candidates for licensure in Quebec submit to an examination conducted by the Board. However, the 1892 measure would have exempted from this provision licentiates and graduates of universities from France, Britain, and the British colonies outside Canada. The reason for including this exemption apparently was to encourage reciprocity of medical registration between Quebec and Great Britain. The exemption clause was not popular with many physicians, who thought it absurd to compel graduates of a school of the caliber of McGill to sit a provincial examination while waiving this requirement for foreign licentiates whose educational backgrounds might well be less rigorous. Nor was reciprocity with Great Britain regarded as particularly desirable. In February, 1893, the *Canada Medical Record* commented:

> For every one of our graduates out of employment here, there are at least a hundred British graduates starving in England. So that if the new medical bill be passed, we might see hundreds of L. S. A. [licentiates of the Society of Apothecaries] granted a license, while our own high class graduates were obliged to pass an examination. It would be far better to abandon reciprocity, and let Canadians desiring to practise in England take a British qualification in the future as they have done in the past.[149]

Support for higher standards

Opposition to its reciprocity clause and the continued hostility of the universities to the creation of a central examining board forced the College to withdraw the bill in early 1893. The profession was not successful in exacting a mandatory provincial examination of Quebec's medical graduates until 1909. Following the death of the bill in 1893, the *Canada Medical Record* remarked that the profession would be better served by vigorous action by the Medical Board in tightening educational standards and in prosecuting unlicensed practitioners than by a new law. The *Record* suggested that the Board

> do well two things which it already has full power to do: First, to limit the number of practitioners by raising the standard of candidates who are about to begin the study of Medicine, so that it would be impossible for those who are uneducated and unrefined to become medical students after a few months' training; and second, to employ a detective and a smart young lawyer to harass and persecute [sic] in every possible way the numerous charlatans who infest the Province....
>
> The raising of the standards by the Medical Board... would only apply to those who desire to practise in this Province; the

universities may safely be left to deal with the question of the entrance examination of those who intend to practise elsewhere. If the miners of British Columbia or the lumbermen of Michigan and the medical boards of these countries are all satisfied with an M.D. who knows nothing of Greek or Metaphysics, that is their affair, and not the business of our Medical Board, which has only to look after those practitioners who are manufactured for use in the Province. As we have often said, each Province or State should see that its own professional men are not subjected by overcrowding to too keen a struggle for existence.[150]

MEDICAL LEGISLATION IN THE MARITIMES AND THE WEST

While physicians were consolidating their monopoly position in Ontario and Quebec, the profession in the other jurisdictions of British North America was not idle. In 1871, Prince Edward Island enacted its first medical act.[151] The act created a Board of Examiners, consisting of five physicians appointed by the Lieutenant-Governor, with the power to grant licenses to practice in the colony. All persons not holding a medical degree from some college in the United Kingdom, Canada, any British colony, or from the universities of Massachusetts, Pennsylvania, or New York, were required to submit to an examination of the Board.

The statute contained an unusual grandfather clause whereby certain physicians could escape examination. A physician practicing in Prince Edward Island for at least five years who was successful in collecting the signatures of at least thirty householders living within five miles of the physician's place of practice testifying to the fact that the doctor should receive a license, could be licensed at the Governor's discretion.

The penalty for practicing in violation of the law was set at £10 for the first offense and £20 for each subsequent offense. Military physicians, midwives, nurses, and "persons treating cases of cancer" were exempt from the statute. The law further provided that homeopathic physicians producing a diploma or other proof of competency, together with the signatures of five householders supporting the applicant's licensure, would be licensed without examination.

There appears to have been little purpose served in enacting this statute. The colony had a population of just 94,000 at the time the act was passed[152] and only thirty-nine physicians seem to have registered under the law after its enactment.[153] A ratio of 2,410 residents per physician was significantly dissimilar to comparable figures for New Brunswick and Nova Scotia in 1871[154] and it is not unlikely that a significant number of practitioners were operating in the province beyond those whose names appeared on the register.[155] The law cannot have been strictly enforced. It appears to have been passed more to provide Prince Edward Island with some medical licensing legislation and thus to bring the colony into line with other Maritime provinces than to effectively restrict competition.

After the colony entered Confederation, however, the regular profession made some attempt to enforce the law, weak as it was. The established physicians of the province immediately brought pressure to strike out the provisions of the law treating graduates of American medical schools on a par with those from the United Kingdom and the rest of Canada. As a result, in 1874, the provincial legislature amended the act[156] to provide that henceforth graduates of medical schools in the United States would be required to both present their degrees and, in addition, to undergo an examination by the Board. At the same time, the grandfather clauses of the 1871 law were repealed.

Nova Scotia

In 1872, Nova Scotia enacted its first comprehensive medical statute.[157] The act created a Provincial Medical Board comprising nine physicians, four of whom were to be appointed by the Nova Scotia Medical Society and the remaining five by the Governor-in-Council. The Board was empowered to conduct preliminary examinations of all prospective medical students in a variety of subjects stipulated in the act. As well, it was authorized to examine all candidates for medical licenses not holding degrees in medicine from those schools designated by the Board as "in good standing." The law further specified both the curriculum and duration of professional study expected of applicants. This was to consist of a minimum of four years' study, of which three years were to have been spent in an approved medical college. Diplomates of approved institutions were not required to undergo an examination but had to register their credentials with the Board.[158] The act contained a grandfather clause permitting the registration of all physicians then practicing in the province licensed under its 1856 act.

The penalty provisions of the law were similar to those contained in the Ontario act of 1869, making it illegal to fraudulently procure or attempt to procure registration or to employ a title or description implying that one were registered. Further, it contravened the act to practice "for hire, gain, or hope of reward" unless registered, under penalty of a fine of $20 per day of illegal practice, plus costs. All monies were recoverable under a civil suit by the Provincial Medical Board. An informer system was encouraged in the law by providing that "where the information leading to such recovery shall have been given by any person unconnected with the medical profession, such person shall be entitled to receive one-half of the sum so recovered."

Provincial penal clauses

Soon after its passage, several physicians expressed the fear that the penal clauses of the act would be declared beyond the powers of the province by the courts. The *Canada Medical and Surgical Journal* noted in 1873 that although "we certainly rejoice to hear that the medical profession in our sister province has obtained an Act of incorporation,

> ... we fear that [the penal provisions] will be difficult to enforce. There will be the same difficulty which has been experienced in Ontario. The clause being penal, it is held by a large number of members of the legal profession in that province that no judge would enforce it, because the Local Legislatures of the provinces do not possess the power of introducing clauses of this nature into any of their Acts. This power alone rests with the House of Commons for the Dominion. If this be the case, then will the Act of the Legislatures, both of Ontario and Nova Scotia, become inoperative.[159]

These fears, in fact, proved groundless, and unlicensed practitioners were successfully prosecuted under this and succeeding laws with similar provisions.[160]

It does appear, however, that the penal provisions of the Nova Scotia act were only rarely invoked during the first decade following the law's passage. Lack of funds and the fear of alienating an unsympathetic public compelled the Board to confine its prosecutions to the most egregious cases of unauthorized practice. One physician, writing of the history of the profession in the province in 1889, observed that

> the effect of the penal clauses has been mainly a moral one. An apparent reluctance on the part of the Board to act upon the penal clauses, has created an amount of dissatisfaction and loss of

confidence, entirely uncalled for. Proceedings so far, have been chiefly carried on against persons who neglected to register, and two or three irregular practitioners, and in all cases with uniform success. The expenditure incurred and the feeble response to an appeal for financial aid from the profession, does not justify the Board in going any further in this direction. In one sense it is not an unmixed evil that the hands of the Board are thus tied, because in enforcing these clauses they forfeit the sympathy of the public and endanger the existence of valuable legislation.[161]

But, despite this policy, it was still possible to conclude that because of the act, "quackery has diminished very perceptibly, and it is rare to observe any manifestations of its grosser forms."[162]

New Brunswick

Of the four provinces entering Confederation in 1867, only New Brunswick had not adopted an effective medical statute by the end of the 1870s. The province's established physicians had made several attempts to gain enactment of a workable law but their petitions were unsuccessful until 1881, despite the encouragement of the profession throughout the Dominion. In 1879, the *Canada Lancet* noted that physicians in New Brunswick were

considering the propriety of making some effort towards medical legislation similar to, or better if possible, than that now in force in Ontario. They are becoming tired of free-trade in medicine, and are now beginning to wake up to the prospective benefits of protection. We shall be very glad to see their efforts crowned with success. All that we shall say at present is that the Ontario Medical Act has done great service to the cause of medical education, and has also diminished to a great extent the evils of quackery.[163]

And, in his presidential address before the Canadian Medical Association in 1880, Dr. R. P. Howard urged the need for legislation in New Brunswick to place the profession in that province on an equal footing with that prevailing in the other original provinces. "Let us hope," he commented, "that the sister province of New Brunswick will ere long, pass a medical bill which shall place the requirements of the medical student and the terms of registration of medical practitioners upon as satisfactory a basis as obtains in the [other] three Provinces."[164]

Legislation enacted

Agitation in New Brunswick for a comprehensive statute finally bore fruit in 1881. In that year the provincial legislature passed a medical law[165] creating the Council of the New Brunswick Medical Society, composed of nine practitioners, four of whom were to be appointed by the Governor-in-Council and the remaining five by the Medical Society.[166] All physicians legally registered in the province were members of the Medical Society. The Council was empowered to set preliminary examinations for all prospective medical students and to register those physicians meeting the educational requirements set out in the act. All applicants were required to have studied medicine for no less than four years, of which at least three years must have been spent at some medical school "in good standing," and to have followed a specified curriculum of study. Those applicants holding degrees from medical schools imposing a mandatory four-year course of study were exempt from further examination by the Council. All others had to sit the Council's professional examinations. The act provided that physicians holding any diploma in medicine already in practice in the province at the time the law was passed were entitled to registration, as were all practitioners, regardless of credentials, operating in New Brunswick since 1861.

The penal provisions of the law were similar to those contained in the Ontario act of 1874. Fraudulently procuring or attempting to procure registration, and employing any title or designation implying that one were registered, were made illegal. Practicing "for hire, gain or hope of reward," unless registered, was punishable by a fine of $20 per day of illegal practice, plus costs. The burden of proof respecting registration was on the defendant. The act provided that suit for the recovery of any fine be brought by the Council or its appointee. In order to encourage prosecutions, the law stipulated that one-half of any fine recovered be turned over to the person responsible for providing the information leading to conviction. Military physicians on active duty, midwives, and "clairvoyant physicians" were exempt from the law.

Council fees

The Council immediately set about its work of examining the credentials of all applicants and registering those physicians who fulfilled the requisite conditions. It was soon found, however, that the fees the

Council was empowered to collect from new registrants were not sufficient to cover its operating costs. As a result, in 1882 an amendment to the law was enacted[167] permitting the Council to levy an annual fee of up to two dollars on all registered practitioners. The amendment proved totally unworkable, however, since no penalty attached to non-payment and large numbers of practitioners simply disregarded the fee. In response to this, a second amendment was passed in 1884,[168] providing that registered practitioners who neglected to pay the annual fee should have their names struck off the medical register, thus subjecting them to the penal provisions applicable to unlicensed physicians. The result of this action was that, while in 1884, 200 names were entered on the provincial register, the number had dropped to 120 in 1885. A New Brunswick physician wrote the *Canada Lancet* in 1885 respecting these amendments to the 1881 act, noting:

> We have sought a reason for this delinquency, and the answer was, "we do not wish to contribute towards the benefit of the few, or pay taxes for which we receive no equivalent." Now, granting that the practitioner fully complies with the Act and its amendments, what are his privileges? He is legally qualified to practice his profession in the Province and to recover fees for his services; nothing more; nothing less. A quack may practice under his notice from day to day and exact exorbitant fees, while the physician is powerless to prosecute him—the power of prosecuting offenders being entirely vested in the Medical Council, the members of which reside in the cities far from the operations of quackery—and hence the result. "Dr." Sewell travels over the country visiting the sick, and prescribing "Morning Glory," and abuses his patients if they do not purchase his remedies; "Dr." Golden, prescribes cajuput oil locally for congenital cataract and receives a fee of $18; another "Dr." professes to heal the sick with roots and herbs, and dupes his patients with a mixture of chloroform, ether and aromatics, inflicting physical injury on some, while others are hastened to the grave. Language fails us in depicting the enormity of this imposition upon our profession and people. As members of the medical profession let us assert our rights, and urge our legislature to amend the Act, empowering every citizen of our Province with authority to prosecute offenders, and otherwise vindicate our Medical Act.[169]

The desired amendments were soon enacted. In 1886,[170] the penalty provisions were revised, allowing for summary conviction of a defendant and permitting an action to be brought by any licensed physician in the province before any "police, stipendiary or sitting magistrate." The effect of these changes in the law was, predictably, to re-establish the integrity of the medical registration system while increasing the number of prosecutions for unlicensed practice in the province.

Manitoba

Agitation for restrictive legislation was no less intense in the west than in the Maritimes. Almost immediately after being created a province, the Manitoba legislature passed its first medical licensing law. The statute was clearly intended to prevent itinerant American physicians from ministering to the Red River community, among whom were a number of American settlers. By 1871, about half a dozen eastern Canadian practitioners had established themselves in the Winnipeg area, including several who were active in the government of the territory.[171] These physicians attempted to consolidate their position through passage of a law restricting competition from across the border. The Manitoba act of 1871[172] set up a Provincial Medical Board, which was empowered to examine the credentials of all prospective practitioners in the province. Candidates were required to possess a competent preliminary knowledge of Latin, history, geography, mathematics, natural philosophy, French, and English, before embarking on the study of medicine and to have obtained a certificate of qualification to that effect from the Board. Applicants then had to undergo four years of medical study, following a prescribed curriculum similar to that set down by the Ontario Medical Council. The Manitoba law provided for a penalty of $20 per day of illegal practice, but it was unlikely that the act was effectively enforced since conviction was obtainable only on the basis of the testimony of two witnesses. Possessors of "a medical degree or diploma from any University or College in Her Majesty's dominions" were entitled to a license without examination as to their qualifications.

A more extensive statute

Responding to the initiatives of a better organized profession, the legislature enacted a more extensive medical statute in 1877. The 1877 act[173] created the College of Physicians and Surgeons of Manitoba and contained a series of effective penal provisions modelled on those of the Ontario act of 1874. The provincial medical board was authorized to conduct preliminary examinations of medical students within Manitoba, to establish a tariff of fees for the province, and to levy an annual tax of not more than five dollars on each registered physician, and in these respects represented a substantial advance, in the minds of the profession, over the 1871 law. The medical board was empowered to examine candidates for registration if their degrees were not from a university or college whose diplomas authorized the practice of medicine or surgery in any part of the British Empire. Diplomates of British and Canadian universities thus remained exempt from examination, while American graduates, who posed the greatest threat to the profession in the rapidly growing area, were required to undergo the Board's examinations.

The first Manitoba medical register, listing licensees through 1882, shows that forty-eight physicians were registered between 1873 and 1882, and that of this number, thirty-seven were graduates of Canadian medical schools, while only three had taken their final medical degree in the United States.[174] The population of the province at that time was slightly over 70,000, providing a ratio of, at best, 1,460 residents per licensed physician, assuming all registrants remained in practice in the area.

The Manitoba Medical College

The establishment of the Manitoba Medical College in 1883, however, made the need for a more restrictive statute imperative if the number of physicians in the province were not to grow at an unacceptably rapid rate. In response to continued agitation for a new law, the legislature enacted the medical act of 1886.[175] The act created a Council of eleven physicians elected by the profession, augmented by three members chosen from the Manitoba Medical College, to direct the College of Physicians and Surgeons. The law provided for the registration of all practitioners previously licensed under the 1877 act, all practitioners duly registered in any other province or in Great Britain, and "every graduate in medicine by examination of the University of Manitoba." The Manitoba act contained an unusual provision linking the Council or the College of Physicians and Surgeons with the University. Under the terms of the act, seven members of the Medical Council, including the three representatives of the Manitoba Medical College, were to become members of the University of Manitoba's Council. The University Council thus constituted was empowered to

act as the sole examining body for all candidates neither previously registered in another province or Great Britain nor holding a degree in
medicine through the University. The law provided that

> the Council of the University shall have the power from time to
> time hereafter to grant to any person or persons a certificate
> under the Seal of the University that the Council of the University
> have been satisfied, that the person mentioned in the certificate is
> by way of Medical education and otherwise a proper person to be
> registered under this Act but such certificate shall not be granted
> until the person or persons making such application shall have
> given such evidence of qualification by undergoing an exami-
> nation or otherwise as the Statutes of the University then in force
> may require, and the applicant shall in all other respects first com-
> ply with the rules and regulations of the University in that behalf.

Towards this end, the University Council could conduct examinations
and set the preliminary and professional educational requirements
necessary for registration. Manitoba thus became unique among the
provinces in turning over these functions not directly to the College of
Physicians and Surgeons itself but to an arm of the provincial University, comprising representatives of the profession.

The new law re-enacted the comprehensive penal provisions contained in the 1877 act and provided for an annual levy on all registered
physicians of up to five dollars. In addition, the Council was empowered to erase from the register the name of any physician judged
to have been "guilty of infamous or unprofessional conduct," thus effectively legislating the profession's code of ethics.

The North-west Territories

Not to be outdone, physicians in the North-west Territories were able
to gain enactment of an ordinance relating to medical practitioners in
1885.[176] The ordinance appears to have been aimed primarily at two
groups: practitioners who lacked formal medical training and American physicians entering the area, both of which were increasing as the
population of the Territories grew. The ordinance limited the practice
of medicine to all new practitioners who held a medical degree or license from some corporate body, college, or university within the
British Empire that empowered the holder to practice medicine or surgery. The practice of midwifery was not exempt from the act, which
provided a penalty of up to $100 for practicing, professing to practice,

or advertising to give medical advice for hire, gain, or hope of reward. The law contained a complicated grandfather clause allowing for the registration of all practitioners already operating in the Territories, provided they met the new registration conditions. In addition, registration was granted those physicians who were British subjects if they had been practicing in the Territories for at least one year, provided they possessed a degree from some medical school in the United States requiring at least a two-year course of study. Physicians who either did not fulfill the two-year educational requirement or were not British subjects were required to sit an examination in a series of specified subjects before two practitioners appointed by the Lieutenant-Governor and to pay a fee of $10.

Public opposition

It soon became apparent that the law was not stringent enough to effectively limit competition. Indeed, only twenty-two physicians registered under the ordinance between its passage and the end of 1886, although many more could have met the requisite qualifications.[177] There appear to have been some half-hearted attempts to invoke the penal clauses of the ordinance,[178] but they were almost certainly unsuccessful. The public was unsympathetic to the profession's attempt to stifle competition and especially resented the ordinance's provision respecting midwifery. Soon after passage of the law, the *Edmonton Bulletin* commented:

> The Medical Ordinance as it now stands is a one-sided affair, having no regard whatever for the peculiar circumstances of this North-West country. As in the case of the legal Ordinance, no one would object to a duly qualified physician being allowed a large percentage of advantage over a quack; much greater even than should be allowed the lawyer over the pettifogger, for in his case life itself, not merely money, is at stake. But that in a country such as this, where for instance, the three hundred miles between Edmonton and Battleford, and for two hundred between Edmonton and Calgary there is no qualified physician, nor is there likely to be for years, it should be made a punishable offence for a person to receive pay for doing some necessary act of medicine or surgery, it is an outrage....
>
> It is nonsense to say that a certificate granted by two ordinary practitioners, who in all human probability would be biased for or against the applicant, should rank as high as the diploma con-

ferred by a first-class university, and yet that is the intent of the
ordinance. The most uncalled for feature of the ordinance, however, is that of classing midwifery with ordinary medicine and surgery.[179]

And when, by April, 1886, only seven physicians had registered under
the ordinance, thereby giving them alone the legal right to practice in
the Territories, the *Bulletin* noted: "An ordinance which gives seven
men a monopoly of the medical practice of the North West is a case of
law making run wild."[180]

Erecting barriers

With the population of the area increasing at a substantial rate and the
market for physicians' services becoming more and more lucrative, the
profession felt it imperative to erect an effective barrier against less
well-trained practitioners. As a result, a new bill was enacted in
1888.[181] The 1888 ordinance created a College of Physicians and Surgeons of the North-west Territories, directed by an elected Council.
The act specified that the Council was to admit to registration anyone
holding a license from any province.[182] Other candidates were
required to hold a diploma from a medical school requiring a four-
year course of study and, "if deemed necessary," to pass a satisfactory
examination set by the Council. Provision was made for the Council
to exact an annual levy of up to two dollars on each registrant. The
penalty clauses of the ordinance, modelled on those contained in the
effective restraints on competition in the Territories.

British Columbia

By the mid-1880s, the profession in British Columbia, disappointed
with the registration law originally enacted in 1867 and impressed with
the legislative gains made by physicians in the other provinces,
organized themselves into a provincial society. In January, 1885, the
British Columbia Medical Society was formed in Victoria and invita-
tions were extended to all registered physicians, about 35 in number,
to join the new organization.[183] Predictably, the first order of business at the Society's first full meeting was the appointment of a committee "to draft an Act to regulate the laws governing the medical
profession of British Columbia." The bill drawn up by the committee
was submitted to the provincial legislature[184] and subsequently passed
into law as the medical act of 1886.[185] The act created the Medical
Council of British Columbia, comprising seven physicians elected by

vote of all registered practitioners in the province. It provided that all physicians licensed under the 1867 ordinance were entitled to registration under the new act; future applicants for licensure were required to hold a diploma in medicine from a medical school requiring at least a three-year course of study and, additionally, to pass an examination before the Council. (In 1893, after passage of the new Imperial Medical Act,[186] it was found expedient to amend the law[187] to allow for the registration of all applicants registered in Great Britain without examination.)

The penal clauses contained in the act were similar to those in place in the other provinces. Falsely procuring or attempting to procure registration, or assuming any title or designation implying that one were registered, were made illegal. Practicing, professing to practice, or advertising to give advice in medicine or surgery, "for hire, gain, or hope of reward" were punishable by a fine of not less than $25 nor more than $100 per offense, plus costs, by summary conviction before any justice of the peace, the burden of proof for registration falling on the defendant. The act exempted midwives from its provisions.[188]

The medical register indicates that 39 physicians registered under the act of 1886.[189] No candidate presented himself for examination at the first meeting of the Council in August, 1886, but the records show that one applicant was examined a month later and duly entered on the register.[190]

The profession's political power

The 1886 act represented a signal victory for the profession in British Columbia. The province had a population of less than 70,000 at the time of the act's passage and had no more than 40 physicians practicing throughout its vast territory. Still, the profession managed to gain enactment of a law giving an elected group of seven practitioners the right to examine all applicants, regardless of the quality of the school from which their degrees issued. Only Ontario had yet enacted such a sweeping statute. The Canadian medical schools, located in the eastern part of the Dominion, were furious that their graduates were not exempt from examination. In 1889, the professor of clinical medicine at McGill University, in his address opening the 57th session of the medical faculty, was sharply critical of the new law. "The Province of British Columbia," he commented,

> has secured the existence of a board. There are some fifty practitioners in that province (I counted 51 in the copy of the register

for '87), and united they form the Medical Council of Physicians and Surgeons of British Columbia. "Now, we have got in, let us keep the others out," seems to be their motto. If they had contented themselves with examining diplomas and rejecting those that came from indifferent colleges, then, perhaps, a useful function would be fulfilled, but, as the law stands at present, there is not one of you who, after graduating, would not become liable to punishment if he dared to give advice in British Columbia. He would be obliged to pass before the members of the Council, or such of them as may be appointed for the purpose, a satisfactory examination touching his fitness and capacity to practice as a physician or surgeon. In other words, the Provincial Board of British Columbia would have to make it its duty to see for itself whether your teachers understood what they were about when they taught you, examined you, and certified on your diploma that you were a fit and proper person to practice medicine.[191]

Divisiveness within the profession

This antagonism between the provincial boards and the medical schools was destined to increase over the following years as, in their search for more restrictive measures to control the supply of physicians, the profession in each of the provinces added more and more requirements for licensure. That Ontario, with its extensive history of medical licensing laws and its powerful and well-organized medical lobby, had found it possible to add an examination as a prerequisite for licensure was not surprising; that British Columbia, with a population no larger than that of a town like Dartmouth, Nova Scotia, today, would have empowered its handful of physicians to examine all prospective practitioners entering the province was no less than astonishing. It speaks to the political power that physicians in British Columbia had in shaping the competitive terms under which they operated.

With passage of the British Columbia act of 1886 and the North-west Territories ordinance of 1888, all the territory comprising the Dominion of Canada west of the Ontario border, with a combined population of only 280,000 and with fewer than 200 physicians, had some form of prohibitory medical legislation in place. The laws enacted in British Columbia, Manitoba, and the Territories were all highly restrictive, especially towards physicians trained in the United States. In areas where examinations were not made mandatory for all applicants, the favored technique for keeping out new physicians was the imposition of substantial, often prohibitively high, initial registration fees.[192] These laws placed Canadian-trained practitioners in general and those physicians already operating in the region west of the Lakehead at an enormous advantage, while guaranteeing them a lucrative potential market for medical services as the population of the area steadily increased.

Chapter 4

The Triumph of the Guild System, 1887-1912

THE ONTARIO MEDICAL ACT OF 1887 AND THE ESTABLISHMENT OF COMPLETE PROFESSIONAL CONTROL OVER ENTRY INTO PRACTICE

In 1887, eighteen years after the creation of the College of Physicians and Surgeons, the ratio of physicians to the population in Ontario was no higher than it was in 1869. Indeed, the medical profession in the province had succeeded so well in restricting entry into medical practice that, between 1871 and 1881, the ratio had actually declined, from 1:1,036 to 1:1,084.[1] The educational requirements imposed by the College had made it far more costly to embark upon the practice of medicine in the province and had effectively eliminated the major source of prospective competition, holders of American medical degrees. Because of the abundance of medical schools in the United States at the time, there was little difficulty in gaining admission to even the better ones.[2] Ontarians who were intent on becoming physicians, therefore, could traditionally turn to the American schools for their training (as did American practitioners eventually immigrating to Canada), provided they satisfied the preliminary and professional course of studies prescribed by the licensing authorities. After 1872, however, this avenue was made far more costly with the introduction of the Medical Council's requirement that all holders of American degrees attend yet an additional year at some medical school in the province. As a result, this means of gaining a medical education was less and less used as the education of Ontario physicians was increasingly confined to Ontario schools. This dramatic shift in the educational background of medical registrants between 1866 and 1887 is presented in tables 4.1 and 4.2.

Exclusion of American degree-holders

The move away from studying medicine outside the province was even more pronounced than suggested by the raw figures in tables 4.1 and 4.2. Between 1866 and 1869, it was not uncommon for prospective

TABLE 4.1

ACADEMIC BACKGROUND OF PHYSICIANS APPEARING IN THE ONTARIO MEDICAL REGISTER, 1878

	Year of Registration													
	1866	1867	1868	1869	1870	1871	1872	1873	1874	1875	1876	1877	1878	Total
Canadian Universities*														
University of Toronto	55	10	8	26	7	1	8	3	9	4	1	2	18	152
University of Victoria College	167	21	31	49	18	13	6	6	10	6	10	5	2	344
University of Trinity College	10			1			1		2	1	2		25	42
Queen's University	76	6	11	26	5	4	9	5	6	4	2	2	9	165
Toronto School of Medicine	2	3		4	1		1		2	1				14
McGill University	68	15	12	30	6	10		4	10	6	3	5	8	177
Laval University								1						1
University of Bishop's College												1		1
Sub-Total	378	55	62	136	37	28	25	19	39	22	18	15	62	896
Foreign Diplomates														
British and Irish Graduates and Licentiates	65	5	2	21	3	6	3	7	6	7	4	2	2	133
American Medical Schools	46			21	4	3	1			5	1	2	2	85
Other Foreign	3													3
Sub-Total	114	5	2	42	7	9	4	7	6	12	5	4	4	221
Homeopathic Practitioners														
American Medical Degree				26					1	2	1		2	32
Degree, if any, Not Indicated	1	1		20			1	1		2		1		28
Sub-Total	1	1		46		1	1	1	1	4	1	1	2	60
Degree, if any, Not Indicated	73	5	7	81	24	31	46	28	64	78	43	83	19	582
TOTALS	566	66	71	305†	68	69	76	55	110	116	67	103	87	1,759

† The large number of practitioners who registered in 1869 is almost certainly the result of passage of Ontario's new medical statute in that year. The 1869 act, unlike its predecessor, provided severe penalties for practicing unless one's name appeared on the province's medical register.

* See notes to Table 4.2.

Source: *Ontario Medical Register, 1878* (Toronto: College of Physicians and Surgeons, 1878).

TABLE 4.2

ACADEMIC BACKGROUND OF PHYSICIANS APPEARING IN THE ONTARIO MEDICAL REGISTER, 1887

	Year of Registration									
	1879	1880	1881	1882	1883	1884	1885	1886	1887	Total
Canadian Universities*										
University of Toronto	4	6	6	15	7	4	9	11	17	79
University of Victoria College	4	15	8	10	14	17	18	35	35	156
University of Trinity College	7	10	6	22	24	33	39	36	48	225
Queen's University	1	5	7	10	8	10	12	21	20	94
Western University							1	5	3	9
McGill University	2	14	9	7	5	4	10	15	22	88
Laval University	1						1		2	4
University of Bishop's College					1		1			2
Victoria University, Montreal		2				1				3
Sub-Total	**19**	**52**	**36**	**64**	**59**	**69**	**91**	**123**	**147**	**660**
Foreign Diplomates										
British and Irish Graduates and Licentiates	3	5	5	9	11	6	4	7	10	60
American Medical Schools	1	5		1		3	1			11
Sub-Total	**4**	**10**	**5**	**10**	**11**	**9**	**5**	**7**	**10**	**71**
Homeopathic Practitioners										
American Medical Degree		1		1	2	2			1	7
Degree, if any, Not Indicated	1		1			2			1	5
Sub-Total	**1**	**1**	**1**	**1**	**2**	**4**			**2**	**12**
Degree, if any, Not Indicated	**47**	**12**	**7**	**6**	**6**	**13**	**7**	**14**	**8**	**120**
TOTALS	71	75	49	81	78	95	103	144	167	863

Notes to Tables 4.1 and 4.2:

* Included in graduates of Canadian universities are holders of American medical degrees who took a second degree in Canada.
Graduates of Queen's University include graduates of the Royal College of Physicians and Surgeons, Kingston, in affiliation with Queen's from 1865 to 1891.
Victoria University, Montreal, refers to the Ecole de Médecine et de Chirurgie, affiliated with the University of Victoria College, Cobourg, for degree-granting purposes.

Source: *Ontario Medical Register, 1887* (Toronto: College of Physicians and Surgeons, 1887).

TABLE 4.3

ONTARIO MEDICAL REGISTRANTS, BY LOCATION OF MEDICAL TRAINING, 1866-1887*

Year	American Schools (%)	American Schools (First Degree) (%)	British Graduates and Licentiates (%)	Quebec Schools (%)	Ontario Schools (%)
1866–1869	8.4	5.3	11.7	15.7	58.4
1870–1873	5.9	3.7	14.0	15.4	61.0
1874–1877	6.6	2.5	15.7	20.7	54.5
1878–1881	4.2	0.0	7.8	18.8	69.3
1882–1885	1.6	0.6	9.4	9.4	78.9
1886–1887	0.0	0.7	5.9	13.6	79.8

* Data exclude homeopathic practitioners and all registrants for whom no degree is shown.

Source: Tables 4.1 and 4.2.

practitioners to train at a medical school in the United States and then to take a second degree in Ontario. Under the 1865 act, only Ontario medical schools possessed the power to examine candidates for licensure and some schools awarded a degree once its examinations were passed. If one includes those physicians who took their first medical degree among American degree-holders, then the percentage of registrants trained in the United States dropped from 13.7 percent in the period from 1866 to 1869 to .7 percent in 1886–1887. Table 4.3, summarizing the academic background of registrants between 1866 and 1887, separates out those registrants who took their first medical degree in the United States.

The decline in the percentage of registrants who had studied outside the province was not compensated for by an increase in the number of graduates from Ontario's medical schools. Between 1878 and 1884, these colleges steadily awarded approximately 100 degrees in medicine, despite the fact that the population of the province increased by about 152,000. The following figures on medical graduates are suggestive:

Increased incomes

The drop in foreign medical graduates combined with steady enroll-

TABLE 4.4

GRADUATES OF DEGREE-GRANTING MEDICAL SCHOOLS IN
ONTARIO, 1878–1884

Year	University of Toronto	Queen's University*	Western University	Trinity Medical College	Total**
1878	41	11		35	87
1879	42	15		30	87
1880	40	12		30	82
1881	36	17		35	88
1882	31	15		38	84
1883	11	13	1	62	87
1884	12	15	—	58	85

* Royal College of Physicians and Surgeons, Kingston.
** Totals do not include degrees awarded by the University of Victoria College, which graduated approximately 15 to 20 physicians a year during this period.

Sources: Number of graduates of Queen's University, Western University, and the University of Toronto are taken from Charles M. Godfrey, *Medicine for Ontario: A History* (Belleville, Ont.: Mika Publishing Co., 1979): 256. Data on graduates of the medical school of the University of Trinity College appear in Illinois State Board of Health, *Report on Medical Education, Medical Colleges and the Regulation of the Practice of Medicine in the United States and Canada, 1765–1889* (Springfield, Ill.: Illinois State Board of Health, 1889): 26.

ments at Ontario's medical schools almost certainly raised the incomes of physicians operating in the province. Despite constant complaints that the profession there was subject to severe overcrowding, the Medical Council appears to have made the struggle for existence comparatively easy for its physicians. In 1886, the *New York Medical Journal,* quoting the Toronto *Globe,* gave a rough breakdown of the 1885 incomes of 106 practitioners operating in Toronto. The figures suggest a median income of between $1,200 and $1,600 per year,[3] or approximately two and a half to three times the income of the average printer, carpenter, or plumber working in the province.[4] Life could not have been too worrisome for most physicians considering that the wages of a female domestic in Toronto in the same year were between $6.00 and $8.00 per month plus board.[5]

Notwithstanding the financial condition of practitioners in Ontario, the profession felt that certain improvements in the medical act were still badly needed if physicians were to continue to enjoy the advantages they had already won. At the 1884 meeting of the Ontario Medical Council, its committee on legislation recommended certain amendments to the medical law, the most important of which would have empowered the Council to discipline any member of the College that it judged guilty of unprofessional conduct. "This power," the *Canada Lancet* observed,

> seems to be greatly needed, in view of the fact that certain members of the College have so far forgotten what is due to their honourable calling as to hire themselves to peripatetic quacks and imposters to do professional work in this Province from which the latter were debarred by the Act.[6]

Disciplinary clauses

The disciplinary provisions requested by the College were incorporated into the medical act of 1887.[7] Most previous medical laws, both in Ontario and the rest of British North America, had allowed for the erasure from the medical register of the name of any physician convicted of a felony.[8] The new law went far beyond this. Not only did it expand the category of offenses that could result in the removal of one's name from the register, but the act was made retroactive in its effects. The relevant section reads:

> When any registered medical practitioner has either before or after the passing of this Act and either before or after he is so registered been convicted either in Her Majesty's dominions or elsewhere of an offence, which if committed in Canada, would be a felony or misdemeanour, or been guilty of any infamous or disgraceful conduct in a professional respect, such practitioner shall be liable to have his name erased from the register.

The Council was thus given authority to deprive any registered physician of the legal right to practice on the basis of any action held to be professionally "disgraceful." The procedures established to prevent abuse of this enormous power were not particularly strong. Hearings were to take place before a disciplinary committee of the Council, at which the physician charged was entitled to attend. The physician was allowed at least two weeks' notice of a hearing, the notice to specify the charges leveled against him or the subject matter of the inquiry.

Although the physician was permitted counsel, so was the disciplinary committee. Both parties were permitted to call witnesses, who were required to testify under oath, and to examine and cross-examine witnesses. In cases where erasure was ordered, the defendant physician possessed the right of appeal to a judge of the High Court of Ontario. Appeals to the High Court, however, were to be based solely on a record of the hearing and the committee's report to the Council, and the disciplinary committee alone was empowered to judge the facts of the case. The disciplinary committee thus combined the functions of both prosecutor and judge.

Suppression of advertising

One of the most immediate concerns of the profession was the suppression of advertising, which contravened the codes of ethics of both the Canadian Medical Association and the Ontario College. Soon after the creation of the disciplinary committee, the *Canada Lancet* editorialized against this evil. "It is a pity," the journal remarked,

> that men belonging to one of the noblest professions, will prostitute it, by even *permitting* such notices to appear in local papers.
> . . .
> No one can contemplate such advertising without condemning it. Let us hope that our Committee of Discipline may, in their wisdom, find some effectual means of combating this evil, and that a healthier professional spirit may soon be found in the land.[9]

Of the four cases originally taken up by the disciplinary committee in 1890, two concerned advertising, which the committee held to constitute "professional misconduct" serious enough to warrant expulsion.[10] However, action against the two physicians, Dr. B. H. Lemon and Dr. Nelson Washington, was temporarily suspended. Dr. Washington had written a letter of apology, promising to desist from all advertising, and this appears to have played a role in the Council's decision.[11] But, lest this leniency be understood by any practitioner as condoning Dr. Washington's behavior, the following was entered into the minutes:

> The Council desire to have it distinctly understood that they do not thereby approve of the form of advertisement contained in

Dr. Washington's letter, nor of any form of advertisements, nor of advertising.[12]

Indeed, both physicians soon found their names removed from the medical register by order of the Council. Dr. Lemon was expelled from the College in the following year for persisting in placing advertisements in the press and for continuing the practice of magnetic healing.[13] Dr. Washington continued to advertise both in the newspapers and by handbills and was expelled in 1892.[14]

The Washington case

Washington's lawyer decided to appeal the decision of the Council to the courts, arguing that, under the law, the College's concern with professional misconduct should primarily relate to the treatment of patients and not whether a physician chose to advertise his treatments.[15] The case was tried in June, 1893, and the action of the Council was sustained. A higher appeal was dismissed, the appellate court holding that though mere advertising in itself could not be construed as infamous or disgraceful conduct in a professional respect, the particular advertisements submitted "were studied efforts to impose upon the credulity of the public for gain," and were utterly disgraceful, "if not in every respect, at all events in a professional respect."[16] During the period of his appeal, Washington continued to practice, although his name had been removed from the medical register. He was finally apprehended by the College prosecutor and fined $50.00 for unlicensed practice.[17]

Letters of apology, in which the offender agreed to cease his "disgraceful" behavior, occasionally resulted in the Council suspending disciplinary proceedings. But if there were evidence that a physician persisted in his ways, the Council was quick to vote expulsion. Thus, in 1893, Dr. S. E. McCully, who advertised regularly in the Toronto press and was a fierce opponent of the College's annual tax — "the Medical Council . . . live now but to degrade the profession and harass and tax honest men to create an irresponsible monopoly," he wrote to one newspaper[18] — submitted a letter admitting his actions were unprofessional and agreeing not to further offend the College by advertising.[19] However, the advertisements and the letters continued to appear and he was ordered to present himself before the disciplinary committee once again. By this time, McCully had relocated in Milwaukee and the Council ordered his name removed from the Ontario medical register.[20]

Unprofessional behavior

The scope and level of activity of the disciplinary committee increased dramatically over the next decade and a half.[21] In 1906, however, the Council received a setback from the courts respecting the sorts of actions that could properly be construed as falling under the definition of unprofessional conduct. The Ontario Council had assumed that the legal definition of the term in Ontario would follow that offered by Lord Esher in *Allinson v. General Council of Medical Education and Registration*. Unprofessional conduct was there held to comprise such conduct performed by "a medical man in the pursuit of his profession ... which would be reasonably regarded as disgraceful or dishonourable by his professional brethren of good repute and competency."[22] The British court's ruling effectively permitted the British Medical Council to define the term in any way it saw fit, and the Ontario Medical Council assumed that the same liberality would be granted it by the courts of the province.

In 1906, Crichton, a registered practitioner, was charged by the Council with advertising the efficacy of a medication for grippe. Although all the testimonials received by Crichton were proved to be genuine and although he had offered to submit the preparation to hospital tests, he refused to disclose its ingredients to the Council. Crichton was thereupon expelled from the College, on the grounds of "fraudulently" advertising his remedy and refusing to reveal its contents, thus violating medical ethics. The court reversed the decision of the Council and ordered Crichton's name restored to the Ontario register. In finding against the Council, the court offered the following definition of unprofessional conduct:

> The meaning of [the Act] is not what is "infamous" or "disgraceful" from a professional point of view or as regarded by a doctor, and as construed in the light of the written or unwritten ethics of the profession; it is whether his conduct in the practice of his profession has been infamous or disgraceful in the ordinary sense of the epithets, and according to the common judgment of men.[23]

Although the power to discipline its membership was thus somewhat curtailed by the court's curious interpretation of the medical act in *Crichton,* the Council continued to take action against physicians engaged in a variety of activities deemed unprofessional, including advertising and consorting with unregistered practitioners. In 1908, the police of Ontario initiated a campaign against physicians in the province who were administering abortifacients or performing abortions, and several doctors were successfully prosecuted.[24] Not to be outdone, the Council proceeded to take disciplinary action against a physician for procuring a miscarriage, despite his having been acquitted of the identical charge in a court of law.[25]

Professional educational requirements

Although it early consolidated its position with respect to disciplining physicians who violated professional ethics after passage of the 1887 act, the Ontario Medical Council did not neglect the question of raising the educational requirements for licensure. When the Medical Council had made a four-year course of professional study compulsory in 1880, it had provided that university graduates be credited with one year's time towards their medical studies. The number of medical students who began their professional education after graduating in arts was rising by the 1880s, however. In 1884, the Council removed this exemption, thus making four years at a medical school, each year comprising a six-month session, compulsory for all candidates.[26]

Many physicians regarded the required six-month session as inadequate and pressed for an extension of the academic year to nine months.[27] The Council agreed with the need to tighten the educational requirments for licensure, but there was some disagreement respecting what new requirements would have maximum effect. At its 1889 meeting, it was decided to require attendance at a ten-week summer session in addition to four six-month winter terms.[28] In the following year the Council appointed a special committee to investigate the medical curriculum of Canadian and British universities and to recommend changes respecting the educational requirements to be exacted of prospective Ontario licentiates.

Preliminary standards

In 1891, the Council succeeded in gaining passage of a series of amendments[29] to the 1874 act. One of these repealed the provision of the earlier law that permitted any matriculant in arts in any university in the British Empire to automatically matriculate in medicine without a preliminary examination. It had been felt that the earlier provision was "opening the door too wide" to entry into the profession, especially since "in some parts of Her Majesty's dominions there might be universities whose matriculation standards might be hardly high enough."[30] The new amendment empowered the Council to determine what the preliminary standard was to be, anywhere up to and including a degree in arts. In the wake of this change in the medical act, the Council, at its 1891 meeting, radically altered both the preliminary requirements and the curriculum and duration of study, along the lines suggested by its special committee on medical education. All prospective candidates were forthwith to have passed the departmental university matriculation examination in arts, with Latin and the science subjects compulsory, before embarking on the study of medicine. The number of years to be spent in medical training was extended from four to five, comprising four winter sessions of six months each and one ten-week summer session. Of the fifth year, six months were to be devoted to working in a scientific laboratory and the remaining six months either in the office of a practicing physician or in a hospital. The number of Council examinations was increased to comprise a primary examination at the end of the second year, an intermediate examination at the end of the fourth year, and a final examination at the close of the final year.[31]

Relieving an overcrowded profession

The new requirements were immediately hailed by physicians as perhaps the best method of relieving the "overcrowding" of the profession. The *Canadian Practitioner* was pleased to report that "altogether the standard, according to the new requirements for a license to practise in Ontario, will probably be higher than that of any other country in the world," and offered its congratulations to the education committee for its "able and complete report."[32] The *Maritime Medical News,* in defending the new standard in Ontario against its detractors, noted:

> It may be urged against the new Ontario regulation that it will make it increasingly difficult for the poor man or the poor man's son to become a doctor, but we are not aware that poor men or poor men's sons make better doctors than the rich or rich men's sons, and on the contrary are of the opinion that the entrance into the profession of the sons of wealthy people will be a positive benefit, by bringing into its fold a more liberally educated and independent set of men than sometimes now find their way in.[33]

But even these requirements appear not to have been sufficiently rigorous in curtailing entry into the profession. In 1893, the *Canada Lancet* decried the fact that so many young men were entering upon the study of medicine, despite the strict requirements imposed by the Medical Council, and suggested a drastic increase in medical tuition fees:

> What this over-crowding is due to is not very easy to determine. It cannot be rightly attributed to any apathy on the part of the Medical Council; that body have been continually at work for the past ten years at the Matriculation Examination, and although it is higher to-day than the Matriculation Examination required by any licensing body in Europe the influx still continues. The Matriculation Examination and the subsequent portion of the curriculum is to-day nearly three times as difficult as it was ten years ago, and yet the number of students entering the profession is thrice as great....
>
> If something could be done to make the fees of the medical student as nearly approach to those of the Old Country colleges, as does the teaching itself, it is quite possible the effect would be beneficial upon the schools of medicine and the entire profession.[34]

An over-ambitious populace

One anonymous physician, in a letter to the same journal, went so far as to blame the educational system in the province for encouraging the young to think that, with sufficient study, any trade was within their reach. The proposed solution to this "overcrowding" was as radical as the choice of cause.

> Education is, in many cases, a curse instead of a blessing. Owing to it, the farms are being deserted. The young men are flocking to the cities to be hangers-on in real estate, businesses, or professions, leaving strangers and aliens to till their fathers' soil. Education, theoretically, is a most excellent thing, and up to a certain point this is the truth; but it remains a fact that the pursuit of happiness and pleasure is the leading passion animating the human breast, and will ever remain so. Therefore, the system of compulsory education of this Province, planting the germ of diseased ambition in hundreds of brains, causing them to regard labor as degrading and unworthy of them, embittering their whole existence in the futile struggle for wealth is wrong, and is doing Canada more harm than any other one thing.

> People don't like to be told this, but it is nevertheless a fact.
> The Government of the country should close up some of the su-
> perfluous medical schools of this Province. One would be more
> than sufficient to cater to the needs of the community.[35]

These sentiments, however extreme they might now appear to be,
were shared by other established physicians at the time. Nor was the
author alone in suggesting that the medical schools and the profession
were working at cross-purposes. The medical schools throughout
Ontario and Quebec had been early supporters of restrictive licensing
laws at a time when these laws had acted to their benefit in limiting the
competition Canadian universities faced from American and British
institutions and from practitioners without the requisite formal training. But once they were secure in their position as exclusive purveyors
of a mandatory medical education, the Canadian schools began to re-
sent the interference of the various provincial licensing boards.

Having been granted a virtual monopoly over the education of prospective physicians in the Dominion by the various medical acts, the
universities found that the interests of the provincial boards were beginning to diverge rather radically from their own. The policy of the
boards was to restrict the number of applicants for licensure by limiting
the number of students who could qualify for a medical degree. The
schools, on the other hand, were primarily interested in increasing
their enrollments and their income from tuition fees.

Reaction of the nation's medical schools

This antagonism between the Dominion's medical schools and the provincial boards was exacerbated by the introduction of separate licensing examinations in Ontario and British Columbia. In 1889, even before the introduction of the Ontario Council's new preliminary requirements, Professor R. L. MacDonnell, in his address opening that
year's session of the McGill medical faculty, gave voice to the bitterness
that many of the schools felt towards the restrictive policies instituted
by the provincial boards, and particularly those of the Ontario Council. "Boards were established," Dr. MacDonnell observed,

> at the instigation of the members of the profession themselves, by
> the provincial governments, with the good intention of regulating
> admission to practice and preventing quacks and charlatans from

exercising their dangerous trade. So far so good. But the boards, like Jupiter's stork, were not satisfied. They have in some provinces assumed the *rôle* of educators, and dictate to teachers what they must teach and to learners what they must learn. They have injured the profession they were intended to protect, and they have hampered and impeded the progress of the medical schools. From their mischievous interference this school suffers to an extreme degree. In particular, the College of Physicians and Surgeons of Ontario imposes upon our students certain very vexatious regulations, and exacts of them pecuniary taxes, wholly out of proportion to the benefits they may ever expect to derive from becoming licentiates. It would seem that but two objects are aimed at by these regulations and impositions. Firstly, the establishment of a barrier to keep out of the field as many competitors as possible, the originators of the movement having affected an entrance before the fence was put up; and secondly, to render it more and more inconvenient and uncomfortable for an Ontario student to seek his education out of his own province.[36]

Criticism from the medical press

Dr. MacDonnell's comments, although unexceptionable to anyone even casually familiar with the operations of the provincial boards, drew a storm of criticism from the medical press. No less a figure than William Osler, writing from Johns Hopkins University, responded with the same arguments reserved for his attacks on the enemies of professional cartelization, wherever they appeared:

> Unrestricted competition between the colleges without state supervision leads to the chaos which is seen on this side of the line; and that the same state does not exist in Canada, is not owing to any virtue on the part of the schools — far from it — but is due solely to the wisdom of the men who organized and have supported the medical boards. We must remember that it is a new thing for the university degree to carry with it the license to practise, and it has only crept in in the case of the Doctorate of Medicine. It is a function of the state to determine whether a man is fit to be entrusted with the lives and limbs of citizens; and to carry out this function through an organised profession, by its representatives, is a thoroughly Anglo-Saxon way.[37]

The *Canada Medical Record* was more forthright in its defense of the provincial boards:

Now, it is no part of the duty of the professors of a school to find honorable livings for its graduates after they have left its halls. Professors, as a rule, don't care how crowded the profession is as long as they get the fees. But, on the other hand, it is the first duty of the profession to protect itself against the disastrous competition which the schools would inflict upon it if the latter were not under state control; the only machinery the profession has at present for this purpose is the Provincial Medical Boards, which have the power of saying how crowded they will allow its ranks to become. As we believe no one is more anxious than [Prof. MacDonnell] to see the status of the profession kept up, and as the object of his attack on the salutary provincial boards may only have been to say something that would please the students, we should not, perhaps, take him too literally as meaning what he said.[38]

Matriculation standards raised

In keeping with its duty, and, doubtless, in a "thoroughly Anglo-Saxon way," the Ontario Medical Council decided to raise the preliminary education requirements imposed on all applicants even further in 1895. Dr. Alexander Sangster, one of the more outspoken members of the Medical Council in his demands to raise the matriculation standards for the purpose of preventing "further overcrowding," introduced a resolution providing that no candidate be admitted to the study of medicine after October, 1896, who had not first passed the departmental senior leaving examination. In presenting his motion, Sangster remarked:

> The profession is overcrowded in Ontario, and unless drastic measures are taken immediately the profession will be brought into disrepute, and will soon be ruined. The great majority of members of the profession in Ontario are not more than making a bare living at the present time, while year after year hundreds of young men are being turned loose as full fledged medical men. Something has to be done. If the present standard for qualifying is not raised within five years, the membership of the profession will be doubled. The public mind is ripe for a raising of the standard. The Local Legislature will second rather than oppose the scheme. I would like to see a degree in arts made necessary, although my resolution has not gone that far.[39]

The Council's preliminary education requirement, in the form of a departmental leaving examination, was interpreted so literally by the registrar that no other certificate, regardless of its equivalence, was accepted.[40] Nor was any student admitted to candidacy by the Council if he had not passed all the subjects in which he was to be examined at the *same* sitting. Indeed, it appears that the Council refused to admit to the study of medicine students who were within a few months of completing a university degree, on the ground that they did not possess the requisite matriculation credentials.[41] The rigidity with which the Council interpreted its pre-professional requirements led even the *Canada Lancet,* traditionally one of the provincial board's strongest defenders, to comment that "the action of the Council seems to be in the direction of making the matriculation examinations, and all the circumstances surrounding registration, more and more difficult and arbitrary."[42] The Council was so intent on reducing the number of medical candidates that, in June, 1895, it even entertained the possibility of temporarily rejecting all applicants for matriculation.[43]

Higher costs of education

The Council's policy of strictly enforcing such a high matriculation requirement deprived those students in modest circumstances of the opportunity to become physicians. It drove many others to study medicine in the United States,[44] despite the substantial additional costs imposed by the Ontario Council on students who took their degrees at American medical schools. In response to the actions of the Medical Council, the Ontario Minister of Education, under pressure from the Patrons of Industry, an opposition party within the legislature,[45] introduced a bill bearing on the subject in 1896. It provided that henceforth all candidates who passed any arts matriculation examination approved by the government would be eligible to embark upon the study of medicine and to sit the Council's examinations.[46] The measure was withdrawn, however, when the Council conceded at its next meeting that it would set its preliminary standard at the province's junior matriculation examination in arts, with physics and chemistry compulsory.[47] The Council yielded little in agreeing to this standard, inasmuch as it remained by far the highest in North America at the time.

In 1896, the representatives of all the medical faculties of Ontario excepting that of Western University, met in Toronto and there proposed that the academic year be extended from six to eight months and that the ten-week summer session be eliminated.[48] The Council agreed to this option at its meeting that year, and in 1898, made an eight-month session mandatory.[49] Finally, at a special meeting in November, 1908, the Council decided to revise its fifth-year requirement to allow students the option of either practical training or formal education at a medical school.[50] At the same time, the minimum passing grade at both matriculation and professional examinations was raised.[51]

Reduction in the number of graduates

The Medical Council's actions in raising the matriculation and professional requirements for licensure seem to have achieved the desired result. The number of graduates from Ontario's medical schools dropped significantly between 1890 and 1901 and did not exceed its 1888 levels until twenty-three years later. Yet, between 1888 and 1911, the population of the province increased by almost 500,000, or 23 percent. The table on the following page gives some indication of the effect of the Council's policies.

Despite these figures, physicians in Ontario, through letters to the public press and editorials in the medical periodicals, complained bitterly about the huge number of graduates pouring into the profession. In 1895, the *Canada Medical Record* took note of a letter appearing in the Toronto *Mail and Empire,* deploring the fact that "the profession in Canada is rapidly becoming filled to overflowing." The *Record* suggested that the solution might lie in exacting a university degree as the matriculation standard. "The Medical Colleges," it noted,

> of course have no interest in curtailing the number of students, so the profession must look to the Medical Council of each province to either raise the license fees or raise the standard of the entrance examinations in order to keep down the number of practitioners to 1 per 1000 of inhabitants. Neither should we admit graduates from other countries who have not complied with the same requirements as are demanded from our own graduates. The simplest and best standard for admission to study is the B.A. degree of a recognized University, simply because it is a guarantee that its possessor has gone through a long course of intellectual training, which is of great advantage to those who are to be the Medical men of the future.[52]

TABLE 4.5

**GRADUATES OF DEGREE-GRANTING MEDICAL SCHOOLS
IN ONTARIO, 1888-1912**

Year	University of Toronto	Queen's University	Western University	Trinity Medical College	Total
1888	61	28	11	85	185
1889	51	36	13	70	170
1890	52	32	20	70	174
1901	52	25*	13	37	127
1902	48	25*	15	29	117
1903	90**	48	15*		153
1904	96	42	15*		153
1909	90	40	27		157
1910	125	30	20		175
1911	143	46	26		215
1912	53	53	38		144

* Estimates
** In 1903, the medical faculty of the University of Trinity College was absorbed into the University of Toronto.

Sources: Data for the period 1888 to 1890, except for Trinity Medical College, appear in Charles M. Godfrey, *Medicine for Ontario; A History* (Mika Publishing Co., 1979): 256; graduates from Trinity Medical College for these years are contained in Illinois State Board of Health, *Medical Education, Medical Colleges and the Regulation of the Practice of Medicine in the United States and Canada, 1765. 1891* (Springfield, Ill.: Illinois State Board of Health, 1891): 11. 12. Data for 1901 to 1912 appear in the annual surveys of medical education in the United States and Canada, *Journal of the American Medical Association*, various issues.

The *Canada Lancet* apparently manufactured its statistics out of whole cloth when, in the same year, it reported that "the proportion of medical men to the population at large in Ontario, is about 1 to 600, and steadily getting worse." It observed:

There can be no doubt that the profession of medicine has become terribly overcrowded in Ontario, notwithstanding the raising of the standard of matriculation by the Col. of Phys. and Surg. Each successive effort made to discourage candidates for the magic M.D., succeeding only in filling the halls of the Medical Colleges with an increased number of school teachers and farmers' sons, who imagine that the profession must have a "good thing" that they are trying to keep others away from.[53]

Trade to profession

The vigor with which practitioners tried to keep their numbers from increasing is perhaps the best indication that they indeed "had a good thing," and that the financial condition of physicians in Canada had improved as the various provincial medical boards erected increasingly effective barriers to entry. Between Confederation and the turn of the century, medicine had transmuted itself from a trade into a profession, not primarily because of advances in the field but because of a highly energetic campaign to employ the political mechanism to achieve this end. That physicians were aware that a well-paying profession was worth more time and effort to protect from competition than was a modest trade, there can be no doubt. It is true that medicine in 1900 was a more advanced science than it had been a third of a century earlier, but it must be borne in mind that the base-point from which its advance is charted was shockingly low. Not only had medical therapy contributed very little, if anything, to the decline in mortality rates before the twentieth century, but clinical medicine had resulted in few significant advances in the postponement of death or in the treatment of the most common non-fatal diseases before World War I.[54] Despite the limitations of medical science, which physicians took great pains to deny, the practice of medicine became steadily more lucrative through restrictive legislation and as per capita incomes and expenditures on health care rose. Physicians in Canada had achieved the enviable goal of determining the conditions under which future doctors might enter the profession. They had everything to gain by discouraging young men from considering medical practice as a career and by convincing the public that, despite the artificial decrease in supply brought about by the provincial boards, most practicing physicians were living in penury.

Too many doctors

At the 1899 meeting of the Canadian Medical Association, held in Toronto, Dr. Irving Cameron devoted the whole of his presidential address to the problem of "overcrowding" in the profession. Much of

Dr. Cameron's speech consisted of extensive quotations from an earlier address delivered by Sir William Mitchell Banks to one of the branches of the British Medical Association, which Cameron felt precisely expressed his own sentiments and those of most physicians in Canada. To the question, "What is the cause of this bitter cry from many of the rank and file of our profession, that they can only make their bread by miserable fees, earned by intolerably hard work?" Banks replied:

> Gentlemen, it requires no royal commission to find this out. The simple fact is that, with us as with many other businesses and trades, there are too many of us for it. That is the sum and substance of the whole thing.[55]

The solution suggested by Banks to this state of affairs, however, was hardly one that operated in the case of other businesses and trades:

> My remedy consists simply in stiffening up the entrance examination. I hold that there ought to be a rough sieve applied at the very beginning and that all who cannot get through this sieve should be cast on one side. As things stand at present any man who gets through an entrance examination will ultimately get a qualification of some kind which will enable him to put "Doctor" on his door plate, with just as much effect as a graduate in honours of the London University. You cannot hinder him from this by any amount of scientific or professional examinations. He will rub through these bit by bit. Any teacher will tell you how futile it is to attempt to turn back a man who has once passed an entrance examination, if that man is determined to go on. Besides, it seems to me unfair to allow an inferior man to enter upon a course of professional studies for which he is obviously unfitted. He ought not to be allowed to get so far. He should be turned back at the very commencement, and not encouraged to throw away years on unavailing work. It has been said that if only those who have had a really good preliminary education are to be allowed to enter the profession, you may keep back many poor but struggling geniuses, who might afterward make great names for themselves. Well, there would be reason in this argument if we were in want of men to join our ranks, but when our object is to keep out applicants, the persons to be kept out are the badly educated, underbred ones. They will be far happier as decent tradesmen, in positions where their manners and their ways of thinking will not be out of place.[56]

A suggested standard for matriculation

Dr. Cameron reiterated these views with enthusiasm and proceeded to delineate the nature of the syllabus he thought necessary to matriculate in medicine and what would constitute adequate medical training in Canada's medical schools:

> The preparation... which I would require of all candidates in the Medical Faculty to have undergone in their own best interest as well as in that of the Profession, would be such a literary training as is involved in what we call in the University of Toronto "the general course," and which comprises, *inter alia*, the subjects of Latin and Greek, French and German, Astronomy and Physics, Biology and Geology, Philosophy, History and Political Economy. Having graduated in this course after three or four years of study, I would have them then proceed to the Faculty of Medicine and devote the first two or three years therein to those branches of science which are immediately ancillary to Medical Knowledge, viz.: – Biology (including Physiology), Human and Comparative Anatomy, Chemistry and Materia Medica; and the final three years should be spent in the clinical laboratory, the hospital and the post-mortem room.[57]

If ten years of university education did not reduce the supply of physicians in Canada, obviously nothing would! Had Dr. Cameron's recommendations been instituted, it is unlikely that more than a handful of physicians could have entered the profession each year, its ranks depleted as quickly as those practitioners already licensed died off. Certainly the proposal would have led to the closing of every medical faculty in the Dominion excepting that one fortunate enough to remain in operation to train the dozen or so students who were prepared to devote ten years to mastering the required curriculum.

It is chilling to realize that Dr. Cameron's suggestions, which would have compelled every prospective physician in Canada to undergo an educational program far more rigorous than that which prevailed at any medical school in any country in the world, were taken seriously by a large proportion of the profession. The *Maritime Medical News* summed up this view when it editorialized:

> Let the course of instruction be as full, as complete, as wide-reaching as it is possible to make it. The more difficult it becomes to obtain a diploma in medicine, the more valuable will that diploma become and the worthier will be the men that seek for it.

No more rational solution of the problem of elevating our profession and preventing its overcrowding could be suggested than
to make the medical diploma so difficult to obtain that only men
of lofty ideals and broad intellect would venture to apply for it.[58]

An oversupply throughout the civilized world

The *Canada Lancet* was no less forthright in its columns. When, by
1906, it became apparent that there was a limit to how stringent the
educational requirements for practice could be made, the *Lancet*
proposed that physicians devote more of their energies to discussing
other ways of reducing competition. "All over the civilized world," it
commented — on what evidence the reader is left uninformed —

> there are too many doctors. In Ontario there are about 3,500
> doctors to 2,000,000 people, or 1 to 700. In the cities, the over-
> crowding is worse. Remedies for this have been suggested in the
> direction of rendering the college term longer, and the entrance
> standard higher....
>   But the most important phase of the subject is that doctors,
> when they meet in conventions, pay too much attention to the dis-
> cussion of disease, and in what way they can give away their time
> by aiding moral reform, and not enough consideration to the
> business side of their calling. Now we are not decrying these
> worthy efforts, but the poor doctor must live if he is going to be
> even a moral force in the community. You may say what you will,
> but so long as the doctor's body is not a delusion of mortal mind,
> he requires shelter, food and raiment. The profession in every
> municipality should form a business association to regulate the
> abuses that threaten them from so many quarters.[59]

One of the "abuses" that was of particular concern to the profession,
and to which the editorial doubtless refers, was the rise in the number
of drugless practitioners operating in the province.

Prosecution of unlicensed practitioners

The College continued to prosecute unlicensed practitioners with the
same vigor that it had earlier shown. For example, at the 1895
meeting of the Council, it was reported that in the previous twelve
months, 59 cases had been brought by the College prosecutor against
unlicensed practitioners and that of these, 29 had resulted in conviction, yielding fines of $1,215.[60] Indeed, as early as 1892, one member

of the Council had remarked at that year's meeting: "I must confess here, that the late prosecutor had done good work; he has chased all the delinquents out of my territory."[61] And another representative noted that "as the years go by these prosecutions are gradually ceasing; they are becoming far less frequent than they were in the past; and we think they are likely to be still less in the future."[62]

In its campaign against unauthorized practice, the College had won a major victory in the courts when, in 1894, it had successfully convicted a druggist for practicing medicine when he had inquired of a customer what his symptoms were before selling him a bottle of medicine. The druggist contended that, since he had several products that might prove suitable to the customer's general complaint, it was necessary to learn what the symptoms were before he could determine which to sell him, and that, in any case, he had gained nothing from his questions since he had charged no extra fee for the medication finally sold. On appeal, the druggist's conviction was upheld. The court ruled, in *R. v. Howarth,*[63] that the druggist had, in fact, practiced medicine "for gain," since the court could not divide the transaction, so as to apply the full consideration solely to the sale of the drugs.

A new threat

The sanguine predictions respecting the eradication of all unauthorized practice earlier made by the Medical Council, however, did not take into account the rise of competitive forms of medical practice that did not rely upon the administration of drugs nor on the legal interpretation of such practice by the courts. In 1900, the College was dealt a severe blow when the conviction it had obtained against a practitioner whose sole treatment consisted in manual manipulation of the patient was reversed on appeal. The appeals court there held, in *R. v. Valleau,* that

> manual manipulation of a patient for reward with the object of curing disease, even where it follows upon a close inquiry from the patient as to his symptoms, is not ... a practising of medicine within ... the Ontario Medical Act.[64]

The court's decision had thus opened the door to chiropractors, osteopaths, and other drugless healers to operate within the province with impunity. Nor was this all the College had to suffer. The rise of

Christian Science practitioners was a further source of outrage to the profession. In 1898, the *Canada Lancet,* commenting on a meeting of Christian Scientists at Albany, New York, who were petitioning the state legislature for exemption from the state's medical licensing law, noted:

> We in Ontario must not be too ready to throw stones, for we ourselves are truly living in glass houses, and it would scarcely be a matter of surprise if the Ontario Government succumbed to an attack of a similar nature made upon it in the name of Christ by some mob of imperfectly sexed vixens and hysterical sufferers from unsatisfied desires, it having in the past shown clearly an animosity whenever any bill has been introduced protecting the medical profession of the Province. The fact is, one often wonders what protection exists. On every hand we find nurses conducting an obstetrical practice, Munyon and Viavi Co. doing gynecology; doctors of refraction in jewellery shops, doing the work of the oculist; and with the sanction of a legislative body that requires a long and costly course of study on the part of those desirous of practising scientific medicine.[65]

Drugless healers

The court's ruling in *Valleau,* which made the prescribing of drugs a requirement for the successful prosecution of unlicensed practitioners, quickly led to demands for a change in the Ontario law that would enlarge the definition of medical practice. In the meanwhile, the profession was left no recourse in dealing with drugless healers except that of exhorting the public to avoid them, a method with which—lacking the compulsion of law—they had little or no experience. At the 1901 meeting of the Ontario Medical Association, Dr. Angus MacKinnon, in his presidential address, spoke of the pressing need for legislation to halt Christian Scientists in particular, whom, he contended, contributed to the spread of infectious diseases. "Our noble profession," he commented,

> which gives its all to the relief of suffering humanity, has attached to its skirts many things which are not clean. I might mention the advertising cancer-curer, the Osteopath, the so-called Christian Scientist, whose religion in claiming to be Christian is as much a fake as his science, the electric belt man, and many others. It is our duty to the public to warn them against these, that they be not deceived. They are all frauds. . . .

The masses of the people even at this day are deplorably ignorant so far as anything relating to disease is concerned. They know nothing beyond the worse than useless things they read in the newspapers and quack advertisements. Many men are woefully ignorant in medical matters, in the knowledge of disease and its treatment, who are in other matters fairly intelligent. Clergymen, lawyers and successful business men are often the dupes of the veriest quackery. . . .

I referred to the semi-religious, "pray-for-hire healers," known as Christian Scientists . . . . Thus far the medical profession has treated these people with ridicule or ignored them entirely. If they continued their efforts to the unfortunates who imagine they have ailments they have not, we could well afford to continue thus to treat them. But when we find them impudently undertaking to treat infectious diseases . . . which they are unable to recognize, we think we have come to a point where toleration and forbearance become criminal. We have a right to insist, in order to protect the people from the spread of these diseases, that no man or woman shall be allowed to treat disease, by any means whatever, who has not had the training necessary to enable him to know the character of the disease he undertakes to treat. These people deny that disease exists and, of course, do not report to the proper officers any case of infection. They go in and out amongst the infected and allow others to do the same; thus criminally and at variance with all health regulations, they are doing all they can to spread these infections.[66]

Christian Science

The implication of Dr. MacKinnon's remarks is, of course, that treatment by a licensed practitioner of any illness should be made compulsory. Since only licensed physicians were in a position to determine if an illness were an infectious disease, not to seek treatment of an illness would have results identical to those engendered by seeking treatment from a Christian Scientist. Similar assumptions did not stop the *Canada Lancet* from advancing its own argument in favor of making the practice of Christian Science illegal. In 1905, it editorialized:

> There is no law to compel a person over 21 years of age to send for a doctor, but there ought to be a law that would render it impossible for a person to take charge of any case who has not the requisite qualifications for such duties. Christian Scientists have no knowledge of medicine, surgery and obstetrics. Indeed, they

declare that the teachings of medical men are all wrong, and there is not such thing as disease, as it is only a delusion of mortal mind. All you require to do to be well is to believe that you are well and there will be no longer any pain or sickness. Persons holding such wild views should be prevented by the most stringent legislation from attending or administering in any way to the wants of the sick or injured.[67]

It is a wonder that the profession did not go all the way and petition for legislation that would prevent for the calling of a priest in times of severe illness!

At the 1904 meeting of the Medical Council, the prosecutor's report noted that, despite "a large number of complaints against osteopaths, Christian Science healers, magnetic healers, and others," he was unable to "protect the public against them" until the provincial medical act was amended.[68] Agitation to broaden the legal definition of medical practice now intensified. The *Canada Lancet,* speaking for an almost unanimous profession, remarked:

> The time has now come when the medical profession should insist upon the medical act being so amended as to render it impossible for those who have received no qualification to assume the charge of medical and surgical cases. It should make no difference whether they charge or do not charge. The most essential feature of the law should be the protection of the citizen. The individual is not always a capable judge as [to] the fitness or otherwise of different classes of "doctors" or "healers." It is, therefore, the duty of the State to protect him against the "unqualified," as much as it is to protect him against adulteration of food or light weights. The condition should be secured under the law that any one who announces himself to take care of the sick or injured should at least have conformed to a standard of medical studies that will ensure [a] reasonable degree of skill.[69]

Even the College's official prosecutor, in his 1905 report, felt compelled to call to the attention of the Medical Council certain facts:

> Year after year I have drawn your attention to the need of a small amendment to the penal clause of the Medical Act, as from the decisions rendered by judges of our higher courts it is impossible to secure a conviction as the Act now stands, against many persons who, I consider, practice medicine, but from the fact that they do not prescribe drugs, the higher court judges have decided

that it is not practising medicine. Many of those who do not give medicine, although practising the art of healing, are more dangerous to the public than he who prescribes medicine. I think it is time for the Ontario Medical Council to lay the facts before the Attorney-General, and I feel sure that if this were done he would see to it that such an amendment was passed, not in the interest of the medical profession, but to protect the public from this class of healing.[70]

As a result, the Council proposed the following amendment to the Ontario act:

It shall be unlawful for any person not registered to practice medicine, surgery, midwifery, or any other method of healing, or to attempt to heal, attend upon, or treat any person the subject or supposed to be the subject of disease, for hire, gain or hope of reward.[71]

Defining medical practice

To the surprise of the profession, the Council's amendment was rejected by the government.[72] In its place, the government offered to refer the question of what constituted medical practice under the province's medical act to the Ontario Court of Appeal for interpretation. The question posed the Court was:

Ought it to be held upon the true interpretation of section 49 of the Ontario Medical Act... that a person not registered under that Act, undertaking or attempting for reward to cure or alleviate disease, does not practise medicine within the meaning of that section, merely because the remedy advised, prescribed or administered by him does not involve the use or application of any drug or other substance which has or is supposed to have the property of curing or alleviating disease, that is to say, do the words "to practise medicine" in the said Section mean to attempt to cure or alleviate disease by the use of drugs, etc., or do they include cases in which the remedy or treatment advised, prescribed or administered does not involve the use of drugs or other substances which have or are supposed to have the property of curing or alleviating disease.[73]

To this question the Court refused to supply a definite answer. The majority opinion, written by the Chief Justice, in part, reads:

The generality of the questions prevents a categorical answer. It would not be possible even by attempting a process of exclusion to cover all cases that might arise.... [U]nless there is a concrete case with the facts proved or known, how is it possible to say whether or not the words of sec. 49 are applicable? If the answer given was that if it were shewn that a person not registered under the Ontario *Medical Act* attempted to cure or alleviate disease by methods and courses of treatment known to medical science and adopted and used in their practice by medical practitioners registered under the Act, or that such person advised or prescribed treatment for disease or illness such as would be advised or prescribed by the registered practitioner, then although what was done, prescribed or administered did not involve the use or application of any drug or other substance having or supposed to have the property of curing or alleviating disease, he might be held to be practising medicine within the meaning of sec. 49, it would still leave the matter to be dealt with in a concrete case in which the ultimate decision must turn upon the facts found.[74]

Garrow, J. A. offered the interpretation of the act most favorable to the monopoly privileges of the College:

The term "practising medicine" need not and does not, in my opinion, necessarily involve only the prescribing or administering of a drug or other medicinal substance, but may well include all such means and methods of treatment or prevention of disease as are from time to time generally taught in the medical colleges and practised by the regular or registered practitioner.... The thing practised must, to be illegal, be an invasion of similar things taught and practised by the regular practitioner, otherwise it does not affect his monopoly, and is outside the statute. And it must be practised as the regular practitioner would do it — that is, for gain, and after diagnosis and advice. And it must be more than a mere isolated instance, which is insufficient to prove a "practice."[75]

Neither the majority nor minority interpretations were of particular value to the profession, which had hoped for a definition of medical practice sweeping enough to encompass anything from chiropractic to faith-healing. The *Canada Lancet* was particularly bitter. It reminded its readers that it had "repeatedly taken occasion to warn the medical profession that it must be alert to maintain such restrictions in the Act as will protect the public," and noted that "it is a poor reward, indeed, at the hands of our legislators to secure such faulty legislation, when one considers all that the medical profession has done for the public along the lines of preventive medicine and hygiene."[76]

Osteopathic practitioners

Within a few months of the Court's decision, the twenty-five trained osteopaths then practicing in Ontario, oblivious to the effect such a move earlier had on eclectic and homeopathic physicians, proposed that they be brought into the College of Physicians and Surgeons. The bill submitted to the provincial legislature would have amended the medical act to include five osteopathic representatives on the Medical Council and to broaden the penal clauses to encompass the practice of osteopathy. Osteopathic applicants were to have complied with the preliminary educational and examination requirements of the Council and to have successfully completed at least three winter sessions of not less than nine months each at some college of osteopathy in the United States or Europe. Additionally, they were to pass all the required professional examinations of the Council—most before osteopathic examiners—except those in materia medica, therapeutics, and pharmacy. Under the proposed bill, registered osteopaths could not prescribe medicines, either internally or externally (except anesthetics, antiseptics, or antidotes) and could not perform major or operative surgery unless they had attended an additional, fourth, year at a school of osteopathy studying surgery and had taken the Council's examinations in surgery before its osteopathic examiners.[77]

Although some members of the Medical Council were somewhat sympathetic to the bill, hoping thereby to contain a competitive practice that allowed for unrestricted entry, most of the profession saw in the proposed measure the beginnings of what could turn into a serious dilution of the College's monopoly over medical practice. The *Canada Lancet* reflected the more popular view. When the bill was first proposed, it noted:

> Such legislation would completely change the Medical Act and the status of the entire medical profession. It must be remembered that there are a number of bodies which are aggressive and self-seeking, while the medical profession is taking no active interest in the acts and doings of the law-makers. It is in this way that these bodies succeed in securing privileges which they are not entitled to and that would be most injurious to the public weal, and that the medical profession may not be able to hold the safeguards for the people which now exist.[78]

Three months later, it returned to the same subject:

> Osteopaths are loud in the advocacy of their so-called system of treatment. It would be just as proper for a body of persons to ask for incorporation as balneopathists, or hypnotists, or manicurists, or electropathists, etc. Some other subsection of therapeutics might equally well be selected for incorporation as a new practice, such as the administration of stimulants, and be called stimulantists, or the use of water in medicine and be dubbed the hydropathists, or, if they preferred a more novel name, the aquariologists. There might thus be no end to the sub-varieties into which medical practice might be broken up, by subdividing that portion of general medicine known as therapeutics. And this brings us back again to the starting point that osteopathy is only massage, and as such is a section of therapeutics and should be under the supervision of a physician. Osteopathy should not, therefore, be incorporated as a system of medicine. It behooves the entire medical profession to take an active interest in this question; but there is every reason to expect that the osteopaths will renew their attempts on a future occasion to secure legal recognition.[79]

Prosecution for unlicensed practice

Osteopaths temporarily abandoned their attempt to gain admission to the College after the failure of their bill. The regular profession, in the meanwhile, continued to take legal action against osteopathic practitioners whenever possible. In 1908, the Medical Council is reported to have begun proceedings for an injunction against the practice of osteopathy, but the action was soon abandoned.[80] And, in the following year, relying on a recent lower court decision that defined the practice of medicine as "the employment of any means to the end of healing," the Council's prosecutors tried to obtain convictions against osteopaths for practicing medicine in violation of the medical act, but without success.[81]

Having failed to gain admission to the Ontario College, osteopaths had a second bill introduced into the provincial legislature in 1910, which would have incorporated the profession and permitted it to license all osteopaths in Ontario. The provisions of the proposal were similar to those contained in the earlier bill, and would have provided for the creation of a separate College, with the power to determine the curriculum and duration of study of all osteopathic applicants and to examine candidates. The proposal raised such a howl of protest among regular practitioners, however, that it was finally dropped.[82] The profession was particularly surprised, therefore, when, only two years later, the Medical Council actually proposed that the medical act be amended to allow for the admission of osteopaths to the College. There were fears that osteopathy would gain in popularity at the expense of regular medicine and that the sect would, in any case, ultimately succeed in becoming legally recognized. This led the Medical Council, with the concurrence of the osteopaths, to recommend that the medical act be altered along the lines of the proposal originally put forward by the osteopaths themselves in 1907.

A large segment of the profession opposed

Most of the profession was stunned and outraged at the measure. The proposed amendment seems to have caused such a commotion in the provincial legislature that its sponsor, himself a physician, withdrew the bill after second reading.[83] The *Canadian Medical Association Journal,* commenting on the bill, observed:

> The Ontario Medical Council, true to the old adage, has in its hour of misery, selected a strange bedfellow. The miracle of the lion and the lamb being found in harmonious relations has been outdone, the puzzle being to say which is the lion and which the lamb. The osteopaths, under the protecting wing of the Medical Council, almost succeeded in passing legislation that would have enabled them to register in the Province of Ontario, and it is by no means certain that, with the encouragement already received, they will not be able to obtain their desire.
>
> A committee of the Medical Council boldly championed the cause of the men and women who had qualified at American colleges of osteopathy, . . . and the argument justifying such a course was that it would enable the council to hold the whip hand in dealing with the irregular practitioners. Just how this control was to be secured has not been made plain, and just how the honest medical student was to be compensated for the outrage inflicted on him is a greater mystery still.[84]

Expanded definition of medical practice

The problem of drugless healers continued to plague the profession in Ontario into the 1920s. It was only with the election of a new government in 1920 that the College was able to gain a sympathetic hearing to its demands that the definition of medicine be expanded.[85] As a result, the 1923 amendments to the medical act[86] contained the following provision:

> Every person shall be deemed to practise medicine within the meaning of this Act who holds himself out as being able to diagnose, treat, operate or prescribe for any human disease, pain, injury, disability or physical condition or who shall either offer or undertake by any means or method to diagnose, treat, operate or prescribe for any human disease, pain, injury, disability or physical condition.

This solution proved temporary, however, since the amended act exempted from its provisions all osteopaths, chiropractors, and other drugless healers who, on January 1, 1923, were operating in the province and who registered their names with the Provincial Secretary. Additionally, the Lieutenant-Governor–in–Council was empowered to make regulations for the admission to practice of future drugless practitioners. Rather than place itself in the position of having to draft regulations respecting drugless healing, the government brought forward a new bill in 1925. The Drugless Practitioners Act[87] created a governing body, the Board of Regents, to license drugless practitioners in Ontario. The Board was empowered to set the qualifications necessary for admission to practice, to maintain a register, and to act as a committee of discipline. Only registered physicians under the medical act were permitted the titles "doctor," "physician," "surgeon," etc., nor could any registrant under the Drugless Practitioners Act prescribe or administer any medication, either externally or internally, use or prescribe any anesthetic, or perform any surgery, however minor. Passage of the Drugless Practitioners Act, although it appeared to grant legal sanction to competing forms of medical practice that did not rely on prescribing drugs, effectively eliminated drugless healers from the province.[88] Thus, while in 1923, 551 chiropractors and 157 osteopaths had registered with the Provincial Secretary in Ontario, the combined total of chiropractors and osteopaths practicing in the province in 1931 had fallen to 254.[89]

Medical prepayment plans

Although regular physicians finally prevailed in their battle against drugless healers, the profession found it somewhat more difficult to contain the proliferation of medical prepayment plans. Such plans took the form of "lodge" or "club" contracts with certain physicians for a specified period of time in return for a flat fee. By the 1890s, lodge practice had reached sufficient proportions to become a common subject of condemnation in the medical journals.[90] Of particular concern was the "cut-rate" fees for services charged by lodge practitioners, with a concomitant reduction in demand for full-priced medical services. In 1891, the *Canada Lancet,* in an editorial attacking the practice as a threat to the character of the profession, noted:

> No one can review the tendencies of modern times and their effects upon the practice of medicine without entering a strong protest against certain modern practices: that of contract work in lodges is perhaps the most pernicious, certainly it is the most general. In this class of practice the regulations which govern ordinary practitioners are overruled, the fees are cut down to the merest pittance and the physician himself made to feel under obligation to the "noble viziers" and tin-capped aristocracy who, by their great influence in the "*lodge*," have succeeded in securing his election as its physician; whereas, in truth, the doctor is the source of benevolence, by whose labors alone such organizations are able to exist. Is it not a lamentable fact that educated and able physicians of refined feeling allow their names to be put in nomination for the office of lodge doctor, in opposition to some other local physician?[91]

In 1894, the Ontario Medical Association, after having discussed the problem, adopted a resolution condemning lodge and contract practice as violative of the profession's code of ethics. It formally requested that the Medical Council construe the practice as "unprofessional" and hence subject to the disciplinary procedures of the College, thereby "purging the profession of all who engage in it." Although the Council was sympathetic to the request, it felt that to include lodge practice within the scope of activities for which physicians could be suspended or expelled from the College would exceed its authority.

> The Council's power in this regard is limited in the statute by the phrase "*grossly unprofessional or infamous.*" To seek for further legislation giving increased prerogative would at the present juncture be perhaps injudicious and possibly would encounter the personal prejudice of a majority in the Legislature. Although contract practice of any kind is strongly to be deprecated and against the best interests of the profession, the conclusion inevitably

arrived at [is] that the remedy is in the hands of the various medical associations, and not within the jurisdiction of the governing body.[92]

Professional opposition

Attacks on the practice continued – one physician is reported to have commented of the practice at the 1897 meeting of the provincial medical association that "a vampire never bled its prey more effectively than do the lodgers their medical attendants,"[93] – but as more physicians became involved in dealing with groups on a contract basis, the arguments put forward against the practice became somewhat less vituperative. In 1899, the *Montreal Medical Journal* lamented:

> While we are firmly of the opinion – and we feel certain that this opinion is shared in by a majority of the lodge physicians themselves – that the doing of lodge or society medical work is degrading both to the medical man and to his profession: still we confess that, as society is now constituted and as the medical profession is yearly becoming more over-crowded, it seems more than likely that the number of physicians will increase.[94]

Three years later, Dr. F. W. Goodwin, Professor of Pharmacology and Therapeutics at the Halifax Medical College and, at one time, guilty of engaging in lodge practice himself,[95] appealed to the self-interest of physicians who continued to work on a contract basis:

> The disadvantages . . . outweigh the advantages. The lodge doctor is on quite a different footing from the private practitioner. The services of the one are *demanded*, while those of the other are *asked*. One is treated cavalierly, the other respectfully. One is spoken of as "only a lodge doctor," the other is referred to as the best in the vicinity. In club practice the doctor is suspected of a tendency to slight his work. This attitude of the patient is not conducive to pleasant relations. In private practice the principle of selection secures confidence. When medicine is furnished the doctor has an additional incubus. He is judged to some extent by the amount of medicine he uses. Many members are well able to pay good fees, yet get treatment for a dollar a year. Thus the profession is robbed. True, many do not take advantage of it but the fact that it is so cheap makes them despise the doctor and they are apt to say so to his injury. Very few employ the lodge doctor in their families. Many young doctors fondly hope they are going to

get a large connection by means of them, but the general experience is they are doomed to disappointment.[96]

Decrease in contract work

What finally appears to have reduced the amount of lodge practice to a minor problem was the threat of disciplinary action against physicians who participated in such programs and the contempt of those members of the profession who opposed this breach of medical ethics. It seems most likely that contract work had effectively disappeared by World War I because physicians who engaged in such practice were subject to substantial pressure both from other medical practitioners with whom they came in contact and from the Provincial College itself. At the same time, the profession continued its attacks on lodge work as, in the end, unremunerative. Thus, the *Canada Lancet,* in commenting on the subject in 1905, noted:

> Just think for a moment how absurd it appears that a doctor should agree to attend a lodge of 200 men for $1.25 per year and supply the medicine! We do not hesitate to say that he would be better off by declining the $250 and take what he can get in the ordinary way. Experience has proven this to be a sound view.[97]

It is true that lodge practice continued for a time,[98] but the ethics of the medical profession and collegial constraints no longer made it an attractive alternative after the outbreak of the World War. By that time it had decreased to the point where it ceased being a major concern to fee-for-service practitioners.

MALPRACTICE SUITS AND THE FORMATION OF THE CANADIAN MEDICAL PROTECTIVE ASSOCIATION

The competition of drugless healers and the rise of contract practice were not the only problems that physicians had to contend with around the turn of the century. As physicians consolidated their monopoly, invoking as their rationale for increasingly restrictive regulations the need for better-trained practitioners, the courts and, in particular, the laymen who comprised the juries became more sympathetic to plaintiffs who brought actions for medical malpractice. The problem was hardly a new one, although it never became as common in Canada as in the United States. A successful malpractice suit, of course, relied heavily on the testimony of physicians who were prepared to swear that the defendant physician had failed to properly discharge his professional duties, either through a lack of reasonable skill or as the result of negligence.

The attack on malpractice suits was three-pronged. The profession aimed to have all actions for malpractice tried solely before a judge, since juries tend to be far more responsive to the plaintiff in such cases. Secondly, it sought to introduce a constrictive statute of limitations on such suits. And, thirdly, it wished to discourage, as far as was reasonably possible, any physician from giving evidence against another. By the first decade of the twentieth century, physicians were successful in all three endeavors.

Early professional complaints

Complaints respecting malpractice suits appeared in the medical press even before Confederation. Thus, in commenting on an unsuccessful action for malpractice brought by a carpenter against a licensed practitioner in Toronto in 1852, the *Canada Medical Journal* speculated that such suits were a measure of rivalry among physicians, at whose instigation they were brought:

> It appears that the Yankee custom of suing for mal-practice is commencing. To such an extent was this carried a few years ago, in the States, that even the most eminent surgeons used to refuse to undertake the management of a case, unless the patient, or his relatives, if he were a minor, bound themselves legally, not to institute proceeding for mal-practice, if the case did not terminate successfully. To pay a medical bill is a great annoyance to many people, but how pleasant to square off accounts with a threat for mal-practice, or to mulct some unfortunate doctor in heavy damages, for not restoring an irremediably shattered limb to a perfect state. We hope, however, that the result of this attempt to persecute a learned and honourable physician, will serve as a warning to all evil doers, and that some of the profession who are ever willing to drag their brother practitioners into courts of justice, and who encourage the public to do so, will likewise take a hint from it. We are satisfied, that the majority of these suits are entered upon, at the instigation of rival practitioners, and we regard their frequency as the best index of the bad state of professional feeling, where they occur.[99]

The case to which the *Journal* referred was tried before a jury, as were most suits of this kind in the nineteenth century. With the transformation of medicine from a trade into a profession, however, the Canadian courts became increasingly sympathetic to the argument put forward by physicians. In their view, juries, unlike judges, were incapable of properly assessing the complexities of medical treatment, of evaluating what constituted reasonable skill, and of determining to what extent the patient had defied the physician's instructions. For these reasons, it was early held by the courts that "judges are generally desirous of impressing on juries the necessity of construing everything in the most favourable way for the defendant, when such actions are brought against a surgeon."[100] And, in 1869, the Ontario Court of Appeal gave judicial notice to the "problem" of jury trials in actions for malpractice. It there held:

> It is notorious there are many cases in which jurors are not the most dispassionate or most competent persons to try the rights of parties, and an action [for medical malpractice]... comes within this class. In such actions the Judge should firmly assume the responsibility of determining himself whether sufficient evidence has or has not been given to compel him to leave the case to the jury.[101]

Opposition to jury trials

Physicians, of course, were strongly opposed to jury trials at all, for the obvious reason that the laymen comprising a jury would be far more likely to identify with the plaintiff, especially when assessing damages, than with the defendant physician. Having deprived the public of low-cost competition and having held themselves up as the sole possessors of the arcana of the human body and its ills, practitioners looked upon juries with suspicion. They saw malpractice suits as attacks on the integrity and sanctity of medical science itself. One physician writing on medical jurisprudence, whose work became a standard reference in the mid-nineteenth century, observed of malpractice suits:

> In the majority of cases these actions are the direct offspring of envy, hatred, malice and all uncharitableness, and when, rocked in the cradle of calumny and nursed by the hand of speculation, injury is often inflicted upon the character of the physician, who is at the same time left without any proper remedy at law. The

effect, also, of such suits upon the public mind is apt to be pernicious, for success in obtaining damages often stimulates others into a repetition of the experiment, and the physician consequently practises his art in chains, being perpetually exposed to the risk of a suit, which may ruin his reputation as well as his fortune. It becomes lawyers, therefore, to consider, when called upon to institute such suits, that little value can be placed on the *ipse dixit* of a layman sitting as critic upon the professional conduct of a physician. And that, aside from such personal delinquencies as drunkenness, or gross negligence, cruelty towards, or abandonment of his patient, the field in which the physician discharges his professional duties is practically *terra incognita* to the unlearned, and one where no lay critic can follow him.[102]

Trial solely before a judge

These sentiments were not lost on the Dominion's judges. In 1899,[103] and again in 1901,[104] Ontario courts held that malpractice suits should be heard before a judge alone. This process of displacing the jury in such actions was summarized in a decision handed down in 1902:

> Actions of this kind were, as a matter of course, formerly tried, both here and in England, by a jury; and it was the almost inevitable result that juries, perhaps innocently and unconsciously, looked more favourably upon the case presented by the patient than on that presented by the physician and surgeon. To remedy this condition of affairs, and not to leave doctors in this country entirely at the mercy of juries, the courts in this country early became astute to lay down limitations and restrictions on the actions of the twelve; or, rather as to what matters ought to be left to them to deal with. . . . The *ratio decidendi* of these cases was, that a medical man ought not to be placed in peril with a jury where their decision would involve the consideration of difficult questions in the region of scientific inquiry. The next step in the practice was the suggestion by the courts that this class of cases ought more properly to be tried by a Judge without a jury. This was the corollary or natural logical sequence of the cases which I have cited, . . .[105]

By 1912, the notion that a jury trial was a totally inappropriate forum in which to hear malpractice suits had become so firmly established in Canada that one Ontario judge could comment:

> I have no kind of doubt that an action of malpractice against a

surgeon or physician should be tried without a jury—and I am strengthened in that opinion by the almost if not quite universal practice for twenty years. . . . I never saw one tried with a jury since about 1887. . . . Shortly before leaving the Bar a case of malpractice in which I was counsel, came on for trial. . . . The sole question (outside of damages) was one of fact. . . . Mr. Justice Meredith, the trial Judge, nevertheless, dismissed the jury and tried the case himself.[106]

The move away from trial before a jury almost certainly led to a reduction in the number of successful malpractice actions and in the damages awarded those few plaintiffs who prevailed in such suits. Indeed, there is every reason to believe that this shift accounts for the fact that malpractice suits have been more frequent and more often successful and that awards are much higher in the United States than in Canada.[107]

Statutes of limitations on negligence

By the last decade of the nineteenth century, physicians had also achieved legislative enactment of statutes of limitations on their liability for negligence or improper or unskilled treatment. Ontario practitioners had attempted to amend the province's medical law in 1878 and again in 1886 toward this end, but both bills were withdrawn for lack of support.[108] Physicians finally proved successful in 1887, however, when the provincial legislature was prevailed upon to amend the medical act to empower the Medical Council to discipline the membership of the College. With respect to suits for malpractice, the College had sought a limitation of one year from the date on which the negligent act was alleged to have taken place—a datum almost impossible of proof, yet crucial to the plaintiff's case. The provision as finally enacted, however, stipulated a limitation period of one year from the date that treatment for the ailment by the physician terminated. In either case, patients were placed at a severe disadvantage in successfully prosecuting a claim for malpractice since, in most instances, the statute would have run before the patient had even discovered that he had suffered an injury. The Ontario provision,[109] later copied almost verbatim in the medical acts of the other provinces,[110] reads:

No duly registered member of the College of Physicians and Surgeons of Ontario, shall be liable in any action for negligence or malpractice, by reason of professional services requested or rendered, unless such action be commenced within one year from the date when in the matter complained of such professional services terminated.

Limitations invariant

Despite the gross injustices arising from a strict interpretation of the statute,[111] it has always been held by the Canadian courts that the limitation period runs whether the patient has learned of the negligent act or not.[112] Thus, in *Miller v. Ryerson*,[113] a physician was sued for administering treatment to a child of six, the effects of which were alleged to have caused her to become deaf and mute. These effects did not appear until three years after treatment but within one year of the commencement of the action. The court held that action against the physician was barred under the statute of limitations. Meredith, J. was candid in offering the reasons of the court behind the decision: "[T]he Medical Act . . . [is not] an Act respecting limitation of actions but one passed mainly for the benefit of the medical profession, and [the section of the medical act limiting suits for negligence] was enacted for the special protection of registered members of that profession."[114]

The court's bias in favor of physicians reached an extreme during this period in *Town v. Archer*. Plaintiff suffered an injury to her ankle and was attended by the defendant physicians in June, 1899. As a result of complications to her injury, she returned to their offices in December, 1899, and January, 1900. In December, 1900, the plaintiff instituted proceedings against the defendants. The court found that action was barred by the limitation period of the medical act, holding that

> when the plaintiff went to see the defendants on the last two occasions she did not go as continuing the relation of patient and medical man, but as a person who had a grievance and who was dealing with the defendants more or less at arm's length.[115]

Complaints of an ailment and its first treatment were thus interpreted by the court as equivalent in law to appearing at the physicians' offices for the purpose of selling magazines or recovering an item left there!

Negligence suits brought out of spite

The profession's successes in the provincial legislatures and the courts did not halt physicians' complaints that malpractice suits were still far too common and were, in almost all cases, brought by ignorant patients out of the basest motives. At the 1900 meeting of the Canadian Medical Association, Dr. R. W. Powell, in his presidential address, spoke of the threat of blackmail under which physicians were forced to practice, and the need to defend the profession from the very people they so selflessly served:

> We continually have our attention drawn to the case of a brother practitioner being forced to defend a suit for malpractice or else submit to blackmail. I am sorry to say that, unfortunately, the conditions in certain individual cases are such that the latter alternative has to be accepted and rather than be ruined, or perhaps have a reputation blemished, a settlement is made out of court.... The plaintiff, often induced by low or sordid motives, or animated by jealousy or spite, perhaps goaded forwards by a hidden enemy of the doctor, takes his course with nothing to lose and everything to gain.
>
> The defendant knowing full well the disastrous results of defeat in the withdrawal from him of public confidence, which is his only stay, uses every means to win. He is forced to employ the best available legal talent to fight for him, and eminent counsel with handsome retainers become necessary. Legal technicalities arise, and he is taken from court to court while the bar and bench wrangle over abstruse questions of law and the original suit is a mere circumstance.
>
> The case finally is disposed of, and may be won or lost; but who do you suppose has supplied the sinews of war? Why, the doctor of course, and it oftentimes happens that he is absolutely impoverished, and has spent the savings or earnings of years in fighting for a principle and to uphold the honour and dignity of himself as a man, and of the profession to which he belongs. ... Unrighteous and unholy suits of this kind must be fought unhesitatingly and unsparingly, and when the public know that they cannot frighten a doctor into paying up hush money, but rather that he will be backed up and supported by his brethren and their action bring down on their own heads publicity and shame and redound in the long run to the credit of him whom they are trying to disgrace, such actions will be few and far between.[116]

Dr. Powell then raised the possibility of a defense association, in which physicians could band together to protect themselves from negligence suits:

This is not the . . . occasion to formulate in detail a scheme for a defence association. Whether it is to be purely local, or larger and more provincial, or whether it should emanate from this Association and be Dominion, are questions well worthy of your consideration and debate. An enlarged scheme, such as I have just hinted at, could be undertaken without any very great difficulty and an executive chosen for each province who would carefully investigate the merits of all cases submitted, and if defensible, bring into operation the forces at their disposal through the various provincial channels.[117]

A defense association

The project for a defense association to which all physicians throughout the Dominion would belong would also serve the purpose of protecting practitioners threatened with "unjustified" malpractice suits from the testimony of medical experts acting for the plaintiff, thus, in many cases, virtually removing the decision of whether negligence had occurred from the courts. Dr. Powell's scheme was immediately hailed by both the country's leading physicians and by the medical journals as a salutary and necessary step to protect the profession against malicious suits. The *Montreal Medical Journal* commented:

> We cannot by any words of ours place more forcibly before our readers the terrible hardship inflicted upon the practitioner who becomes the victim of a scheme of blackmail than did Dr. Powell. . . . The practitioner so persecuted is bound in self-defence to preserve his honor, professional reputation and his standing in the community, even if in doing that he, through the machinations of disreputable lawyers — and only disreputable lawyers take up such cases — is harrassed for long months, as the case passes from court to court. He preserves that reputation and standing in the community at a terrible personal cost and at a risk, it may be, of being rendered penniless.
>
> So terrible is this trial that all of us sympathise with the victime of blackmail and, as a matter of principle, are agreed that the profession as a body, rather than the individual, should undertake the defence in cases of this nature. It is not right that the individual should suffer so greatly in maintaining along with his honor, the fair fame of the profession as a whole. Nay more, we all recognise that the essence of blackmail lies in this, that those who bring suits of this nature against practitioners, rely upon the isolation of the practitioner; they know full well the pecuniary

loss involved in defending a case and the horror felt by right-minded individuals in being even suspected of malpractice, and they expect that rather than go before the courts the practitioner will consent to be fleeced, knowing that if he does not so consent, he runs the chance of social and financial ruin. The very union of the profession to contest such a case, the knowledge that a corporation adequately endowed with funds and able to summon to its aid the best legal advice is prepared to fight the case, would largely put a stop to blackmail.

From every point of view, therefore, we acknowledge the advisability of establishing in this country a scheme of Medical Defence.[118]

The Medical Defence Union

Within weeks of Dr. Powell's address, the St. Francis District Medical Association, in Lennoxville, Quebec, took the first steps towards the establishment of a Dominion-wide defense association. The Medical Defence Union, to which every registered physician in Canada was invited to join, put forward as its objectives:

> 1. To support and protect the character and interest of Medical Practitioners practising in the Dominion of Canada.
> II. To promote honorable practice, and to suppress or prosecute unauthorized practitioners.
> III. To advise and defend or assist in defending members of the Union in cases where proceedings involving questions of professional principle or otherwise are brought against them.
> IV. To consider, originate, promote and support (so far as is legal) legislative measures likely to benefit the Medical Profession, and to oppose all measures calculated to injure it. And for these purposes aforesaid to petition Parliament and take such other steps and proceedings as may be deemed expedient.[119]

Arguments that such an organization should be a national body, especially since its intended scope was national,[120] prompted the district association to turn the direction of the defense union over to the Canadian Medical Association. As a consequence, it was unanimously resolved at the 1901 meeting of the CMA in Winnipeg that a Physicians' Protective Association be created, with Dr. R. W. Powell as its first president.[121] The establishment of a defense union was warmly greeted by the medical journals, who urged all licensed practitioners to enroll by paying the annual $2.50 fee.[122]

Enormous value of such an organization

In its last issue of 1902, the *Canada Lancet* editorialized on the enormous value of the organization, noting that "it would be difficult for the members of the medical profession in Canada to imagine any organization that would be of greater use to them than a powerful and well managed protective or defence association."[123] The advantages of membership were substantial, it argued:

> In the first place, if an action for damages is brought against a member, he receives financial assistance. This makes him bold in resisting an unjust attempt to extort money from him. Another advantage is to be found in the fact that such an organization would go a long way towards preventing malpractice suits. Most suits of this kind are unjust and known to be so to the plaintiffs. If it was known that they would have the entire profession to fight, instead of a single member thereof, they would count the costs with much more care before they embarked on their suits. And, again, the costs would fall lightly on the defendant member. It is not beyond the truth to say that, though an action may be unjust, and could be successfully defended, the doctor against whom it may be brought could ill afford to defend himself, or, if he did, he might be well nigh ruined in doing so. This can all be avoided by being a member of the Canadian Medical Protective Association. But there is one more reason for joining this organization. Nothing will bind the profession together like that of mutually helping each other.... We know of some cases where doctors have been early ruined by the expenses involved in their own defence. Recently three cases of malpractice have been tried in Ontario courts, and, in every instance, the doctors won. Their victories, however, cost them heavily. Let the profession of this country adopt the national motto of the great country to the south of us, *E pluribus unum.*[124]

Membership in the Association appears, indeed, to have been worthwhile. The annual reports indicate that the Association came to the aid of any of its members threatened with litigation, both with advice and legal assistance. Beginning with a membership of 242 practitioners in 1902,[125] the organization was able to report that 622 physicians had enrolled in the Association by 1909, of which 382 were from Ontario.[126] Dr. Powell, who continued as president until his death in 1935, noted with pride in the 1909 report of the Association that, since it began operations in 1902, every case against a physician defended by the Association had been won and that not one was appealed.[127]

Expert testimony

By 1910, it became virtually impossible to successfully prosecute a claim for medical malpractice in Canada, except when the grossest and most palpable forms of negligence were clearly evident. The following observations from a text on medicine and the law published in 1978 gives some indication of the effect the organized profession has had on a prospective plaintiff's ability to gain the expert testimony of physicians when prosecuting an action for malpractice:

> Physicians' reluctance to testify in malpractice actions probably has some basis in their distaste for adversarial methods and reflects a general abhorrence of the courtroom.... However, ... defendant doctors do not as a general rule have difficulty in obtaining expert testimony....
>
> Members of the medical profession, knowing the frailty of the craft and fearing public rebuke where the health and welfare of a fellow human being has been diminished, seek to protect their image lest unreasonable controls be placed on the profession in response to adverse public sentiment....The consequences of medical associations discouraging members from testifying may have even a greater impact on doctors than pressure from insurance companies.
>
> There was a time when insurance companies inserted a clause in a malpractice policy which terminated the contract if the insured took the stand against another physician. Although the existence of this policy is denied in Ontario, a Canadian writer has submitted that the insecurity of Ontario physicians with respect to the Canadian Medical Protective Association [the insuring agency for Canadian physicians] does bear on the problem of obtaining expert testimony.[128]

THE PROFESSION IN QUEBEC

The most pressing problem confronting physicians in Quebec at the end of the nineteenth century was the absence of any legislation that would have permitted the College's Board of Governors to discipline licentiates who engaged in "unprofessional" conduct. As a consequence, the College was virtually powerless to take action against physicians who were prepared to violate the profession's code of ethics by advertising. The problem had reached sufficient proportions by 1889 to prompt the *Canada Medical Record* to print a blistering attack against these "quacks" who, in advertising their services, were robbing other physicians of between $15,000 and $25,000 per year in the city of Montreal alone. "It is a very generally expressed feeling among a great many of our readers," it editorialized,

> that the medical authorities of this province are a protection, not to those that do well, but to the evil doers. For the evil doer can come here and obtain a license to practice... and forthwith become rich in a very short time by resorting boldly to the most unprofessional conduct, while the well doer, the honorable and strictly professional man, forbidden to advertise even the truth, may be pretty sure to see himself growing thin while the quack grows fat. Of course virtue is its own reward, but it is discouraging for the regular practitioner to see the charlatan drawing patients to him by thousands by means of lying advertisements, while he himself cannot even insert his card in the papers to notify the public that there is such a person as he in existence. We have spoken to some of the officials to whom we pay a tax for the express purpose of being protected, and in reply are told that the fact of these charlatans taking away from fifteen to twenty-five thousand dollars a year from the city of Montreal alone does not injure the regular practitioner; in fact they tell us that we are even benefited thereby, because our patients will be sicker than ever after having passed through the hands of these quacks. That they will be sicker we admit to be true, but that it benefits us any to have our patients come to us and ask to be treated gratuitously because they have just paid twenty-five dollars to an imposter, certainly does not help the practitioner much in his endeavor to obtain an honorable living.... If the law as it at present stands is not sufficient for the purpose [of disciplining these practitioners], then it should at once be altered. We feel sure that the depredations of these professional pirates are a more serious thing than the officials of the College seem to think. The majority of the public consider them as medical men, and their conduct, no matter how disgraceful, is reflected more or less on the whole profession.[129]

Despite numerous complaints of a similar nature, however, it was not until late 1897 that the Board of Governors formally petitioned for changes in the medical law that would establish a disciplinary committee with the power to censure or suspend any member of the

College who had violated the code of ethics adopted by the College some twenty years earlier.[130] At its meeting of September, 1897, the Governors approved the following recommendations for submission to the legislature:

> 1st. The nomination of a Council of Medical Discipline, composed of four governors, elected by the Bureau [Board of Governors], and of the President who shall be *ex-officio* President of this Council.
> 2nd. The duties of the Council shall be to hear any complaints which may be brought against any members of the College, to make any enquiries it may judge necessary, and to give its decision in conformity with the code of etiquette adopted by the College of Physicians and Surgeons on the 25th September, 1878.
> Of pronouncing, according to the gravity of cases—1st. censure. 2nd. The deprivation of all office and the right of voting for a discretionary term not exceeding six years. 3rd. The deprivation for a given time of the right to practice the profession of medicine. 4th. The Council of discipline shall have the right to condemn one or other of the parties to defray expenses, or to divide it between them. 5th. It may appeal to the Medical Bureau for decision.[131]

The provincial legislature took action on these recommendations almost immediately. At the beginning of 1898, the medical act was amended along the lines suggested by the College, and a Council of Discipline was duly created.[132]

Elections to the Provincial College

This change in the medical law, however salutary, was not sufficient to satisfy the English-speaking members of the profession. The 1879 law, under which the membership of the forty-man Board of Governors was chosen for three-year terms, provided that thirteen members be elected at large from the District of Quebec, thirteen from the District of Montreal, three from the District of Trois Rivières, and three from the District of St. Francis, representing the Eastern townships. (The other eight members were to be chosen by the province's four medical schools). Because of the demographics of Quebec's anglophone population, and especially because members of the College were permitted to vote by proxy for their Governors, English-speaking physicians—and not a few French-speaking practitioners as well—

viewed the College as a purely francophone institution. They regarded it as oblivious to the real interests of the profession, having fallen under the control of one man, its Registrar, Dr. J. M. Beausoleil. It was felt that the College's primary concern centered on the question of inter-provincial reciprocity, a particular interest of Dr. Beausoleil, while the demands of the profession for much-needed legislation were neglected. Specifically, the profession had hoped to gain passage of an amended medical act that would broaden the definition of medical practice and that would empower individual practitioners to initiate prosecutions against unregistered practitioners, rather than going through the College's prosecutor. Most importantly, there was growing sentiment against the prevailing method of electing the members of the Board. In its place, a number of physicians proposed that the province be divided into thirty-two electoral districts, the practitioners of each district empowered to elect their own representative. Under such a system, similar to that prevailing in Ontario, proxies would, of course, have been forbidden.[133] The *Montreal Medical Journal* summed up the attitude of the English section of the profession in an editorial in March, 1898:

> There is, we know, a disposition on the part of the English speaking members of our profession, to be callous with regard to the College, and to "let sleeping dogs lie." We are in so small a minority, that what we do appears to be of little influence; in short, the general disposition has been to let the French members run the College their own way, and only to think of agitating when the French representatives of the College appear by their legislation to be encroaching upon our prerogatives. This attitude of mind is inexcusable.... It is to our advantage to support the reform movements, for such support cannot weaken the English representation in the College; it may possibly improve it. It is, for example, utterly indefensible, that under existing conditions, the large body of English speaking physicians in this city, has no direct representation upon the Governing Board. To put the condition of affairs plainly, as matters at present stand, while nominally the mass of members of the Board of Governors of the College is elected by the profession at large, the truth is that the profession absolutely plays no part in the election. With few exceptions, including the university representatives, the members are elected upon one ticket and under the present regulations whereby members of the profession in this Province can vote by proxy, it is possible for any one who is politically minded, to col-

lect together such a number of undated and indefinite proxies simply signed by the names of practitioners in the Province, that at the election he can produce all these proxies and completely swamp the votes of those present. Thus it is possible for one man who has been sufficiently energetic in the matter of collecting proxies, and who has sufficient influence, direct or indirect, to do this work, to elect a working majority upon the Board of the College, a majority completely subservient to him. We grant freely that under certain conditions this power might be utilised to the advantage of the profession in general; indeed we know from history that autocratic rule has been at times fraught with great advantage, but we know also that it can be fraught with most serious evils. Without beating about the bush, we may say that the autocrat in this case is the Registrar of the College, Dr. Beausoleil.[134]

Attacks on the Medical Board

In early 1898, the Montreal Medico-Chirgurical Society, representing the anglophone physicians of the city, launched a campaign against the governing body of the College. The Society, in a circular to the profession, attacked the current composition of the Board and urged the election of a reform slate at the forthcoming elections that would dedicate itself to establishing territorial representation on the Board.[135] English-speaking physicians in the province thereupon lent their active support to reformist elements in the French camp, who also supported changes in the method of representation. In one of its election circulars, the Society's election committee noted that the profession in Quebec, both French and English-speaking, had agitated for these reforms for a decade, but without success:

Nine years ago, at the election for 1889, a Board of Governors was elected pledged to obtain this representation by districts; in 1892 the Board repeated this promise to the profession, and at the last election in 1895 the then Board once again placed this reform upon its programme. Once the elections have come and gone no regard has been paid to the promises thus made, and what is more, the Board, or those controlling the Board, have always rejected every motion brought forward asking for the fulfillment of these promises. Only this last December [1897] a small group of the members of the Board did not hesitate to employ every means possible to prevent the legislature at Quebec bringing in an amendment to the law which was in accordance with the desire of the profession. Now, only three months later, they again, for the fourth time in nine years, have the audacity to promise the desired reform, relying, no doubt, on their being able by some means or other to baulk us later.

It is the object of this committee to obtain the election of those pledged to bring in this system of district representation by ballot. If we succeed in electing a Board of Governors favourable to our object, that Board will immediately apply to the Government to so modify the present law as to give representation to each district — the districts to correspond as nearly as feasible with the parliamentary electoral districts of the Province.[136]

Thanks in part to this cooperation between a large segment of the French-speaking profession and virtually all English-speaking physicians in the province, the reform slate was elected to the Board of Governors in July, 1898.[137] The Board thereupon petitioned the provincial legislature for the necessary amendments to the medical act respecting district representation and its suggestions were drafted into law in 1900.[138]

Legislative exemptions

The provincial legislature was not always as compliant with the wishes of the College. In 1898,[139] and again in 1904, 1908, and 1911,[140] it had circumvented the examining provisions of the medical act by permitting students then enrolled in the province's medical schools to sit their preliminary examinations without loss of any time previously spent in the study of medicine. The medical act, as originally enacted in 1876, was explicit in specifying that all candidates studying medicine were to have first successfully completed the College's preliminary examination. The Board of Governors had interpreted this requirement quite literally. It had refused to credit any candidate with any time already spent in the study of medicine unless he had first completed these examinations. Thus, graduates in medicine had actually been refused licenses by the College, despite their having met all the other requirements for registration, because they had failed to take their preliminary examinations prior to commencing their medical studies. The injustices caused by this policy prompted the legislature to amend the medical act in 1900, to permit the College to exempt any candidate from its preliminary examinations "whenever they consider that the circumstances justify their so doing."[141] Needless to say, the College never concluded that circumstances warranted such a departure from policy. The position of the College was set forth in a letter to the *Montreal Medical Journal* by Dr. E. P. Benoit of the Board of Governors:

> A student who has not registered in the books of the College by presenting... his *brevet* (Provincial Board matriculation) has *no legal existence*, that is to say, is recognised neither by the law nor by the College of Physicians, and would not obtain the license even though he passed his university examinations....
>
> The non-registered student leaves the university with a worthless diploma so far as his license is concerned. To be recognized by the College of Physicians he must do what he should have done at the very first, namely, have his name inscribed in the official register of the candidates for the license, and for that purpose pass the proper examinations before the examiners of the College. Moreover, as the law prescribes that a student only has a right to a license, inasmuch as he has obtained his diploma after four years of medical study from the date of his admission to study, the non-registered student must, after undergoing his preliminary examination or *brevet* before the College of Physicians and registering his name with the Registrar, wait four years more before he be allowed to pass an examination before the examiners of the Board to obtain a license. It is in a way a penalty imposed on those who have not observed the rules.[142]

The matriculation examination

The Board of Governors was particularly anxious to preserve its right to examine candidates at the matriculation level, since it did not yet possess the power to exact a professional examination of prospective licentiates. The passage of the Pineault law of 1898 struck the College as an unwelcome intrusion into College procedure since it appeared to disallow the rejection of a certain group of candidates who had neglected to pass their matriculation examinations four years earlier. The law provided that:

> [T]he College... is authorized to admit to practice the medical students who on the first of November, 1896, had commenced attending a medical course in a duly incorporated university of the Province of Quebec before having obtained a certificate of admission to the study of medicine, and grant them the necessary license to practice medicine, surgery, and obstetrics after having

passed the examinations required for admission to study and those required for admission to practice.[143]

It thus seemed that the most the Board could exact of applicants to whom the law applied was a matriculation examination *after* they had received their medical degrees from a Quebec university, an examination these candidates presumably would have had no difficulty in passing. Thirty-four medical graduates presented themselves to the Board for licensure in the spring of 1900, and requested that they be exempted from the examinations for admission to study, having already passed professional examinations at their universities.[144] To this request the Board consented, but only on the condition that these applicants take a second professional examination before the Board of Governors.[145] A graduate of Laval University, Joseph Gosselin, refused to comply with the Board's demand and brought suit against the College. In December, 1900, the court found for Dr. Gosselin and the judgment was affirmed by the Quebec Court of Revision.[146]

Reaction of the College

The College and the profession were predictably furious. Dr. Benoit commented that

> the fifteen hundred physicians of the Province of Quebec, who at present lawfully practise their profession, and who for that purpose have imposed upon themselves all the sacrifices of work, time, and money demanded by law, are entitled to the protection of the Medical Board and of the Courts, by requiring that all irregular candidates at least comply with the law as amended.[147]

And the *Montreal Medical Journal* editorialized of the judgment:

> The high standing of medical training is not promoted by lowering the matriculation examination, nor by allowing students to begin their professional studies before passing it. The regular course of medical study is quite sufficient to absorb all the energy of the student.
>
> The regulations of the study of medicine in Canada is the result of years of experience in this and other countries, and the laws governing it should be respected. It is always unwise to have rules that are not enforced. To let a few students through the examinations, matriculation or professional, without requiring from them

the same proficiency demanded of others is to sow seeds of discontent and ill-feeling. The Governors of the College of Physicians and Surgeons will, we feel sure, have the sympathy and loyal support of the profession in their endeavour to maintain the standards of study of medicine in this Province as established by law, and to oppose the entrance into the profession of any student through other than the regular and legal portals.[148]

Partly in response to this setback, the College renewed its agitation for the power to compel all graduates to sit its own professional examinations before being licensed. Further, in late 1903, the College recommended that the medical act be amended to require that the course of professional study be extended from four years to five years, each year to comprise a session of at least nine months. It further moved that the preliminary education requirements be raised to that of the "cours classique complet" (somewhat similar to the senior matriculation examination in Ontario).[149]

The Medical Act of 1909

Support for a provincial professional examination was not unmixed. In September, 1905, the Board of Governors, meeting at Laval University, discussed the subject at length and supported the measure despite the objections put forward by Laval's representatives.[150] The majority of members felt that "the profession had to safeguard the competence of physicians wishing to practice in Quebec and that this duty could not be properly discharged unless [the College] controlled the examinations."[151] Finally, in 1908, Laval consented to the proposed change.[152] Thus, with the concurrence of the province's medical schools, the College was in a position to exert pressure on the provincial legislature to make the necessary alterations in the medical act respecting both preliminary and professional educational requirements and a mandatory province-wide professional examination. The result of their lobbying was the Quebec Medical Act of 1909.[153] Not only did the new law require that all candidates for licensure sit the College's professional examination, but it also incorporated the suggested alterations respecting professional studies, extending the required period of study to five yearly sessions, each comprising nine months. Additionally, the act broadened the definition of medical practice.[154] The effect of these changes on the number of graduates from the province's medical schools was almost immediate:

TABLE 4.6

GRADUATES OF DEGREE-GRANTING MEDICAL SCHOOLS IN QUEBEC, 1901–1918

Year	McGill University	University of Bishop's College	Laval University Montreal	Quebec	Total
1901	106	8e	40e	24	178
1902	96	7	45e	19	167
1903	100	5	45	20e	170
1904	86	10	45e	20e	161
1909	71		55		126
1910	79		29	13	121
1911	31		51	19	101
1912	46		34	10	90
1913	61		35	22	118
1914	63		22	14	99
1915	60		15	13	88
1916	28		17	10	55
1917	63		29	7	99
1918	62		43	19	124

e Estimate.

The medical faculty of the University of Bishop's College fused with that of McGill University in July, 1905.

Source: Data are taken from the annual medical education issues of the *Journal of the American Medical Association,* 1901 to 1904 and 1909 to 1918.

Between 1909 and 1914, the number of graduates dropped by over 20 per cent and did not return to its 1909 levels until the end of World War I. Yet, during the period 1909 to 1914, the population of Quebec increased by over 177,000, or 9.2 per cent.

THE MARITIMES AND NEWFOUNDLAND

The greater laxity respecting entry into the profession that had traditionally prevailed in the Maritimes throughout most of the nineteenth century was, by the 1890s, no longer tolerable to the physicians of that area. At the urging of its practitioners, Prince Edward Island, whose statute was the weakest, made some attempt to enact a comprehensive medical law in 1890. The 1890 act[155] established a Medical Council of seven physicians elected by the profession. The Council was empowered to conduct matriculation examinations covering a specified curriculum of preliminary study of all future applicants for licensure. Candidates were required to have devoted at least four years to the study of medicine, "one of which may be with a regular practitioner," and to possess a diploma or license to practice from any "accredited" college or school of medicine in Canada, the United States, or Europe. In addition, the Council was given authority to conduct "practical" examinations of candidates "as the Medical Council may think necessary for the public safety." Unregistered practitioners, including those qualified physicians who failed to register, were liable to a fine of not less than $25 nor more than $100 for each offense. The use of any title or designation implying that one were a registered practitioner unless one's name appeared on the register was also punishable under the act.

From the standpoint of the profession, the law was totally inadequate. Although the population of Prince Edward Island had remained almost constant between 1881 and 1891, census data indicate that the number of physicians in the province had increased during this period by over 40 per cent, from 63 to 90. The Medical Council did not conduct "practical examinations" of prospective registrants, nor did the 1890 law provide that an applicant's matriculation examination be passed before he was credited with any period of medical study. Finally, the act required that candidates undergo only three years of formal medical training. These provisions did nothing to close the door to American-trained physicians who were still able to settle in the province at will.

As a result, the profession submitted a second bill to the legislature two years later, incorporating most of the provisions it found wanting in the 1890 law.[156] The 1892 act[157] made a professional examination before the Council mandatory and required that any applicant for licensure pass a matriculation examination "equivalent to that of the College of Physicians, London," before commencing the study of medicine. The Council was further empowered under the new act to levy an annual fee of up to $5.00 on each registrant and to erase from the register the name of any practitioner it found guilty of "infamous or disgraceful conduct." Finally, by amendment in 1894,[158] attendance at a medical school requiring a four-year graded course was made compulsory.

New law welcomed

The profession welcomed these changes, which promised to effectively halt the inflow of new physicians into the province. That each applicant was required to sit a professional examination before the provincial Medical Council was regarded with particular favor. The *Maritime Medical News* took note of this provision and expressed the hope that New Brunswick and Nova Scotia would soon follow Prince Edward Island's lead:

> It is generally looked upon now that a diploma alone is not sufficient to legalize the practice of medicine. In England the teaching bodies do not grant diplomas. Ontario has many years ago started on the right road in this matter. British Columbia followed suit. Prince Edward Island comes third with the progressive van, and we trust that New Brunswick and Nova Scotia will insist on getting their laws amended, to enable them to appoint or join in the appointment of an interprovincial board of examiners as the *sole qualification* to legalize the practice of the profession. . . .
>
> Quackery can never be suppressed or held in abeyance so long as we accept the colleges as the sole authority for legalizing degrees for practice. Is it not a notorious fact that England and Scotland and Ireland have produced their quota to the army of quacks, as well as any other country? We have heard these men boasting of their diplomas as being superior, ignoring the fact that the diploma is only an evidence of having pursued a certain course of studies. Canadian, and certainly American universities, rank also very high; for instance, the University of Pennsylvania has a compulsory course of four years of nine months each, but still the great State of Pennsylvania has declared that their own diplomas will no longer be sufficient to legalize practice, but must pass the examination of the state, in addition, for a license. When will men give up this nonsense about the value of diplomas? Some men, we fancy, are like the child that takes great delight in handling a *bauble* when this question is up. We hope the dawn of a better era is upon us, and that great progress will be made towards bringing the whole Dominion into line on this question. If we stand firm and boldly for our position we will succeed; if we vacillate and halt between two opinions, we leave ourselves at the mercy of every wind that beats to and fro.[159]

Public reaction

The public does not appear to have been as enthusiastic about this additional requirement as were physicians in the Maritimes. The editors of the *Presbyterian Witness* used the occasion to attack the profession as a monopoly and the institution of a compulsory provincial examination as unjust. In a letter reprinted in the *Maritime Medical News,* one physician responded:

> It is a mistake... to assume that the possession of a diploma or degree ought to constitute a legal right to practice anywhere. That so-called legal right places or puts all so-called doctors, regulars or irregulars, men of learning or charlatans, wise practitioners ready and competent to use every rational means and method in the never ending combat with disease and death, or Christian scientists, faith curers, hydropaths, electropaths, and all the other humbugging "paths" on the same level before the great mass of the people, who always assume that the possession of a degree or some euphonious title implies not only an authority to practice but the *ability* to practice. Higher medical education is in the true interests of the people and the profession, and I fail to see wherein it can be regarded in any case as a "monopoly."...
>
> For years in this province we had no law, and were made the dumping ground for the rejected material of schools and councils, until an effort was made to pass a law requiring a certain standard of qualification.... The tendency is in every country to confine the colleges to teaching and instruction and conferring degrees as evidence of their curriculum, but the authority to practice is placed in different hands. Times change, Mr. Editor, and we must move on apace or be left behind.... A conjoint application to the different legislatures should receive the united support of the press, because we are not monopolists or speculators, but men believing in a code of ethics that requires a high state of morality to carry it into effect.[160]

In 1899,[161] Prince Edward Island's medical act was revised once again to provide the Medical Council with a greater degree of flexibility in determining the curriculum of professional study required of applicants, and to formalize the status of candidates admitted to the study of medicine with the creation of a "medical students' register." And in 1910,[162] the profession successfully petitioned the legislature for a further amendment, lengthening the required term of professional study from four to five years. Thus, by the first decade of the new century, the seventy-five or so physicians practicing on this tiny island had managed to bring its medical law into line with the most restrictive statutes in the country.[163]

Heterodox systems

The need to change New Brunswick's fairly thorough medical act of 1881, as amended through 1886, was not regarded as particularly pressing by the profession in the province. The 1881 act and its amendments had provided comprehensive disciplinary provisions whereby the Council was empowered to remove the name of any practitioner found guilty of "infamous conduct in a professional respect" from its register. This, together with an effective campaign to prosecute unregistered practitioners, appear to have satisfied the physicians of the province. Minor adjustments permitting the New Brunswick Medical Council to alter the content of its preliminary examinations were made in 1895 and 1899.[164]

Probably the most important provision added to the law before its major revision in 1920 was a clause legally recognizing heterodox systems of practice. In 1895, despite the vigorous protests of the Medical Council and the profession, the law was changed. The provisions respecting the professional examination given graduates of certain medical schools — those whose curriculums did not meet the Council's requirements — were amended with the addition of the following clause:

> [I]n the event of any person applying for registration as a practitioner of any system of medicine, the registered practitioners of the system shall have the right to appoint an examiner or examiners on the subjects peculiar to that system, namely, materia medica, pharmacy and therapeutics, and if they should neglect so to do the council shall have the power to appoint such examiner or examiners.[165]

Increased standards

In 1920, the medical act was revised[166] to extend the required period of professional study at a medical school "in good standing" to five years of eight months each and to make a professional examination mandatory. However, the offending clause respecting special examinations for heterodox applicants was left in the act. And, to the profession's chagrin, yet another provision was included, stipulating that "nothing in this Act shall prevent any person from practising methods of treatment which are commonly recognized as distinctly osteopathic."[167] Although few osteopaths practiced in New Brunswick over the years,[168] regular physicians found the clause offensive and constantly petitioned for its removal. Nevertheless, it was only with passage of the medical act of 1958 that osteopaths were required to meet certain educational requirements and to pass the Council's examinations.[169]

Nova Scotia

New Brunswick's physicians were the last in Canada to institute a mandatory professional examination of all candidates for licensure. The Nova Scotia profession was more fortunate, having succeeded in gaining enactment of a revised medical act granting its Medical Council the power to examine applicants in 1899.[170] The law provided that, as of July 1, 1902, all applicants had to sit the Board's professional examinations before registration. The legislature felt that fairness demanded that, in enacting the bill as recommended by the profession, it include a clause allowing a candidate who "intimates his intention to practice the system of homeopathy" to be examined by homeopathic practitioners in the usual array of subjects, i.e., materia medica, therapeutics, and the theory of medicine and surgery. This provision respecting homeopathy seems to have been little, if at all, used but remained as part of the province's medical act until 1969,[171] when it was rephrased to require that the homeopathic applicants pass the standard examinations in addition to those respecting homeopathy.

With the coming into force of the compulsory examination provision, the number of applications for licensure dropped substantially.[172] The *Maritime Medical News* reported that no candidate presented himself for examination at the September, 1902, meeting of the Board, and that in April of the following year, only seventeen applicants, most newly graduated from Dalhousie, took the examination.[173] Indeed, the provision seems to have been particularly effective in limiting the number of physicians entering the profession, since the number of practitioners operating in Nova Scotia remained almost constant between 1904 and 1918.[174] In addition, there appears to have been a shift away from practitioners trained outside the province to those graduating from Dalhousie. Colin Howell, referring to the Nova Scotia register for 1890 and 1910, gives the following figures respecting the academic background of the province's physicians:[175]

Location of Medical School	1890	%	1910	%
Canada (outside Nova Scotia)	63	19.3	149	27.1
Nova Scotia			151	27.5
United States	236	72.4	208	37.9
British Isles and Other	27	8.3	41	7.5
Total [176]	326		549	

The decrease in the percentage of practitioners trained outside the province follows that which had earlier occurred in Ontario after enactment of its compulsory professional examination provision. It thus appears that one effect of this policy was to reduce the mobility of applicants for licensure and to encourage inbreeding.[177]

Unprofessional conduct

The 1899 act also set up an internal disciplinary procedure whereby the Medical Board could regulate the conduct of the membership of the profession. Any practitioner adjudged guilty of "infamous conduct in a professional respect," and this was interpreted to encompass any infringement of the profession's code of ethics, could have his name erased from the register. In defending this provision, the president of the Nova Scotia Medical Association, and a member of the province's Medical Board, commented:

> In duty to ourselves and to the public, we should have some authority competent to deal at least with prominent offenders. There are certain well recognised offences against the Code of Ethics, and the tribunal to decide on these, the tribunal to carry into effect the judgment of the general conscience of the Profession is the Medical Board.[178]

It was with some annoyance that physicians in Nova Scotia greeted the news that, in 1908, the legislature altered the language of this provision to permit a practitioner to appeal the erasure of his name from "the conscience of the profession" to a judge of the Supreme Court in instances other than those involving "infamous conduct."[179] The incident that precipitated this minor alteration in the law involved one Dr. Ira T. Dyas. Dyas claimed to hold a medical degree from Tufts Medical School and was duly registered on the basis of his professional credentials. The Medical Board, however, suspicious of Dyas' documents, communicated with the school, whose registrar and secretary trekked to Halifax to inspect Dyas' diploma. They were pronounced forgeries and Dyas' name was consequently erased from the register in 1907. Dyas, who had set up practice in Amherst, was both well-liked and regarded as perfectly competent to practice by his patients. He also seems to have had a number of highly influential friends, including the Attorney–General of the province, who acted as his legal adviser. The Attorney–General was apparently unsuccessful in having a private bill passed by which Dyas would be granted a license. However, he did manage to insert an amendment into the medical act allowing the courts to hear appeals on both questions of fact and law from the decisions of the Medical Board that resulted in a practitioner's name being removed from the register, except in cases where the Board had determined that the physician had been guilty of "infamous conduct in any professional respect."[180]

The bill that incorporated the appeal clause contained yet another amendment to the medical act, one that proved far more welcome to the physicians of the province. The 1908 law added physics to the list of compulsory subjects comprising the professional curriculum and extended the required period of professional study at a medical school in good standing to five years, comprising sessions of at least eight months each.

Definition of medical practice

In 1921, the Nova Scotia medical act was once again revised[181] to reflect the further demands of the Medical Board. The profession had succeeded, in 1899, in changing the language of the medical act so that it was made illegal to practice medicine, surgery, or midwifery without being registered — whether for payment or the hope of payment or not. However, this provision appeared to contradict the penalty section of the same act, the language of which remained unaltered from earlier statutes and which provided that practicing, professing to practice, or advertising to give advice in medicine, surgery, or midwifery "for hire, gain or hope of reward" was punishable by a fine of up to $20.00 per day.[182] The contradictory provisions made it almost impossible to convict anyone not registered who practiced medicine solely for charitable purposes. Thus, in 1908, one member of the Board complained:

> As to the difficulty of securing convictions against irregular practitioners, I may mention the case of a clergyman no great distance from Halifax, who practises among the people of his neighbor-

hood, and against whom we failed to secure a conviction, even although the words "for hire, gain or hope of reward" have been struck from the section dealing with such cases.[183]

The 1921 law rectified this problem by removing all references to "hire, gain or hope of reward" from its penalty clauses. Additionally, the definition of medical practice was expanded to read:

> Any person shall be held to practise medicine within the meaning of this section who shall—
> (a) by advertisement, sign or statement of any kind, allege ability or willingness to diagnose or treat any human disease, defect, deformity or injury;
> (b) advertise or claim ability or willingness to prescribe or administer, or who shall prescribe or administer any drug, medicine, treatment or perform any operation, manipulation or apply any apparatus or appliance for the cure or treatment of any human disease, defect, deformity or injury;
> (c) act as the agent, assistant or associate of any person, firm or corporation in the practise of medicine as hereinbefore set out.

Thus, after 1921, even to *claim* that one were competent to diagnose or treat a scratch or a hangnail was a violation of the letter of the medical act.[184]

Disciplinary provisions

The 1921 law also expanded the disciplinary powers of the Board, permitting it to suspend "for such time as the board may determine" any practitioner found guilty of "unbecoming or improper conduct." No appeal procedure from the decision of the Board to the courts was provided for anyone so suspended and it was left to the profession alone, through its Medical Board, to determine what constituted "unbecoming conduct." Finally, the examination clauses of the medical act were slightly altered by the 1921 amendments. The special provisions that applied to homeopathic applicants were enlarged to include osteopathic candidates. Henceforth, those intending to practice homeopathy or osteopathy in the province were permitted to undergo examinations that "relate to the subject-matter included in such other system" by exponents of their system of medicine.[185] These applicants were to otherwise meet all the educational requirements and pass all the examinations, preliminary and professional, which applied to the exponents of regular medicine.

Newfoundland

Medical conditions appear to have remained extremely primitive in Newfoundland throughout most of the nineteenth and well into the twentieth century. The colony did not possess a hospital until 1813, and for the first sixty years of its operation had no resident physicians. It is reported that as late as 1893, the institution still had no operating room nor any qualified nurses.[186] Indeed, in 1902, only sixty-seven physicians were listed as practicing in Newfoundland, serving a population of approximately 230,000 residents. Despite the dearth of medical personnel that traditionally plagued the colony, practitioners in St. John's and Conception Bay had banded together towards the end of the nineteenth century to form medical societies with the aim of restricting further entry into the profession. In 1893, the colonial legislature enacted Newfoundland's first medical licensing law. The act[187] created the Newfoundland Medical Board, composed of three physicians appointed by the Governor-in-Council and four others, two elected by the St. John's Medical Society, and two by the Conception Bay Medical Society. All candidates for licensure were henceforth required to sit the Board's preliminary examinations and to have obtained a degree from a medical school "in good standing."

The Board was further authorized to examine and grant licenses to those not holding a medical degree to practice in specified localities in which no qualified practitioner resided. The penalty for unregistered practice, falsely pretending to be a physician, or taking any title or designation implying that one were licensed unless one's name appeared on the medical register, was set at $20.00 per day or twelve months' imprisonment. Informers who were "not connected with the medical profession" were entitled to one-half of any fine collected. Additionally, the Board was empowered to expel any practitioner "for acts of mal-practice, misconduct or immoral habits."

The act's limitations

The Board created under the 1893 act almost immediately began complaining that the law's provisions were not sufficiently extensive to adequately protect the public from "poorly trained" practitioners. The act had neither specified that applicants had to take their preliminary examinations before completing their medical studies, nor did it require that candidates for licensure complete their professional training at a medical school imposing a minimum four-year period of formal study. As a consequence, the medical act was revised in 1896[188] to effect these changes. In addition, the disciplinary powers of the Board were expanded to allow either for the suspension or expulsion of any registrant it found guilty of "professional misconduct" or "conduct unbecoming a practitioner." At the same time, the penalties were altered to a fine of $50.00 or, in default of payment, at least a three-month term in jail, depending upon the specific offense. While still empowering anyone to act as a complainant under the act, the new law also permitted the Board to appoint a prosecutor to initiate legal action against unregistered practitioners and to "allot such portion of the penalties recovered as may be expedient toward the payment of such prosecutor."

In 1906,[189] the medical act was again amended to provide that holders of medical degrees from outside the United Kingdom, Canada, and the British colonies who were not registered practitioners in any of these jurisdictions would be required to sit a professional examination before the Board before becoming licensed in Newfoundland. Thus, only thirteen years after enactment of its first licensing law, physicians had managed to bring the colony's licensing provisions substantially into line with legislation in the several provinces of Canada.[190] This, despite the pressing need to attract medical personnel to the area. Why a trained practitioner would choose to set up practice in Newfoundland when the requisite credentials would have allowed him to operate almost anywhere in Canada or the United States does not appear to have concerned the colony's legislature. But, doubtless, the Newfoundland Medical Board was keenly aware that limiting the number of physicians entering the colony was of significant advantage to practitioners already operating there. That its licensing laws contributed to limiting the number of physicians practicing in Newfoundland is evidenced by the fact that in 1904 the ratio of physicians to the population of the colony was 1:2,642, while, almost half a century later, in 1950, it was 1:2,639.

THE PROFESSION IN WESTERN CANADA

The development of legislation in western Canada on the whole paralleled that in the east. Manitoba's 1886 law[191] had been quite comprehensive. Not only had it permitted the Council of its College of Physicians and Surgeons to erase from the medical register the name of any practitioner judged guilty of "infamous or unprofessional conduct in any respect," but it had placed in the hands of the University of Manitoba the power to set both the qualifications and examinations of applicants for licensure. In 1888, the Manitoba legislature, under some pressure from the few heterodox practitioners operating in the province,[192] amended the medical act[193] to provide for homeopathic representation on the Council — one representative for each fifteen licensed homeopathic practitioners — and to recognize degrees issued by homeopathic medical schools in the United States and Europe which met those standards set by the University of Manitoba. Examinations in the theoretical aspects of materia medica, therapeutics, the practice of physic, and in the theory of surgery and midwifery, were to be set by homeopathic physicians for those applicants intimating their wish to practice homeopathic medicine. Finally, the statute incorporated a provision whereby no physician's name could be removed from the medical register solely because of his adopting or refraining from adopting a particular theory of medicine or surgery.[194]

In 1904,[195] the medical act was again amended to set the minimum period of professional study necessary for licensure to that equivalent to the requirements of the University of Manitoba, and, in 1905, the University extended the compulsory medical course to five from four years.[196]

Osteopathy in Manitoba

By the turn of the century, several osteopaths had begun practicing in Manitoba.[197] It therefore became a matter of pressing importance to the profession that the definition of medical practice be enlarged sufficiently to encompass both osteopaths and other drugless healers, who posed a threat to the College's monopoly. After several unsuccessful attempts to have the law altered, the profession managed to again prevail upon the legislature to amend the medical act in this regard in 1906.[198] The penalty provision respecting the practice of medicine was revised to read:

> If any person, not registered pursuant to this Act, for hire, gain or hope of reward, practises or professes to practise medicine, surgery or osteopathy, or treats or professes to treat another, or prescribes or recommends or professes to prescribe or recommend, any drug, medicine, appliance, application, operation or treatment for any injury to, or any physical or mental ailment of, or any disease, infirmity or deformity of, another, or if any person, not registered as aforesaid, advertises to give advice in medicine, surgery or osteopathy, or midwifery, or advertises to treat, or prescribes any drug, medicine, application, operation or treat-

ment for, any injury to, or any physical or mental ailment of, or any disease, infirmity or deformity of, another, he shall, for any and every such offence, be liable to a penalty not exceeding one hundred dollars nor less than twenty-five dollars.

With enactment of the 1906 amendments, the practice of osteopathy — and chiropractic — were made illegal in the province, unless performed by fully licensed physicians.[199] Osteopaths attempted to gain passage of an osteopathic bill in 1914 and again in 1920, but opposition from the regular profession proved overwhelming. It was not until 1945, in the face of stiff and unremitting resistance from the College and orthodox physicians, that the Manitoba legislature enacted both an Osteopathic Act[200] and a Chiropractic Act,[201] legally recognizing these systems of treatment.

The North-west Territories

The North-west Territories medical ordinance of 1888 had undergone several revisions during the decade and a half after its passage. The profession, now organized into a College of Physicians and Surgeons, found that it could successfully apply pressure on the newly-established legislative assembly for more restrictive provisions to the Territorial medical statute. Thus, in 1894, physicians prevailed in gaining enactment of an amendment to the ordinance by which a professional examination was made compulsory for all applicants other than licentiates from the United Kingdom.[202] The effect of this provision was two-fold. First, it contributed to stemming the flow of prospective practitioners into the Territories, which was obviously beginning to tell on physicians' incomes. And, second, the $50.00 fee that examinees were required to pay brought in funds that could be used to prosecute the large number of unregistered practitioners still operating in the area.

Hilda Neatby reports that, by 1898, "the prevention of illegal practice was becoming almost routine business at any council meeting."[203] In its campaign against unlicensed practitioners, the Council, in April, 1898, placed at the disposal of each member of the Council the sum of $50.00 for the purpose of obtaining the necessary evidence to secure convictions. The funds were to be used in any manner thought appropriate towards this end, including the hiring of detectives. At the same time, a concerted effort to procure the registration of otherwise qualified physicians who had neglected to pay their registration fees was begun. Both these attempts appear to have been at least partially successful.[204] In 1901, the Council stepped up its efforts against illegal practitioners. In that year, an agent was appointed to collect evidence in the Edmonton area and the funds allotted each member of the Council were increased to $150.00. By 1903, a law student was hired to interview practitioners from Calgary to Edmonton and to institute prosecutions where possible.[205]

Disciplinary powers

Another area over which the Council was given control was the disciplining of the membership of the College, but here it apparently found much less to occupy its time. In 1892,[206] the College had been empowered to erase the name of any practitioner found guilty of "infamous conduct in any professional respect." These powers were broadened in 1898,[207] and provided that an inquiry was to be conducted on the basis of complaints from any three registered physicians. Neatby notes that only three cases before the College's disciplinary committee were heard between 1899, when the committee was created, and 1905. All involved gross incompetence and negligence and all resulted in no action being taken against the defendant physician other than censure. The most egregious case, heard in 1903, involved a physician who had misdiagnosed an obvious case of smallpox, immediately after which he attended a public meeting.[208] Had the same practitioner undertaken to advertise in the public press or breach the profession's code of ethics in some other manner, he would almost certainly have been expelled from the College but, under the circumstances, the Council felt that censure was sufficient punishment.[209]

Saskatchewan

With the creation of the provinces of Alberta and Saskatchewan in 1905, the task of drafting medical legislation for the two new provinces was placed in the hands of the registrar of the Territorial College.[210] As a result, the medical laws of the two jurisdictions reflected almost everything the profession could have reasonably asked. Saskatchewan's law of 1906[211] established a College consisting of all licensed physicians in the province, directed by an elected Council, with representation on the Council by district. Applicants for licensure were required to have attended a school of medicine "recognized by the College" which had exacted at least a four-year course of study of six months each and to pass a professional examination before the

Council. The Council was given extensive authority to discipline its membership, either by suspension or expulsion, for "unbecoming, improper or criminal conduct, professional or otherwise." Practicing, professing to practice, or advertising to give advice in medicine, surgery, or midwifery "for hire, gain or hope of reward" unless registered was punishable by a fine of up to $100.00. It was further made illegal to assume any title or description implying that one were registered unless one's name appeared on the provincial register. Engaging in medical practice, for purposes of the act, was specified to encompass the furnishing of medicine or the treating of any disease or ailment "by medicine, drugs, or any form of treatment, influence or appliance." The definition seems to have served its purpose; the courts in Saskatchewan ruled that a chiropractor providing "adjustment treatment" was held to be practicing medicine under the terms of the statute.[212]

In 1917,[213] the medical act was amended to turn over the conduct of examinations to the University of Saskatchewan and the period of required professional study was extended to five years. In addition, the following clause was inserted at the urging of the College:

> The council may order to be paid out of any funds of the college for all members of the college in good standing the annual dues of such members to The Canadian Medical Protective Association.

Opposition to osteopathic practice

Despite fierce resistance from the regular profession, the Saskatchewan legislature had, in 1913,[214] enacted an osteopathy act, establishing an osteopathic board to examine, license, and register practitioners in the province. Under the act, osteopaths were permitted to treat patients, subject only to the limitation that they were neither to employ or prescribe drugs for internal use nor to perform "any operation requiring the use of a knife." Passage of the law came as a severe blow to regular physicians, who saw it as seriously compromising their professional monopoly. Although it appears that only a few osteopathic doctors were licensed under the statute,[215] the College worked unceasingly to repeal or, at least, alter the law in such a way as to limit the number of osteopathic practitioners who became licensed and, above all, to strictly circumscribe their right to treat patients.

The regular profession's sustained lobbying finally proved successful and in 1917 the osteopathy act was repealed. In its place, the provincial legislature enacted a law governing all drugless practitioners.[216] Examinations for those wishing to register under the new act, including osteopaths, were placed in the hands of the University of Saskatchewan, which was also empowered to set the preliminary and professional educational requirements of all applicants. Candidates for licensure were required to hold a diploma from a school or college recognized by the University of Saskatchewan, at which they had attended a course of study of not less than four years embracing at least five months in each year. Thus, the determination of which osteopathic degrees were acceptable was taken out of the hands of osteopaths themselves and placed under the control of a group hostile to their method of treatment.

Limitations on heterodox practice

More significant, drugless practitioners were prohibited from prescribing or administering any drugs or medicinal preparations or treating any venereal or communicable disease, and from performing any and all surgical or obstetrical operations. A series of amendments to the act[217] did not improve the situation for osteopathic physicians in the province, who found that the requirements imposed on them for licensure were almost as rigid as those applying to orthodox physicians but that they were severely limited in the treatment they could give.

In 1927, they petitioned the provincial legislature to revise the Saskatchewan medical act to provide for the admission of osteopathic practitioners into the College of Physicians and Surgeons, but their efforts in this regard failed.[218] The Saskatchewan legislature seems to have been totally unsympathetic to complaints respecting any of the inequities contained in the drugless practitioners act. When the statute was amended in 1929, counsel for the osteopaths and other drugless healers petitioned for a change in the examination provisions. They asked that the professional examinations at least be conducted by proponents of drugless methods of treatment, rather than by a committee of the University hostile to such practitioners. The *Canadian Medical Association Journal* reports that this modest request was summarily dismissed by the Attorney–General since

> other professions treating the human body were examined under
> the auspices of the University and he could see no reason why the
> drugless healers should not conform to a university standard. He

suggested that the drugless healers' council and the University officials get together to agree on a standard for the profession and on the textbooks for the examination.[219]

Such advice could hardly have been given in good faith since, in 1928, eleven candidates had undertaken the University's examinations under the act and only one had passed![220]

It was not until 1944 that the Saskatchewan legislature once again enacted an osteopathy law,[221] creating an "independent" osteopathic board. The act, however, continued to provide the University of Saskatchewan with a role in determining both the content and conduct of professional examinations. The effect of this train of legislation was that, by 1962, a total of two osteopaths were practicing in the province.[222]

Restrictions in Alberta

Alberta's medical statute of 1906[223] was, predictably, similar in most respects to that of its sister province. The Alberta College was to be directed by a Council of seven physicians, elected by the membership of the province, divided into seven districts. As in Saskatchewan, all applicants were to have taken a degree from a medical school requiring at least a four-year course of study of which each session was to be no less than six months, and to sit a professional examination before the Council. Extensive disciplinary powers were conferred on the Council to either suspend or expel any physician found guilty of "unbecoming, improper or criminal conduct, professional or otherwise." The penalty provisions of the act, including the definition of medical practice, were the same as those provided in Saskatchewan's law of 1906.[224]

It appears that one of the highest priorities of the new Council involved the prosecution of those practitioners still operating in the area who had not received the College's license. Additionally, as one historian coyly observes, the Council devoted a substantial portion of its time to investigating "complaints of unethical conduct in centres where two or more medical men were in practice."[225]

The large number of qualified physicians entering Alberta during the first five years after its establishment as a province seems to have more than kept pace with the rise in population.[226] In 1906, 156 practitioners were listed as practicing in the region; by 1912, this number had grown to 384.[227] The profession viewed this development with some alarm, but there was little the College could do except to increase the severity of the professional examinations that all applicants had to undergo. Towards this end, the medical act was amended in 1911[228] to turn over conduct of the College's examinations to the University of Alberta, whose professors, presumably, were able to be more exacting both in testing candidates and in grading their responses. At the same time, lest there be any confusion about the matter, the act was revised to explicitly refer to osteopaths and homeopathists, who were subject to any examinations prescribed by the University as necessary for the proper practice of their systems.[229]

Practicing medicine defined

The University was also given the authority to determine those medical schools whose diplomas would be recognized as adequate, regardless of the system of medicine involved, and to conduct preliminary examinations in any subjects it might prescribe of any candidate appearing before it. Finally, the definition of medical practice was enlarged to include any act which one could conceive as possibly touching on the health of another. Payment or the hope of payment was no longer a necessary condition of medical practice. The definition, as revised, reads:

> Any person shall be held to practice . . . who shall —
> (a) by advertisement, sign or statement of any kind, allege ability or willingness to diagnose or treat any human diseases, ills, deformities, defects, or injuries;
> (b) advertise or claim ability or willingness to prescribe or administer any drug, medicine, treatment; or
> (c) perform any operation, manipulation or apply any apparatus or appliance for the cure or treatment of any human disease, defect, deformity or injury;
> (d) act as the agent, assistant, or associate of any person, firm or corporation in the practice of medicine as hereinbefore set out.[230]

The medical act was again amended in 1920.[231] It was reputed that relations between osteopaths and regular physicians remained "workable" after passage of the 1911 amendments, with osteopaths holding hospital privileges and the two groups even occasionally referring patients to each other.[232] However, in 1920, the College succeeded in revising the medical law to distance heterodox practitioners from the regular profession. The language of the provisions relating to the University's professional examinations was expanded to encompass the testing of candidates not only in regular medicine, osteopathy, and homeopathy but also those seeking to practice "chiropractic, or any other non-drug science, therapy or system of practice." At the same time, applicants examined for the purpose of practicing any heterodox system of medicine were restricted to the practice of that system alone, under penalty of violating the provisions of the medical act respecting unauthorized practice. Not only did these provisions sharply curtail the methods of treatment previously permitted osteopaths, but they served to further mark them off from regular physicians. Finally, the 1920 bill increased the penalties for illegal practice. Henceforth, practicing in violation of the act was punishable by a $50.00 fine for the first offense and by a fine of not less than $50.00 nor more than $200.00 and three months' imprisonment for each subsequent offense, "and in default of immediate payment of the fine and costs [of] six months' imprisonment."

These amendments appear to have served the profession well. Osteopathy in the province quickly declined and no longer posed any threats to the regular profession's monopoly. More importantly, between 1916 and 1958, the ratio of physicians to the population of Alberta not once reached its level of 1912, when it stood at 1:1,020.

British Columbia

The population of British Columbia during the decade 1881–1891 grew by over 98 per cent and by close to that amount again between 1891 and 1901.[233] As a result, the number of physicians operating in the province increased substantially during this period. Census data indicate that in 1881, thirty-one doctors were operating in British Columbia and by 1891 this had increased to 114 practitioners. If A. S. Munro's figures respecting the number of medical registrants in 1886[234] are a fairly accurate reflection of the number of physicians then practicing in the province, then most of this increase in the physician population occurred between 1886 and 1891. This growth rate appears to have accelerated over the next half-dozen years. In 1892, eleven physicians are reported as having registered; in 1898, the number had grown to twenty-six.[235]

The profession in British Columbia was, until 1898, governed by the medical act of 1886. It appears that, in addition to examining candidates for licensure, the main task of the Medical Council during its first years involved the identification and suppression of unlicensed practitioners, of whom, it is reported, "there were a great many."[236] The Council also turned its attention to the question of tightening the requirements for licensure in response to the large number of practitioners entering the province. In 1890, the legislature had amended the medical act,[237] over the objections of the Council, to provide for the licensing of homeopathic practitioners on the same terms as applied to regular applicants, except with regard to these candidates' professional examinations in certain specified subjects. This change, although unwelcome, appears to have made no difference to the composition of the profession in the province.

Requirements respecting professional study

Of primary concern to the Council was an extension of the minimum period of required professional study which, under the 1886 act, was fixed at three years. Despite the fact that the Council could increase the severity of its professional examinations at its discretion, the educational requirements were such that graduates of almost all American medical schools could qualify to sit the examinations. In 1898, the profession finally prevailed in gaining enactment of a new medical act,[238] whereby the period of compulsory professional study was extended from three to four years. In addition, the new law set up certain disciplinary procedures, permitting the Council to erase the name of any practitioner whose conduct was found to be "infamous or unprofessional in any respect" from the medical register.

In 1909, after much agitation from the organized profession, the legislature enacted a far more comprehensive statute governing medical practice in the province. Both the College and the province's medical societies — and particularly the most powerful of these, the Vancouver Medical Association[239] — had complained that the 1898 law, although an improvement over its predecessor, was inadequate to prevent less qualified practitioners from registering in the province, whose laws were looser than those in eastern Canada. To add to the problem, several osteopathic physicians had set up practice in British Columbia. Given the lack of a comprehensive definition of medical practice, however, the College was incapable of prosecuting them. Members of the regular profession had attempted to gain enactment of a bill prohibiting osteopathic practice altogether in early 1909, but public opposition to such a measure forced its withdrawal.[240] The medical act finally passed in 1909[241] attempted to deal with these issues in a manner at least acceptable to the profession. It provided for the inclusion of osteopathic physicians into the College. Osteopathic applicants were to have graduated from a recognized school of osteopathy and to have passed the Council's examinations, except in medicine and therapeutics, where an examination on the principles and practice of osteopathy was substituted. At the same time, the provisions respecting homeopathic applicants were revised to conform to those applying to candidates in orthodox medicine, save that the Council's examinations in materia medica and the principles and practice of medicine were to be conducted by homeopathic adherents. Henceforth, osteopaths and homeopathic physicians were restricted solely to the practice of their respective systems of treatment, under penalty of engaging in unauthorized practice.[242]

Medical practice rigorously defined

The new law also extended the period of professional study required of applicants. From the start of 1912, all candidates were to have received their degrees from schools requiring at least a five-year course of study for graduation. In addition, the Council's disciplinary powers were further broadened to include under the category of "unprofessional conduct," the placing of any druggist's or drug-store's name on any prescription blank.[243] Finally, the definition of medical practice was greatly expanded, in language later incorporated into the Alberta medical act of 1911.[244]

The courts in British Columbia appear to have had no difficulty in interpreting the medical act to the profession's liking. As early as 1895, a court had held that a patent medicine drummer was engaged in the practice of medicine when, at an outdoor meeting, he invited proposed purchasers to announce their symptoms before applying his remedy. It was here held that, although the defendant had every right to sell his medicines, "he was not entitled to call upon people to submit to his personal manipulation or inspection . . . asking their symptoms, diseases or complaints."[245]

Under the expanded definition contained in the 1909 law, the courts found no difficulty in holding a chiropractor's rubbing the spinal column or twisting the head of a client seeking relief from asthma as practicing medicine.[246] Even giving a massage was held to fall under the definition of medical practice. The 1909 act had specifically exempted "the ordinary calling of bath attendant" from its provisions. The appeal court, however, ruled that, although this exemption might apply to a bath attendant, it did not apply to the defendant masseur, who worked in a room with a portable Turkish bath, inasmuch as "here the primary object is the treatment or manipulation [i.e., the massage], and the bath, generally speaking, an incident."[247]

Besides facilitating the prosecution of possible competitors, the new act apparently served to limit the flow of practitioners moving to the west coast.[248] From a low of one physician to each 783 residents in 1914, the competitive position of physicians gradually improved so that by 1921 the ratio had reached 1:1,066 and remained above 1:900 through the mid-thirties. This drop is reflected in the figures for the city of Vancouver where, between 1898 and 1920, the physician-population ratio reached its peak in 1914 and gradually declined until the end of the decade.[249] By 1930, the ratio in greater Vancouver appears to have fallen to about 1:1,000.[250]

DOMINION RECIPROCITY

As is evident from the foregoing discussion, by the first decade of the twentieth century physicians throughout the Dominion had succeeded in gaining enactment of laws in each of the provinces limiting entry into the profession except through the mediation of medical boards answerable only to the profession itself. These boards, in all cases, were armed with the power to regulate both the preliminary and professional educational qualifications of all applicants for licensure and, in addition, vigorously enforced a policy of prosecuting all unlicensed practitioners. Physicians were thus placed in the enviable position of determining the competitive conditions under which they were to operate.

The constitutional structure of Canada made it necessary to achieve these ends at the provincial level, inasmuch as questions relating to health and education were delegated by the British North America Act to the provinces rather than to the federal authority. This provision worked a disadvantage on physicians to the extent that their licences were invalid beyond the borders of the province in which they were authorized to practice. It had been a long-standing goal of the profession, particularly that portion resident in the eastern provinces, to effect dominion-wide reciprocity. Indeed, as has been shown, one of the first acts of the newly organized Canadian Medical Association in 1867 was the creation of a committee to investigate the feasibility of instituting a dominion-wide system of licensure through the federal government. However, the jurisdictional problem and divisions among physicians themselves surrounding the question of removing control of licensing from the provincial to the federal level led to the issue becoming dormant in 1874. Nonetheless, it was never completely abandoned. At the 1893 meeting of the Association, the CMA's Committee on Inter-Provincial Registration once again recommended the formation of a Dominion Medical Council,

> to take general surveillance of the medical curriculum, and of all matters affecting the general public and profession of the whole Dominion, formed either by representatives (one each) from the members of the various Provincial Medical Councils, or elected by the medical population of Canada, irrespective of Provincial lines; or on the line of the British Medical Council. Its duties should be the equalization of the medical curriculum to a just and high standard; to secure inter-provincial reciprocity; to have the power to withhold or take away a Dominion license from a candidate for just cause; to approve all provincial examination papers before they were presented to candidates. There should be one examination for the Provincial and Dominion licenses, an extra fee for the latter. If it followed the British Medical Council in its formation, the British Medical Council regulations should be operative, as applicable to the Dominion.[251]

Objections were again raised that standards of medical education differed from province to province — e.g., unlike Ontario, Quebec still did not require applicants to sit an examination before its medical board — and that the recommendations appeared to conflict with the jurisdictional authority accorded the provincial legislatures. The membership concluded that reciprocity was neither practicable nor desirable unless the standards for licensure in effect in the various provinces were first raised to the level of that of the most exacting provincial board.[252]

Attempts at establishing reciprocity

At the following meeting of the Association, held at St. John in 1894, and despite the reception accorded the proposal of its Committee on Inter-Provincial Registration the year before, the CMA voted to strike a committee whose function was to establish and assist in securing a uniformly high standard of medical education and registration in each of the provinces, towards the end of achieving reciprocity in licensing throughout Canada. Dr. (later Sir) Thomas Roddick was appointed chairman of the committee and over the next decade and a half worked tirelessly to create a Dominion medical council, both through the Canadian Medical Association and, after 1896, as a member of the federal parliament. At the 1898 meeting of the Association, Roddick's Committee on Dominion Registration issued a series of detailed recommendations respecting the matriculation standards and educational requirements to be exacted of all candidates for licensure in each of the provinces. Additionally, the committee advocated the institution of a mandatory professional examination of all applicants before a provincial board of examiners. Finally, although it strongly supported continued efforts at the Dominion level to establish a national medical board, it proposed a scheme that would provide for interprovincial reciprocity without recourse to federal legislation. The committee recommended

> that the various [provincial] councils of the Dominion shall estab-
> lish an examining board for the Dominion conducted by
> examiners appointed by the medical councils of the several
> provinces, [and that] candidates passing a successful examination
> before said board and obtaining a certificate to that effect, shall
> be entitled to registration in the several provinces of the
> Dominion on payment of the registration fee, . . .[253]

Proposals welcomed by the profession

The proposal was warmly received by a large segment of the profession. The *Montreal Medical Journal* commented:

> The scheme is bold and masterly, and we fail to see why any ob-
> jection should be made to it on the part of our profession. The
> powers and the resources of the provincial colleges are retained —
> the colleges themselves are given a voice in the appointment of the
> Dominion Board of Examiners, and the profession throughout
> Canada becomes a united body. By the act of Confederation, the
> various provinces are given supreme control of all educational
> matters. In medicine the control of educational matters in each
> province is entrusted to the profession, acting through the Prov-
> incial Councils. It is wholly within the rights and powers of the
> Council, to agree upon one common course of education leading
> up to a Dominion examination, while further, it is at least a moot
> point whether the provincial control of educational matters of
> necessity, and implicitly, includes the power of conferment of
> licenses to practice in the various professions.[254]

There is no question that nationwide reciprocity was attractive to most physicians. The population of the Dominion west of Ontario had been growing at a substantial rate, increasing from 168,000 in 1881 to almost 650,000 twenty years later. By 1911, the population of the region had risen to 1,750,000. Practitioners licensed in the eastern provinces, where medical education was most readily available, were prevented from serving this new market without first satisfying the requirements set down by the several western provincial and territorial medical boards and paying a substantial registration fee. Physicians already authorized to practice in these fast-growing areas, on the other hand, were not nearly as supportive of Roddick's proposal, which — once enacted — would have denied them a quasi-monopoly over physicians' services in the west. Thus, the *Manitoba and West Canada Lancet* editorialized in early 1899:

> Few could question the desirability of a Dominion Registration in the future, but the doubt will arise whether this step, so far as the younger Provinces are concerned may not now be somewhat premature. It would certainly let loose in these sparsely settled portions of the Dominion the surplus medical men of the east. The North West is showing immense vitality in the manufacture of Physicians and Surgeons, and the openings available for the practice of their profession are yearly becoming more restricted. How would it be when the various colleges of eastern Canada poured their recently graduated men into Manitoba and the North-West. It is with difficulty bread and butter is secured by the medical man at the present time, but, with such competition as would undoubtedly arise if this system was now to come into force, the butter would probably become an unattainable luxury.... If Manitoba, the North-West and British Columbia are not prepared for the scheme of Dominion Registration, it is time they should be up and stirring in the matter, or they will awaken some day in the near future to find it law.[255]

Roddick's bill

Roddick, however, was undeterred by these reservations, which reflected the views of only a small proportion of the profession. He and large numbers of his supporters were especially motivated to work for the establishment of a national medical board since they saw it as opening the way to reciprocal registration with Great Britain and, via Great Britain, with the rest of the Empire. In speaking of the advantages of a dominion-wide board before the Montreal Medico-Chirurgical Society in March, 1898, Roddick noted that

> another important result of the establishment of such a system would be that Medical practitioners registered under it could claim registration under the Imperial Medical Act of 1886, without undergoing further examination. By this Act ... where parts of a British possession are under both a central and a local legislature, the authority of the central legislature is requisite to entitle a colonial practitioner to British registry. Under the existing systems of provincial registration, Canadian practitioners are debarred from entering the extensive field of medical employment in the various departments of the Imperial service, such as for example, the army and navy, the Indian medical service, the colonial medical services, medical service under the Board of trade, including ships' surgeons, etc., also from employment as sanitary officers in the United Kingdom.[256]

The opening up of such employment opportunities should be particularly welcome to the profession, Roddick concluded, since "the provinces are all congested, the number of medical men being far too numerous in proportion to the population. This scheme would not only lead to a more equable distribution, but it would throw open the entire British Empire to our Canadian youth who have adopted medicine as a profession."[257]

In 1900, after extensive consultation with the medical boards of the various provinces and with physicians' organizations throughout Canada, Roddick drew up a bill creating a dominion-wide registration board with the intent of submitting it to the Commons. The proposal called for the establishment of a Medical Council of Canada, "to promote and effect the assimilation and unification of the various standards of qualification established by the several Provinces of Canada as conditions of admission to the study and practice of Medicine." The Council, comprising three physicians from each province, would, under the terms of the bill, be empowered, among other things, to determine

> the qualifications to be required from all persons desirous of being registered either as practitioners or students under the authority of this Act, including the establishment, maintenance and effective conduct of examinations for ascertaining whether such persons possess the qualifications required; the number,

nature, times and modes of such examinations; the appointment of examiners; the terms upon which matriculation and other certificates from universities, colleges and other educational institutions, or from the governing bodies of other professions, shall be received as evidence of qualification; the recognition of degrees or diplomas granted by any British, Canadian, colonial or foreign school, college or university; the arranging and bringing into effect of any scheme or schemes of reciprocity as to registration with any British, Colonial or foreign medical licensing body or authority; the dispensation of candidates from undergoing examinations either wholly or partially and generally all matters incident to such examinations or necessary or expedient to effect the objects thereof; provided, however, that the requirements of the curriculum shall not at any time be lower than the requirements of the most comprehensive curriculum established at the same time for the like purpose in any Province, nor shall the standards of examinations either preliminary or professional be lower than the highest standard for the like purpose established at the same time for the purpose of ascertaining qualification for registration within any Province.[258]

Protests from Quebec

To the surprise of many, the phrasing of the bill brought strong protests from the French-speaking profession in Quebec, who saw in it an attempt to usurp the traditional privileges of the provincial profession to determine the qualifications for practice within Quebec. The *Bulletin Médical* particularly objected to the language of article 4(c) of the bill, which provided that the proposed Council determine "the qualifications and conditions necessary for registration, including the courses of study to be pursued, the examinations to be undergone, and generally the requisites for registration." Even though the bill's provisions applied only to those candidates seeking licensure through the dominion-wide board and not through any provincial board, all of which would remain autonomous, this clause was interpreted as preempting the existing power of the province to set the educational requirements necessary for licensure within their borders.[259]

The *Montreal Medical Journal* was quick to point out that this interpretation was by no means intended by the drafters of the bill and that "if any of the clauses of the projected measure can be shown to be harmful to any vested interests or to endanger any branch of the profession, [Roddick] will be the first to so modify the clause as to remove all possibility of harm or of misconstruction."[260] The *Journal*—traditionally one of the strongest supporters of restraints on entry into the profession—defended interprovincial reciprocity by appealing to the value of freeing the profession from the fetters of restrictive legislation. "Were medicine," it commented,

> a trade, adventure, or other mercantile concern, the case might be different. It might then be defensible to organize the medical men of each province into a closed corporation and to rigorously prevent all outsiders from poaching upon the provincial preserves. But the first aim of the physician is to be of service to his fellow men; commercial conditions are of right but secondary. Ours is *par excellence* the liberal profession, and this being so, regulations regarding practice should be most liberal.[261]

First moves in the Commons

Roddick had been elected to his seat in the Commons as a Conservative representing the constituency of St. Antoine in Montreal in 1896, the same year in which the Conservatives were swept from office in a Liberal landslide. The cabinet post that had been promised Roddick did not, of course, materialize and the Laurier government was less than sympathetic to any measure aimed at enlarging the privileges of a protected profession or of supporting a bill that might appear to infringe the area of provincial autonomy. Consequently, Roddick felt it fruitless to draw up a proposal for a national medical board until 1900. In March, 1901, despite the objections of many of the French-speaking physicians in Quebec, Roddick introduced his proposal in the Commons as a private member and it was given first reading without discussion. The bill proceeded no further that year,[262] despite the lengthy plea for passage with which Roddick introduced his measure.[263] Between the 1901 and 1902 sessions of Parliament, Roddick had again consulted widely on the language of the proposal and, in an attempt to appease those physicians who saw in it a threat to their prerogatives, altered several of its provisions. When Parliament again met in 1902, a revised version of the bill was introduced. In moving its second reading, Roddick offered an explanation of the new bill's most important substantive change, the composition of the proposed council. Roddick conceded that this aspect of the measure has been a great puzzle to those of us who have had to do with the framing of this Bill. It has occasioned me, personally, a great deal of thought and consideration. We have tried two or three schemes, which have all given more or less satisfaction, but, which have not quite met the requirements. When I addressed this House a year ago, I stated that the plan which seemed to satisfy all the provinces was that three members of the council should be taken from each province — one appointed by the Governor-General in Council, one elected by each provincial medical council, and, the president of each provincial medical council. That, we found, gave dissatisfaction in the larger provinces. The province of Ontario, with its 2,300 odd doctors, said, "It is unfair to us to give us the same number only as the little province of Prince Edward Island with something like 96 doctors." Pressure was brought to bear so strongly that I looked for another scheme, and I think I have found one which will give general satisfaction. It is, that for the first 100 or fraction of 100 practitioners in each province, there shall be one member. That will let in Prince Edward Island, and will also let in the Yukon when it has a central board established. For the second 100 or fraction thereof over 50, there will be one member; and for every 600 above that, one member. That principle can be continued *ad infinitum*. Then there will be appointed members— one appointed by the Governor-in-Council from each province. There will also be university representatives, each university having a teaching medical faculty being entitled to send one, and there will be three homeopathic representatives from the entire Dominion.[264]

Second reading

Despite his having apparently solved the thorny problem of representation on the Council, Roddick was still confronted with a great deal of opposition to the bill in the Commons.[265] Opponents of the measure insisted that it was beyond the jurisdictional purview of the federal government to legislate in this area, and— although it passed its second reading— Roddick moved referral of the bill to a select committee, composed primarily of physicians sitting in the House. When it was objected that this committee was too heavily weighted in favor of members of the medical profession, Laurier is reported to have commented: "Should there not be a sufficient number of lawyers on the committee to kill the bill, then the names of a few lawyers might be added."[266]

Between its second reading and the point at which the bill was again brought before the House, the Prime Minister apparently dropped his opposition to the measure, having concluded that, since the proposal provided that each province could freely opt into the new Council, no trespass on provincial rights was involved.[267] The bill thereupon received third reading in May, 1902, and became law.[268]

The Medical Act of 1902

The statute, as enacted in 1902, embodied a number of changes from Roddick's original draft of 1900. Unlike Quebec's and Manitoba's medical graduates, who could obtain provincial licenses upon completion of their studies in the province without further examination, the medical graduates of Ontario's universities were required to pass an examination before the province's Medical Council in order to practice in Ontario. This disparity in provincial requirements for licensure led the various medical faculties in Ontario to demand the insertion of the following clause, which was incorporated into the act as legislated:

> The possession of a Canadian university degree alone, or of a certificate of provincial registration founded on such possession, obtained subsequent to the date when the Council shall be first duly constituted under this Act, shall not entitle the possessor thereof to be registered under this Act.[269]

It appears that Roddick was aware that such a clause would make it most unlikely that Quebec would pass the enabling legislation necessary to make the act operative in that province, and he so warned the representatives from Ontario when they insisted on its inclusion.[270] The question was discussed by the Montreal Medical Society soon after the bill containing the offending clause was given third reading. The Society's report recommended that the measure be amended to provide that all holders of provincial licenses, irrespective of the particular requirements each province might impose, be permitted to sit the federal board's examinations. The Ontario profession, however, remained adamant. The *Canada Lancet* reported on the suggested amendment and concluded that it was unacceptable:

> [The amendment] would provide that a graduate in medicine of any of the three universities of Quebec would, after registration in the College of Physicians and Surgeons of that Province, be entitled to proceed at once to take the examinations of the

Dominion Medical Council, while graduates in medicine of the other universities, that of Manitoba excepted, would only be allowed to take the same examinations after they had passed the examinations of a Provincial Medical Council.... This suggested amendment aims at preserving to the universitiés of Quebec the privileges they now enjoy, and of which the Roddick Act would deprive them.

If this amendment should be adopted, it would impose on every medical student in a university of Ontario three series of examinations, one for his degree, one for his Provincial license, and the third for that of the Dominion; while the student of Laval, McGill or Bishop's College would have to undergo two only, the first and the last. This would involve a very serious discrimination in favor of the Quebec universities, and it would result in compelling the student of an Ontario university to spend about two months out of every session of eight months in undergoing medical examinations. To escape the burden and the number of these, all in this Province proposing to study medicine would go to the medical teaching institutions of Quebec. This would not, it is certain, make for an elevation of the medical standard.

It is obvious, therefore, that the suggested amendment cannot be accepted in Ontario.[271]

The profession in Quebec

The line was thus drawn between the professions in Ontario and Quebec, each jealous of its own prerogatives. The attitude of Ontario's physicians appears particularly petty, in using the Roddick law — the intent of which was to facilitate interprovincial reciprocity — as a means of raising the requirements for licensure in Quebec and thus to further restrict the supply of medical personnel practicing in Canada. Indeed, it was to have had just this effect. The 1902 Canada Medical Act provided that the requirements for federal registration were to be at least as high as those in effect in that province imposing the most exacting standards for licensure. As a result, at the October, 1902, meeting of the Board of Governors of the College of Physicians and Surgeons of Quebec, it was decided to extend the period of mandatory professional training to encompass a five-year course of study and to raise the matriculation standard to the "complete or classical course of study," that is, to graduation in arts.[272] However, the Board of Governors also passed the following resolution at the same sitting:

That while recognizing as desirable reciprocity in diplomas and licenses in medicine between the different provinces of Canada..., as well as the free access for the purposes of practice between these same provinces by all regular holders of these diplomas and licenses, the governors of the College of Physicians and Surgeons of the province of Quebec believe it their duty to oppose any intervention or organization made to the end above enumerated, which has for its effect the curtailment of the privileges or acquired rights of this board, of compromising its autonomy, or of relieving it of a part of its control of medical studies guaranteeing actual conditions, and for all these reasons the governors believe it to be their duty to refuse their approval of the Roddick Bill as passed by the Federal Parliament; but they are prepared to suggest and to accept a system of reciprocity of diplomas and licenses in medicine between the provinces of this Confederation, provided that this reciprocity shall be put into effect under the direct control of the provincial boards, or of a medical council deriving its initiative from these boards and sanctioned by the Provincial Legislatures.[273]

The need for provincial unanimity

Probably the greatest weakness of the 1902 law was the inclusion of a provision that prevented the act from becoming operative until all the provinces had passed the necessary enabling legislation.[274] Quebec's recalcitrance was thus a serious blow to those members of the profession who saw in the law the best hope for opening up the rapidly-growing western regions of Canada to eastern practitioners, while also achieving reciprocity with Great Britain. The *Montreal Medical Journal* expressed disappointment that the act incorporated a unanimity clause, noting that "we can see no satisfactory reason why the Bill should not have been so drawn as to afford a means by which, say, a majority of the provinces could enter into an agreement to accept the diploma of the Council as adequate for admission to practice within those provinces."[275] But, despite this drawback, the *Journal*, in appealing to the profession throughout Canada to press for adoption of enabling legislation in their home provinces, was convinced that the benefits of the act were clear and substantial, while its disadvantages were minor. "As matters are at present," it noted,

though we are all Canadians and of a common nationality, it is forbidden to us under pains and penalties to cross the provincial boundaries and minister to other Canadians seeking our help, unless we have fulfilled every exaction of the licensing board of the province we seek to enter, – in other words, unless during our undergraduate days we happened to have followed the exact course demanded by that province. The British Columbian whose interests call him east is absolutely debarred from settling in Ontario and there practicing his profession unless he has in the past completed the course and taken the examinations demanded by the Ontario Board, or unless he is willing to spend years repeating his undergraduate work, in the process of taking the exact course required. Our French-speaking compatriots settling in Ontario, Manitoba, or New Brunswick, cannot obtain the services of a fellow-countryman as a village doctor because of these same embargos, save in the rare case of a bilingual French physician who has ventured to enter, and has succeeded in passing examinations in a language not his own, and upon subjects taught in a manner different to that in vogue at Laval. For undoubtedly the French tradition in medicine differs from the English.

That this should be the case is preposterous, and the only way to overcome the difficulty is that proposed in the measure before us.[276]

What is particularly striking about the *Journal's* editorial is that the parochial regulations of which it complains were enacted in the first instance because of intense pressure from physicians themselves, whose goal was to limit the number of new entrants into the profession. And in this task the medical press, the *Montreal Medical Journal* among them, was at the forefront in focusing professional efforts towards gaining enactment of each specific ordinance, the cumulative effect of which was a hodge-podge of petty restraints on those wishing to enter medicine in each of the provinces. Having succeeded in holding down the number of practitioners throughout Canada, the profession now sought release from the provincial constraints aimed at newcomers.

Enabling legislation

The legislatures of several of the provinces were quick to enact the necessary enabling statutes recognizing Dominion registration. The *Maritime Medical News* remarked in June, 1902, that

it is not likely that any opposition will be offered to the Act in the

Maritime Provinces, and the necessary legislation can be obtained without difficulty. Hearty approval of the measure, by the various medical societies which meet next month, would strengthen the hands of the medical boards and materially lessen the risk of hostile opposition in the local legislature.[277]

The profession in the Maritimes did indeed endorse the proposal and, as a consequence, both Nova Scotia and Prince Edward Island altered their medical acts to accommodate the federal law in 1903.[278] Nor was there any real opposition in the prairie provinces. Manitoba's legislature acted in 1903,[279] and both Alberta and Saskatchewan included provision for recognizing federal registrants in their original medical acts.[280]

The situation in Ontario was somewhat more complex. The Ontario Medical Council had withdrawn its earlier objections to Roddick's proposal when it was altered to deny recognition to those applicants whose certificates of provincial registration were based solely on possession of a Canadian medical degree.[281] After passage of the 1902 act, the Ontario Medical Council is reported to have enthusiastically supported the measure and proceeded to appoint a committee whose function was to gain enactment of the necessary legislation in the provincial parliament.[282] However, opposition from elements within the Ontario Medical Association led the Council to drag its feet. Some Ontario physicians feared that the recognition of licenses issued by a dominion-wide board would result in large numbers of Quebec physicians setting up practice in Ontario, where the economic climate for physicians' services seemed more favorable. As a result, the Council, fearful of acting precipitously in recommending enactment of a law that might increase competition within the province, was reluctant to take the lead in pushing for passage. The medical schools, on the other hand, were avid supporters of the measure. In 1905 a delegation representing the medical faculties of Toronto, Queen's, Western, and McGill met with the provincial minister of education to press for action in the Ontario legislature.[283] However, the deputation appears to have done little to effect any change in the attitude of either the Council or the provincial government.

Definition of medical practice

One issue that was to remain of concern to many physicians in Ontario was the definition of medicine provided in the Roddick act. The law went no further than to specify that "medicine shall be held to include surgery and obstetrics."[284] In 1909, the Ontario College of Physicians and Surgeons, troubled by this lack of a sufficiently broad definition, referred the matter to their solicitor, who suggested the following:

> Medicine shall include surgery and obstetrics, and shall mean the art of healing, and relieving and attempting to heal or relieve human diseases, injuries, ailments and complaints by advice, direction, operation, influence or suggestion, with or without the use of medicine or drugs.[285]

The proposed definition appears to have gone some way in reducing antagonism to the federal statute, but the provincial government remained hesitant to introduce an enabling bill until the Quebec legislature had first acted.

French-speaking practitioners had, since the late 1870s, been the dominant force in the College of Physicians and Surgeons of Quebec. The College, consequently, had less to gain from dominion-wide reciprocity than did the profession in the English-speaking provinces. In addition, both the College and the provincial government were particularly disturbed that the Roddick bill contained a provision empowering the proposed Dominion Council to determine "the terms upon which matriculation and other certificates from universities, schools and other medical institutions, shall be received as evidence of qualification."[286] This and like clauses referring to the medical curriculum were viewed as direct infringements of the province's traditional control over the educational qualifications of its licensed professionals.[287] Quebec's anglophone practitioners, on the other hand, viewed these conflicts with provincial autonomy as illusory since, under the Roddick act, the provincial medical board retained the power to determine the qualifications of those physicians seeking licensure solely within the province. The medical faculty of McGill University was especially eager that the Quebec legislature enact enabling legislation, thus opening up the whole of the Dominion to its graduates.

Agitation for provincial adoption

In 1905, the medical students at McGill extended their campaign of support to the other provinces. Acting unanimously, they circulated a letter to each member of the provincial legislatures of Ontario, British Columbia, and New Brunswick, urging adoption of the federal law and outlining the benefits of Dominion reciprocity. While the petition appears to have occasioned no response in Ontario or British Columbia, the New Brunswick Medical Council replied to the communication to the effect that no further legislation in that province was required to implement the terms of the federal law and that the New Brunswick Council was prepared to act under its provisions as soon as a federal medical council was established.[288] Indeed, the New Brunswick profession was overwhelmingly supportive of Dominion reciprocity. In July, 1908, Dr. J. P. McInerney, addressing the New Brunswick Medical Society, reiterated the advantages of dominion-wide registration and castigated those members of the profession — throughout Canada — who were working against the scheme:

We have been seeking for years under the judicious guidance of Dr. Roddick, of McGill University, to transform our *legal status*, which is still but provincial, into a condition with possibilities and powers as wide not only as the Dominion, but as wide as the British Empire itself. It is unnecessary to discuss the many advantages that would come to us as a result of Dominion registration, and affiliation with the profession in Great Britain. In the first place, it would empower a medical man, after having passed the necessary examination before a central examining board, that might be appointed, to practice his profession in any province or locality over which flies the British Ensign. It would have the effect of widening our horizon and our *watchword* for the profession would be *Imperial* and not *Provincial*. By some it may be said that the prevention of successfully carrying Dominion Registration into effect is brought about by the profession itself. That the professional jealousy in certain provinces has caused the law-givers in these provinces to meet the views of their constituents, and to save their skins from a political standpoint, they have voted in parliament to please their narrow-minded friends and against the best interests of the profession. Herein lies a grievance on this point not only against our legislators, but against certain members of the profession, who have failed to make good in advancing the interests of medical science. We believe it to be the bounden duty of all — both legislators and members of the profession — to rise superior to any petty jealousy and for the general welfare of the profession, their trend of action should be Imperial in character. If this province of New Brunswick and this Canada of ours is to be a land of liberty and freedom, it seems but meet and just, that a man after receiving the *Imprimatur* of a recognized University, should be allowed to pitch his tent on any vantage ground he desires on that broad stretch of Canadian territory extending from the Atlantic to the Pacific.[289]

The attitude in British Columbia

McInerney's reference to professional jealousies in certain provinces had particular relevance to the profession in British Columbia, which was sharply divided on Dominion reciprocity. The *Canada Lancet* reported that in British Columbia,

> we are well informed that those in the rural districts favor the Act, while those in Vancouver and Victoria are in favor of the protection to be secured under a provincial system of examination. They fear that these cities would be flooded with doctors under the Dominion Act.[290]

Even as late as January, 1910, Roddick himself, in a letter to H. W. Powell, one of his most loyal supporters and later the first registrar of the Medical Council of Canada, complained of the inaction of the British Columbia Medical Council and of continued opposition to his bill in that province. "I can get absolutely nothing from Fagan [of the British Columbia Medical Council]," Roddick wrote.

> I don't believe they have taken the first step to have a meeting of their Council. . . . A patient of mine, who has just returned from the Coast, tells me that he overheard two doctors discussing the question of Dom. Regis. and one stopped the argument suddenly by remarking that "he wished Roddick and his Bill were both in hell."[291]

It is not surprising that the majority of physicians in British Columbia should have had reservations about supporting a dominion-wide registration system. Protected by legislation that required each applicant to pass a professional examination before its medical board, the profession was not anxious to allow creation of a second portal of entry over which it had no control into what promised to be Canada's fastest growing market for physicians' services. Consequently, opponents of the Roddick bill were able to stall any attempt at passage of an enabling statute in the provincial parliament.

Despite antagonism to the act in British Columbia, Quebec, and, to a lesser degree, in Ontario, Roddick persisted in his struggle to win support from the several provincial boards and professional organizations. These efforts, often frustrating, were not fruitless. In November, 1909, Roddick was able to assemble a committee representing all the provinces at Montreal to discuss possible amendments to the act. These discussions continued on into the following year. Finally, at a meeting held in Toronto in June, 1910, Roddick's efforts proved successful; agreement was at last reached among all the provinces respecting amendments to the 1902 act which, once enacted, would satisfy the various provinces that had not yet brought themselves under the provisions of the federal law.[292]

Changes in the act

Roddick was anxious to submit the proposed changes to the federal parliament at its 1910 sitting, but a request from the British Columbia Medical Council that a draft of the proposed changes be circulated among the whole profession in that province delayed action until the following year.[293] Eventually, in 1911, at Roddick's request, the amended bill was put before the Commons by Dr. J. B. Black. In moving passage, Black noted:

> I do not anticipate any opposition to this Bill at all. These amendments have been submitted to the medical councils and associations of every province, and have been approved by them all. These associations and councils represent between six and seven thousand medical men in the Dominion. When this Bill was introduced in 1902, it met with a good deal of opposition, but all that opposition has passed away, and from Vancouver to Halifax, as far as the profession is concerned, they are in favour of it.[294]

There was indeed little opposition to the bill in the House and it was enacted in May, 1911.[295] Over the next few months, New Brunswick and British Columbia both passed the requisite enabling legislation and, finally, in April, 1912, after the legislatures of Quebec and Ontario had acted, the Canada Medical Act came into force.[296]

The amended statute

The amended act to which the provinces unanimously agreed deleted all reference to any matriculation requirements, a subject acknowledged as being solely within the purview of the provinces.[297] In their place, the following clause was inserted:

> The council shall not determine or fix any qualifications or condi-
> tions to be complied with as preliminary to or necessary for
> matriculation in the study of medicine and for the obtainment of
> the provincial licenses, these being regulated as heretofore by the
> provincial authorities.

In response to complaints from British Columbia that the method
of representation originally devised was too heavily weighted towards
Ontario and Quebec, the Council's composition was altered. Under
the amended act, the Council was to consist of two members from
each province's medical board. In addition, homeopathic physicians
were entitled to three representatives and each of the universities
having medical faculties to one representative. Finally, three members
of the profession were to be appointed by the Governor-in-Council,
each from a separate province, of which two were to come from the
three western provinces until such time as a medical school was established in the region. The original council thus consisted of thirty-two
members, eighteen representing the medical boards of the nine
provinces, eight representatives of the medical faculties then operating
in Canada, three homeopathic members, and three appointees of the
Governor-in-Council.[298]
In order to assure Quebec that the Dominion Council would not sup-
plant the authority of the provincial medical boards in determining
which candidates could sit its examinations, the Roddick act was further amended to provide that:

> No candidate shall be eligible for any examination prescribed by
> the council, unless he is the holder of a provincial license, or un-
> less he presents a certificate from the registrar of his own provin-
> cial medical council that he holds a medical degree accepted and
> approved of by the medical council of the said province.

Thus, the provincial boards retained ultimate control over those applicants admitted to the Medical Council's examinations through their
power to withhold enabling certificates.
Finally, the grandfather clause that appeared in the 1902 act was
altered. The original bill provided that anyone who had been engaged
in active practice in any one or more provinces for a period of at least
six years prior to the establishment of the Medical Council of Canada
was entitled to federal registration without examination. Under the
terms of the amended act, the minimum period of prior practice was
extended to ten years.[299]

THE MEDICAL COUNCIL OF CANADA

Given the amount of bargaining, bickering, and effort necessary to bring the Dominion Council into existence, its early years were disappointingly placid.[300] The inaugural meeting, held in November, 1912, was solely an organizational one and it was not until 1913 that any physician was registered on its rolls. Seventy-one candidates sat the first examinations, held in Montreal in October, 1913, of which forty-four passed.[301] In addition, eighty-five physicians registered under the Act's grandfather clause.[302] By 1920, the Council's register listed a total of 636 licentiates, of which only 311 were by examination.[303] Yet, between 1913 and 1919, the Dominion's medical schools had graduated slightly over 2,000 doctors. Thus, only 15 percent of newly-graduated physicians chose to sit the Council's examinations. More surprising was the small number of practitioners who elected to take advantage of the statute's ten-year clause. Close to 1,500 physicians were eligible to register under this provision when the Council was established, yet only 325 had requested registration by 1920.

Two factors appear to have militated against Dominion registration during this period. The first related to the fact that students newly graduated from most Canadian medical schools were confronted with the prospect of having to sit three sets of examinations if they wished to become licentiates of the Medical Council of Canada, those of their medical faculty, those before the provincial board, and, finally, those of the Medical Council itself.

The second element working to the disadvantage of dominion-wide registration was that arrangements had been made soon after the establishment of the Medical Council of Canada by which each province could, if it so chose, enter into reciprocal registration with Great Britain. When the British Medical Act had been revised in 1886, it empowered the British Medical Council to enter into agreements whereby practitioners duly licensed in any British possession or foreign country which extended the same privileges to British registrants could be entered on the British register without further examination. The statute, however, provided that "where parts of [a British possession] are under both a central and a local legislature, all parts under one central legislature are for the purposes of this definition deemed to be one British possession."[304] This clause effectively forestalled any of the several Canadian provinces from establishing reciprocity with the United Kingdom. Indeed, one of the principal objectives in establishing a dominion-wide Council was to effect reciprocity under the terms of the 1886 law. As matters were to turn out, this proved unnecessary; in 1905, the British legislature once again amended its medical act to include a provision that "where any part of a British Possession is under central and also under a local legislature, His Majesty may, if he thinks fit, by an Order-in-Council declare that the part which is under local legislature shall be deemed a separate British possession."[305] As a consequence of the 1905 amendment, all the provinces except British Columbia had extended reciprocity to British registrants by 1917.

World War I

The First World War did much to promote the movement toward reciprocity with Great Britain. Canadian physicians were legally prevented from practicing either in the British armed forces or in British hospitals unless their licenses were first officially recognized by the General Medical Council of Great Britain. In consequence, those provinces that had not entered into reciprocity prior to the outbreak of the war were encouraged to do so.[306] It quickly became apparent to the profession, however, that reciprocity was a Trojan horse. Inasmuch as all the provinces excepting British Columbia had entered into agreements with Great Britain, it became possible for physicians to employ the British Medical Council as a medium of interprovincial registration. By entering his name on the British register, a Canadian practitioner from one province was free to apply for registration, via such enrollment, in another, thus bypassing the Medical Council of Canada altogether. There were attempts by some provinces to word their agreements with Great Britain in such a way that they extended only to those applicants who could prove British residence, but this condition proved unenforceable and was effectively disregarded. In gist, the effect of British reciprocity, as one professional spokesman complained in 1924, was that

> provincial licentiates avoid the examination of the Medical Council of Canada. They send to Great Britain their certificate of provincial registration together with a fee, obtain British registration thus, and then register in any province. It is a real money order business in registration certificates, and is resented by many of the provinces. It works out practically as interprovincial registration without any equality of standard of preliminary education or of medical education.[307]

Nor was this the only objection to British reciprocity. The British

Medical Council, under the authority granted it by the Medical Act of 1886, had entered into reciprocity with a number of other British possessions, among them Ceylon, Hong Kong, and India,[308] and with several foreign countries, including Italy[309] and Japan.[310] Canadian physicians thus found themselves in the position of having to recognize the credentials of practitioners educated to what they regarded as a much lower standard of medical knowledge. Although the actual effect of reciprocity with these countries was insignificant, the profession was affronted that the British Council should have drawn no legal distinction between doctors who had qualified in Canada on the one hand, and in these other nations, on the other.[311]

The unwanted effects of British reciprocity led several provinces to withdraw from their agreements with Great Britain in the 1920s. In 1924, the Saskatchewan legislature amended its medical act to limit reciprocity only to those registrants of the British Medical Council who were registered by examination.[312] Since the British Council did not hold examinations, the effect of this provision was to deny British registrants legal recognition in Saskatchewan.[313] Two years later, in 1926, New Brunswick's Medical Council, under the authority accorded it by the province's medical act of 1913, permitting the Council to set the terms and conditions regarding reciprocity with Great Britain, revoked its agreement and ceased licensing British registrants without examination.[314] Ontario's Medical Council, accorded similar authority by its medical statute, followed suit in 1927.[315] And, in the same year, the provisions of the medical act of 1909 that had set down the conditions under which reciprocity with Great Britain had been established, were repealed in Quebec.[316] Thus, after 1927, only four provinces continued to admit physicians enrolled on the British register without examination: Alberta, Nova Scotia, Prince Edward Island, and Manitoba.[317]

Conjoint Examinations

The problems occasioned by requiring new medical graduates from the Dominion's universities to sit several series of examinations appears to have been solved by the end of the 1920s, coincident with the effective end of reciprocity with Great Britain. Soon after the establishment of the Medical Council of Canada in 1912, most provincial medical boards adopted a policy of issuing enabling certificates — permitting the holder to undergo the Medical Council's examinations — to newly graduated residents without requiring that these applicants first be examined for a provincial license. By the mid-1920s, the Quebec board alone continued to withhold enabling certificates from candidates appearing before it unless they had first passed the province's own examinations.[318]

During the first years of the Medical Council's operation, potential candidates for the Council's license were faced with yet a further difficulty, the effect of which was to discourage numbers of new graduates from sitting the Council's examinations. These examinations were scheduled soon after the conclusion of the academic year. In consequence, it commonly occurred that the provincial boards felt themselves unable to issue the necessary enabling certificates to medical students who had completed their studies in time for them to sit the Medical Council's examinations that year. Not having yet received the results of the universities' examinations and ignorant of whether an applicant had met all the requirements for a professional degree, the provincial boards waited until they had received this information from the applicant's university, which often was unavailable until after the Council's examinations had taken place.

Postponing the date on which the Medical Council's examinations were to be held would not, apparently, have proved of much help. Since the Medical Council justifiably chose as its examination sites the cities in which the Dominion's medical schools were located,[319] if too long a time were allowed to elapse between the two sets of examinations—those of the university and those of the Council—then graduating medical students would return to their homes and spare themselves the expense of waiting to hear the results of the first examination and of writing the second. Thus, to take an extreme example, a student from Alberta studying at McGill would be encouraged to return to his home province and there take Alberta's licensing examination, rather than wait for several months in Montreal to sit the Medical Council examinations.

The solution to this problem proved, in fact, to be a simple one, although it was not generally adopted by the various provincial boards until the beginning of the 1920s. Rather than wait to receive official word from the applicant's university respecting whether the applicant had passed his university examinations, the boards would issue a temporary certificate, permitting the candidate to sit the Medical Council examinations, later forwarding to the Council formal notice that the applicant had, in fact, obtained his medical degree. The effect of this measure was to substantially increase the number of new graduates applying for the licentiate of the Medical Council of Canada and to enlarge the number of physicians listed on its register.[320]

Disappearance of Provincial Examinations

The prestige and popularity associated with registration with the Medical Council of Canada was significantly advanced in 1919, when British Columbia's medical board decided to discontinue its own licensing examinations and recognize the Medical Council examinations as the only acceptable qualification for practice in the province.[321] Henceforth, all physicians registered in British Columbia would be licensed solely by virtue of their being licentiates of the Medical Council.

In actual fact, British Columbia had been preceded in this policy by Saskatchewan, whose medical board had effectively ceased holding its own examinations shortly after the establishment of the Dominion Council. Under the terms of Saskatchewan's medical act of 1906, the province's medical board had been legally able to delegate its function of setting licensing examinations to the Dominion Medical Council.[322] However, when the Saskatchewan legislature enacted its drugless practitioners act in 1917, it amended the province's medical law to explicitly provide that the University of Saskatchewan hold two licensing examinations each year,[323] thus paralleling the structure of registration requirements that appeared in the statute respecting the licensing of drugless practitioners.[324]

In 1924, the provincial College petitioned the legislature to amend the reading of Saskatchewan's medical law to permit the University "if deemed advisable [to] accept the examiners of the Medical Council of Canada appointed for a similar purpose."[325] This amendment, apparently, was not acted upon and the province's medical law continued to provide for examinations conducted by the University of Saskatchewan. Despite this provision, however, by the late 1920s, the overwhelming majority of provincial residents chose to receive their licenses under the Dominion Council rather than sit Saskatchewan's provincial examinations.[326]

The 1920s marked a crucial period in the fortunes of the Medical Council. Whereas at the beginning of the decade only about 7 percent of all Canadian physicians were listed on the Dominion register, by 1930 this had increased to almost 27 percent.[327] One indication of the growing popularity of national registration is that in 1929 and again in 1930 all newly graduated medical students from the University of

Alberta chose to sit the Medical Council examinations rather than the province's own licensing examinations.[328] This trend appears to have been nation-wide since in 1931 the New Brunswick medical council reported that only one candidate presented himself for the provincial examinations, while all other graduates from the province opted for application to the Dominion Council.[329] The effect of this decline in the number of applicants for provincial licenses led the New Brunswick board to cease offering its own examinations in 1932.[330]

A similar pattern had developed in Ontario where, in 1929, only twenty students had chosen to undertake the provincial examinations.[331] This, even though 189 students were graduated from Ontario's medical schools in that year. As a result of the decline in the number of graduates applying for provincial licensure, the Ontario council recommended that the province follow the lead of British Columbia and New Brunswick and abrogate its right to set its own professional examinations. In consequence, the provincial parliament amended the Ontario medical act in 1934[332] to empower the province's board to require all future candidates to have taken the Medical Council of Canada examinations. In that same year, the Ontario Medical Council passed the necessary by-law officially recognizing the Dominion examinations as the sole portal of entry into practice in the province.[333]

Modern profession as medieval guild

With the creation of the Medical Council of Canada and its establishment over the following two decades as the primary means by which prospective physicians entered the profession, the structure of medical licensure in Canada took its final form. If, on the eve of Confederation, a doctor had referred to himself as belonging to a profession, he could have been thought of as putting on airs. Indeed, medicine could not, with justification, even lay claim to possessing a truly scientific foundation until the germ theory of disease had been decisively accepted in the 1870s.

Physicians, of course, had laid claim to a body of recondite knowledge that warranted protection from ignorant pretenders ever since the fourteenth century, when the first physicians' guilds restricting entry into medical practice were formed on the Continent. But the medieval notion of a community or fellowship protected from competition cannot be translated into the free-market concept of a profession, which the term connoted by the eighteenth century. (A profession in the modern sense, contrary to the views of many sociologists, need not, *by definition*, bear the same characteristics as a profession in the medieval sense.[334]) Historically, what in fact appears to have occurred was that when the protections afforded practitioners of medicine by the medieval guilds disappeared, medicine became a trade, as did so many of the other occupations that had previously held guild status. By the end of the nineteenth century, however, the vocation had regained its standing as a profession, not by devices consistent with a free market but through government intervention to restrict entry into practice. It thus became a profession only in the sense that medieval guilds of physicians were professions.

This is not to suggest that medicine would have continued to remain a trade without being granted a host of government privileges. Indeed, there is every indication that it would have earned its standing as a profession in the free-market designation of the term — that is, as an occupation requiring a substantial amount of specialized knowledge and intensive formal training — by the 1920s, even in the absence of legislative protection. By the end of the first quarter of this century, medical therapeutics had begun to play a major role in reducing the mortality rates from both infectious diseases and, to an even greater extent, from conditions not attributable to micro-organisms.[335] Certainly since the end of World War II, the decline in mortality and morbidity rates for a whole range of diseases can, with justification, be ascribed to medical measures.

It should not be assumed, however, that because medicine was destined to become a profession, it was thereby bound to become a licensed one, with the power to impose entry requirements and to prohibit all those not meeting these requirements from offering their services to the public. There are, after all, unlicensed professions: the clergy, university teaching, pharmacological research, and so on. It is unfortunate that we have become so used to linking the notion of a profession with the powers of a government-enforced cartel that we tend to regard professions whose members are not possessed of these powers as only quasi-professionals or technicians. The truth is that they are as much professionals as are doctors or lawyers, without having their callings protected by intricate systems of licensure.

I point this out in order to show that medicine as a vocation would have eventually transmuted itself from a trade into a profession even in the absence of government prerogatives. But the prestige attached to being a member of a profession was neither the sole nor even the primary, goal of physicians. What an unlicensed profession could *not* bring doctors was the higher incomes that they were able to achieve by virtue of restricting the number of future practitioners with whom they had to compete. Beyond this simple restriction of supply, physicians sought and obtained the power to raise the costs of entry into medical practice above what it was for incumbent practitioners, thus permitting those physicians already licensed to collect what economists call "quasi-rents" on their own less costly professional training. And, because of the nature of this device, the pressure to continue raising the standards (and costs) of entry never really ceases,[336] even after the structural arrangements by which physicians are licensed are finally in place.

This monograph has attempted to trace the history of physicians' efforts to establish a monopoly in the area of medical practice. That they eventually were successful in their endeavors there can be no doubt. By the beginning of the twentieth century, they had effectively restricted the number of prospective practitioners entering the market, substantially expanded the definition of medical practice, thereby prohibiting to non-physicians a host of activities that previously had been permitted them, and raised the code of ethics of the profession— which had as a primary aim the elimination of price competition among licensed practitioners—to the status of law.[337] The evidence that these practices work to the disadvantage of consumers of medical services while at the same time benefiting physicians is decisive.

Given the findings of economics respecting the effects of licensing, and in light of the historical evidence here presented, the following conclusions drawn by a leading student of the medical profession in Canada are, at best, superficial. "In its policies," he writes,

> the profession has tended to live up to "the public expectations in such matters as ethical standards and dedication to improving the lot of men." In short, although few probably would go all the way with the 1934 statement of the C.M.A.'s Committee on Economics ... that "what is best for the medical profession must be best for the public," most must obviously believe that the point at which the medical interest and the public interest begin to diverge is farther along the scale than in the case of most other interest groups.[338]

Alas, the point at which the interests of the profession and those of the public diverged began some two hundred years ago and this divergence has widened to such a degree that only the most radical alterations in the nation's licensing laws will bring the two together again.

Statistical Appendix

The following tables present data relevant to various aspects of this study.

Tables A.1 and A.2 are self-explanatory. Of the two sets of figures on the number of physicians in the various provinces, those obtained from medical directories, and presented in table A.1, are almost certainly more reliable for the period before World War II, since they refer to doctors in active practice during the year in question. Census data before 1941, on the other hand, do not appear to exclude retired or semi-retired practitioners from their totals.

Table A.3 offers a statistical comparison of the physician-population ratios in the United States and Canada and provides some insight into the effects of medical licensing on the number of practitioners in Canada. Effective licensing legislation was not enacted in the United States until the last decade of the nineteenth century but these laws were not instrumental in severely curtailing the number of physicians entering the profession until after the release of the Flexner report on medical education in 1910. Between 1906 and 1918, the number of medical schools in the United States dropped from 162 to 90 and the number of graduates in medicine, from almost 5,400 to less than 2,700. These data are reflected in the precipitate rise in the ratio of population to each physician between 1901 and 1921. In Canada, on the other hand, effective restrictions on entry were in place in all the provinces by 1891 and, as a consequence, the ratio of physicians to the population remained close to constant, at about 1:1,000, for the next half-century. Indeed, as late as 1970, Ontario, with the largest number of active physicians per population, had still not caught up with the physician-population ratio prevailing throughout the United States in 1890.

Tables A.4 and A.5 summarize the statistics on medical education in Canada from the end of the nineteenth century. Unfortunately, no accessible data exist for the 1890s, but it is likely that the number of students and graduates showed little variation during this period. Enrollment in Canada's medical schools was held fairly constant at below 1,800 prior to the final years of World War I and, except for a surge between 1920 and 1923, most likely in response to the War, did not rise above 3,000 until after World War II. Enrollment did not reach the 4,000 level until 1965. The number of graduates in medicine reflects similar trends. Because of the small numbers involved, a three-year average of medical graduates is a better indication of long-run changes than are annual figures, which tend to show broad fluctuations. If these three-year averages are plotted against the population base, as in table A.5, it becomes clear that there was a sharp decline in the number of M.D.s produced by the Dominion's medical schools between the late 1880s and the end of the First World War. Outside of the aberration of the 1924–1926 period, the medical graduates-to-population ratio remained fairly constant at below 5 per 100,000 until after World War II, and did not return to its 1888–1890 levels until the late 1970s.

One further note. There is strong evidence suggesting that the size of the entering class and, consequently, the number of graduates emerging from Canada's medical schools, was not simply a reflection of the limited number of qualified applicants attempting to gain admission to the profession. MacFarlane's claim that "there was little restriction in numbers of students in any of the medical faculties of Canada until the latter years of World War II," [1] has no foundation in fact. Consider the following data for the period 1927 through 1930:

Canadian Medical Schools	1927[a]	1928[b]	1929[c]	1930[d]
Number of applicants matriculating for the first time:	434	390	362	395
Meeting all standards for admission, but refused admission because class full:	203	133	385	218
Credentials not examined, but unofficial statements indicate applicant met all requirements of the Association of American Medical Colleges:		71	24	111

Multiple applications screened out.

(a) Does not include the University of Montreal or Laval University.
(b) Does not include the University of Manitoba.
(c) Does not include Queen's University, Laval University, or the University of Manitoba.
(d) Does not include Queen's University, Laval University, the University of Montreal, or the University of Alberta.

Source: Burton D. Myers, "Report on Applications for Matriculation in Schools of Medicine of the United States and Canada, 1929–1930," *Journal of the Association of American Medical Colleges*, V (March, 1930): 65–89.

There appears to be no question that constraints on the number of medical graduates entering the profession were in part the result of limited educational facilities and were not due to a lack of qualified students who wished to become physicians.

Tables A.6 and A.7 are based on the seminal work of Dr. Thomas McKeown[2] and indicate that the dramatic decline in mortality in Canada between 1871 and 1921 cannot be attributed to advances made in medical treatment or prophylaxis. Before the introduction of the sulfonamides in 1935, clinical medicine was incapable of either effectively preventing or treating most conditions attributable to micro-organisms, especially the leading causes of death, tuberculosis and respiratory and diarrhoeal infections. Yet these diseases accounted for almost 40 percent of the decline in Canada's death rate during the half-century covered. Indeed, the fall in mortality between 1871 and 1921 was almost totally due to a reduction in deaths from infectious causes for which no immunization or medical therapy existed. There is no evidence to support the claim often made by physicians that advances in medical therapeutics accounted for the decline in mortality during this period. The most likely factors responsible for the substantial drop in the death rate during the fifty years following 1871 involve improvements in sanitary conditions, personal hygiene, and nutrition, and the reduced exposure to micro-organisms brought about by these improvements.

Tables A.8, A.9, and A.10 are concerned with physicians' incomes and a comparison of these incomes with those of other non-salaried professionals. Unfortunately, income statistics are not available prior to 1946, and even these figures are of less utility than would data on median incomes have been. There are greater problems respecting the incomes of other professionals, since it is difficult to determine what percentage of active lawyers, accountants, engineers, and architects, are self-employed. Available income figures do, however, indicate that physicians have consistently earned more than a weighted average of other self-employed professionals. This differential reached its lowest point in 1949, when it was less than 9 percent, to a high of over 61 percent in 1971, after the introduction of national health insurance. Indeed, if anything is indicated by these data, it is that the imposition of a mandatory health-care system covering physicians' services represented the single largest boost to doctors' incomes since the end of World War II. Between 1966 and 1971, physicians' incomes increased by over 58 percent, while the consumer price index rose by less than 20 percent. The data also give credence to the claim that doctors' incomes have not kept pace with their 1971 levels, dropping to approximately 116 percent to the weighted average of other professionals' incomes by 1975. Indeed, leaving aside the effects of tax-indexing, to have remained at 1971 levels in constant dollars, the mean net income of physicians would have had to have risen to over $93,700 in 1981, or 37 percent higher than shown. By 1981, doctors' real incomes had dropped back to their 1965 levels, while the real incomes of dentists had increased by about 35 percent during the same period.

Table A.11 presents data on the median salaries of selected full-time university teachers. Since university teaching is an unlicensed profession, the effects of medical licensure appear especially dramatic when the incomes of self-employed physicians are compared to those of full professors and holders of doctorates teaching at Canadian universities. It is unfortunate that no figures on the median incomes of physicians are available; it is not unlikely that the mean incomes of self-employed medical practitioners tend to be somewhat biased downward, inasmuch as the incomes of semi-retired physicians are included in the averages shown. In addition, income data for physicians refer to the calendar year that ends mid-way through the academic year for which university teachers' salaries are presented. However, despite these factors that might tend to lessen the differences in incomes between the two groups, table A.11 shows that self-employed physicians consistently earned approximately twice as much as Ph.D.s teaching full-time at Canadian colleges and universities and that doctors' incomes were about 50 percent higher than were the salaries of full professors.

TABLE A.1

NUMBER OF PHYSICIANS AND RATIO OF PHYSICIANS TO POPULATION, BY PROVINCE, 1902 TO 1958, MEDICAL DIRECTORIES

Year	Alberta		British Columbia		Manitoba		New Brunswick		Nova Scotia		Ontario	
	Number	Ratio	Number	Ratio	Number	Ratio	Number	Ratio	Number	Ratio	Number	Ratio
1902	*		183	1:1056	217	1:1248	237	1:1406	398	1:1163	2,257	1: 982
1904	*		176	1:1285	226	1:1349	261	1:1292	427	1:1099	2,257	1:1011
1906	156		209	1:1267	298	1:1152	235	1:1543	450	1:1057	2,653	1: 885
1909	264		297	1:1129	401	1:1022	260	1:1337	434	1:1119	2,700	1: 922
1912	384	1:1020	452	1: 894	426	1:1114	258	1:1377	439	1:1128	2,864	1: 896
1914	429	1: 999	547	1: 783	444	1:1130	256	1:1415	433	1:1158	2,911	1: 907
1916	449	1:1045	537	1: 845	463	1:1146	257	1:1438	446	1:1139	3,032	1: 898
1918	475	1:1082	505	1: 952	465	1:1207	249	1:1513	443	1:1161	3,192	1: 898
1921	474	1:1241	492	1:1066	467	1:1306	258	1:1503	512	1:1023	3,124	1: 939
1923	530	1:1119	561	1: 989	497	1:1245	265	1:1468	452	1:1146	3,594	1: 838
1925	562	1:1071	610	1: 964	524	1:1206	271	1:1450	457	1:1127	3,839	1: 810
1927	547	1:1157	641	1: 972	532	1:1224	268	1:1485	449	1:1147	3,852	1: 836
1929	585	1:1169	671	1: 982	573	1:1182	262	1:1542	464	1:1110	3,959	1: 842
1931	588	1:1244	720	1: 964	601	1:1165	275	1:1484	436	1:1176	4,028	1: 852
1934	620	1:1223	775	1: 938	638	1:1111	290	1:1459	463	1:1147	4,436	1: 799
1936	623	1:1240	808	1: 922	650	1:1094	286	1:1514	476	1:1141	4,573	1: 788
1938	627	1:1246	883	1: 878	661	1:1089	297	1:1488	490	1:1133	4,682	1: 784
1940	629	1:1256	930	1: 866	670	1:1087	296	1:1527	497	1:1145	4,836	1: 775
1942	673	1:1153	1,015	1: 857	722	1:1003	307	1:1511	529	1:1117	5,086	1: 764
1950	852	1:1074	1,454	1: 782	803	1: 956	353	1:1450	582	1:1096	5,580	1: 801
1956	1,074	1:1046	1,901	1: 736	878	1: 968	390	1:1422	605	1:1148	6,458	1: 837
1958	1,175	1:1026	2,087	1: 737	914	1: 957	408	1:1400	644	1:1101	7,046	1: 826

TABLE A.1 — Continued

NUMBER OF PHYSICIANS AND RATIO OF PHYSICIANS TO POPULATION, BY PROVINCE, 1902 TO 1958, MEDICAL DIRECTORIES

Year	Prince Edward Island Number	Prince Edward Island Ratio	Quebec Number	Quebec Ratio	Saskatchewan Number	Saskatchewan Ratio	Territories Number	Territories Ratio	CANADA** Number	CANADA** Ratio	Newfoundland Number	Newfoundland Ratio
1902	82	1:1247	1,382	1:1217	*		125		4,881	1:1133	67	1:3328
1904	73	1:1374	1,490	1:1174	*		161		5,071	1:1157	86	1:2642
1906	76	1:1294	1,635	1:1112	185		30		5,927	1:1050	79	1:2931
1909	77	1:1241	2,000	1: 964	299		21		6,753	1:1006		
1912	76	1:1226	1,912	1:1066	373	1:1378	6	1:2454	7,190	1:1022	97	1:2522
1914	79	1:1167	1,940	1:1086	427	1:1312	6	1:2358	7,472	1:1024	105	1:2367
1916	74	1:1232	1,859	1:1170	489	1:1249	6	1:2265	7,612	1:1045	95	1:2659
1918	71	1:1269	1,984	1:1133	480	1:1387	6	1:2177	7,870	1:1052	93	1:2761
1921	68	1:1303	1,968	1:1199	474	1:1598	6	1:2050	7,843	1:1120	93	1:2828
1923	67	1:1299	1,945	1:1258	520	1:1496	4	1:3000	8,435	1:1068	95	1:2807
1925	72	1:1194	2,274	1:1121	512	1:1572	5	1:2400	9,126	1:1018	96	1:2816
1927	71	1:1225	2,430	1:1093	505	1:1665	4	1:3250	9,299	1:1036	107	1:2562
1929	63	1:1397	2,605	1:1064	557	1:1585	9	1:1444	9,748	1:1029	114	1:2438
1931	63	1:1397	2,764	1:1040	577	1:1598	7	1:1935	10,059	1:1032	117	1:2408
1934	65	1:1400	2,916	1:1034	595	1:1560	9	1:1556	10,807	1: 994	113	1:2445
1936	71	1:1310	3,053	1:1015	618	1:1507	10	1:1600	11,168	1: 980	114	1:2567
1938	74	1:1270	3,151	1:1010	612	1:1493	12	1:1333	11,489	1: 971	107	1:2793
1940	72	1:1319	3,267	1:1003	611	1:1473	13	1:1308	11,821	1: 963	120	1:2556
1942	79	1:1139	3,382	1:1002	647	1:1311	11	1:1545	12,421	1: 938	111	1:2837
1950	77	1:1247	4,102	1: 968	645	1:1291	18	1:1333	14,596	1: 939	133	1:2639
1956	86	1:1155	4,735	1: 977	760	1:1159	11	1:2864	17,906	1: 954	198	1:2096
1958	87	1:1149	5,091	1: 963	803	1:1110	12	1:2750	19,355	1: 882	213	1:2028

Notes: * Included in North-West Territories.

** Canadian totals exclude physicians in Newfoundland until 1950. Full-time Dominion government physicians included in Canadian total for 1956 and 1958, but not in provincial totals, as in prior years. They numbered 810 in 1956 and 875 in 1958.

Sources: 1902 and 1904: *The Standard Medical Directory of North America* (Chicago: G. P. Engelhard & Co., 1902 and 1904).

1906 to 1958: *American Medical Directory* (Chicago: American Medical Association), various years.

Population figures are from census data. Intercensal estimates from 1902 to 1918 assume constant rates of change between 1901 and 1911 and 1911 and 1921.

TABLE A.2

NUMBER OF PHYSICIANS AND RATIO OF PHYSICIANS TO POPULATION, BY PROVINCE, 1871 TO 1980, CANADIAN GOVERNMENT DATA*

Year	Alberta		British Columbia		Manitoba		New Brunswick		Newfoundland		Nova Scotia	
	Number	Ratio	Number	Ratio	Number	Ratio	Number	Ratio	Number	Ratio	Number	Ratio
1871			31	1:1595	41	1:1519	185	1:1544			262	1:1480
1881			114	1: 861	113	1:1350	230	1:1397			289	1:1524
1891							238	1:1350			353	1:1276
1901												
1911	369	1:1014	416	1: 945	433	1:1065	281	1:1253			408	1:1206
1921	548	1:1073	609	1: 862	557	1:1095	268	1:1448			457	1:1147
1931	583	1:1256	729	1: 952	666	1:1051	269	1:1517			445	1:1153
1941	603	1:1320	810	1:1010	659	1:1108	270	1:1693			428	1:1350
1947	719	1:1147	1,097	1: 952	754	1: 980	298	1:1638			483	1:1273
1948	758	1:1127	1,188	1: 911	745	1:1001	334	1:1491			516	1:1211
1949	788	1:1123	1,264	1: 881	723	1:1047	350	1:1451	141	1:2447	542	1:1161
1951	840	1:1118	1,375	1: 847	838	1: 926	357	1:1445	143	1:2424	588	1:1094
1961	1,356	1: 982	2,150	1: 758	1,120	1: 823	455	1:1314	230	1:1991	706	1:1044
1968	1,994	1: 775	3,032	1: 673	1,336	1: 730	596	1:1052	379	1:1348	994	1: 776
1969	2,129	1: 742	3,242	1: 650	1,353	1: 724	577	1:1083	428	1:1206	971	1: 802
1970	2,256	1: 716	3,471	1: 625	1,401	1: 702	568	1:1109	466	1:1114	1,032	1: 761
1971	2,384	1: 690	3,624	1: 614	1,533	1: 645	609	1:1048	479	1:1101	1,081	1: 733
1972	2,444	1: 686	3,850	1: 592	1,573	1: 631	656	1: 981	504	1:1060	1,147	1: 699
1973	2,526	1: 677	4,004	1: 587	1,597	1: 627	677	1: 962	605	1: 892	1,301	1: 622
1974	2,662	1: 660	4,151	1: 583	1,629	1: 620	726	1: 910	660	1: 828	1,320	1: 619
1975	2,737	1: 663	4,328	1: 568	1,732	1: 588	741	1: 909	732	1: 758	1,388	1: 595
1976	2,911	1: 644	4,470	1: 555	1,769	1: 580	773	1: 885	779	1: 721	1,404	1: 594
1977	3,014	1: 640	4,684	1: 538	1,811	1: 569	781	1: 887	803	1: 707	1,478	1: 568
1978	3,167	1: 627	4,837	1: 528	1,841	1: 559	786	1: 890	809	1: 708	1,539	1: 549
1979	3,241	1: 634	5,011	1: 522	1,839	1: 559	767	1: 920	822	1: 702	1,572	1: 541
1980	3,406	1: 627	5,265	1: 511	1,878	1: 547	786	1: 903	866	1: 674	1,588	1: 539

TABLE A.2 — Continued

NUMBER OF PHYSICIANS AND RATIO OF PHYSICIANS TO POPULATION, BY PROVINCE, 1871 TO 1980, CANADIAN GOVERNMENT DATA*

Year	Ontario Number	Ontario Ratio	Prince Edward Island Number	Prince Edward Island Ratio	Quebec Number	Quebec Ratio	Saskatchewan Number	Saskatchewan Ratio	Territories Number	Territories Ratio	CANADA** Number	CANADA** Ratio
1871	1,565	1:1036	63	1:1728	780	1:1528					2,792	1:1248
1881	1,778	1:1084	90	1:1212	1,065	1:1276			10	1:5645	3,507	1:1233
1891	2,266	1: 933			1,220	1:1220			54	1:1833	4,448	1:1087
1901											5,442	1: 987
1911	3,053	1: 828	72	1:1306	2,000	1:1003	379	1:1298			7,411	1: 970
1921	3,459	1: 848	68	1:1309	2,216	1:1065	524	1:1445			8,706	1:1008
1931	3,934	1: 872	63	1:1397	2,747	1:1046	584	1:1579			10,020	1:1034
1941	4,197	1: 903	67	1:1418	3,162	1:1054	527	1:1700			10,723	1:1072
1947	5,138	1: 813	69	1:1362	3,580	1:1036	586	1:1427			13,098	1: 958
1948	5,025	1: 851	70	1:1329	3,723	1:1017	619	1:1354	17	1:1412	13,259	1: 967
1949	5,058	1: 866	75	1:1253	3,850	1:1008	600	1:1387	17	1:1412	13,726	1: 980
1951	5,363	1: 857	73	1:1342	4,097	1: 990	651	1:1278	18	1:1394	14,343	1: 977
1961	8,040	1: 776	91	1:1149	6,167	1: 853	951	1: 973	24	1:1542	21,290	1: 857
1968	10,239	1: 717	92	1:1207	8,428	1: 707	1,086	1: 883	29	1:1552	28,209	1: 740
1969	11,200	1: 669	94	1:1170	8,499	1: 706	1,129	1: 840	34	1:1382	29,659	1: 714
1970	11,851	1: 646	97	1:1144	8,831	1: 681	1,152	1: 805	41	1:1220	31,166	1: 689
1971	12,506	1: 621	98	1:1145	9,455	1: 639	1,128	1: 813	45	1:1182	32,942	1: 659
1972	13,364	1: 589	105	1:1082	9,677	1: 627	1,140	1: 795	47	1:1209	34,508	1: 636
1973	13,723	1: 583	105	1:1091	10,149	1: 601	1,186	1: 759	47	1:1274	35,923	1: 619
1974	14,125	1: 575	114	1:1023	10,603	1: 581	1,251	1: 721	55	1:1093	37,297	1: 605
1975	15,121	1: 544	120	1: 983	10,846	1: 573	1,305	1: 702	53	1:1179	39,104	1: 585
1976	15,251	1: 545	140	1: 854	11,262	1: 556	1,315	1: 708	55	1:1171	40,130	1: 577
1977	15,692	1: 536	141	1: 862	11,545	1: 543	1,390	1: 679	59	1:1098	41,398	1: 565
1978	16,033	1: 529	147	1: 832	11,606	1: 542	1,404	1: 678	69	1: 954	42,238	1: 559
1979	16,309	1: 524	153	1: 810	11,981	1: 526	1,433	1: 674	64	1:1016	43,192	1: 552
1980	16,664	1: 516	152	1: 816	12,160	1: 520	1,442	1: 677	68	1: 946	44,275	1: 544

Notes:
* After 1941, active civilian physicians only. Data from 1947 to 1980 include interns and residents. *Territories* refers to both the Yukon and the Northwest Territories. 1871 figures include New Brunswick, Nova Scotia, Ontario, and Quebec only. Totals for 1911 figures do not include 1,150 physicians serving in the armed forces. Number of practitioners listed occasionally total more than provincial figures because of the inclusion of physicians thought to be in Canada but for whom no exact location was determined. These are: 1947: 374; 1948: 264; 1949: 318; 1968: 4; 1969: 3; 1972: 1; 1973: 3; 1975: 1; 1976: 1.

** 1871 through 1941, 1951, 1961: Canadian census data. 1947, 1948, and 1949: Research Division, Department of National Health and Welfare, *Survey of Physicians in Canada, June, 1951* [Memorandum No. 2 (Ottawa: Department of National Health and Welfare, 1951)]: 9. 1968 through 1978: Health Information Division, National Health and Welfare, *Canada Health Manpower Inventory, 1979* (Ottawa: National Health and Welfare, 1980): 181–182. 1979, 1980: Health Information Division: National Health and Welfare, *Canada Health Manpower Inventory, 1981* (Ottawa: National Health and Welfare, 1982): 185–186.

Sources:

TABLE A.3

RATIO OF PHYSICIANS TO POPULATION, COMPARATIVE
CANADIAN-UNITED STATES RATES, 1871 TO 1980*

Population per Physician

Year	Canada	United States
1871	1,248	667[a]
1881	1,233	614[b]
1891	1,087	629[c]
1901	987	637[d]
1911	970	685[e]
1921	1,008	746
1931	1,034	793
1941	969[f]	754[g]
1949	980	741
1951	977	751
1952	968	755
1953	960	757
1954	955	758
1955	934	758
1956	928	758
1957	920	756
1958	905	752
1959	893	748
1962	799	756
1963	786	727
1964	791	718
1965	771	700
1966	754	697
1967	740	686
1968	740	674
1969	714	664
1970	689	658
1971	659	643
1972	636	626
1973	619	622
1974	605	604
1975	585	583
1976	577	568
1977	565	568
1978	559	544
1979	552	527
1980	544	514

272

TABLE A.3 — Continued

RATIO OF PHYSICIANS TO POPULATION, COMPARATIVE
CANADIAN-UNITED STATES RATES, 1871 TO 1980*

Notes: * Data for the period 1962 to 1980 refer to active civilian physicians only. Active civilian physicians are defined as all civilian physicians, including interns and residents, whether or not in private practice, and whether or not involved in direct patient care, neither living abroad nor retired. Doctors of osteopathy are not included in American totals. Had they been included, the ratio of physicians to the population in the United States would be: 1965: 669; 1970: 629; 1971: 615; 1972: 599; 1973: 596; 1974: 580; 1975: 559; 1976: 549; 1977: 544; 1978: 522; 1979: 505; 1980: 493.

(a) 1870 figures; (b) 1880 figures; (c) 1890 figures; (d) 1900 figures; (e) 1910 figures; (f) physician total includes members of the Canadian armed forces; (g) 1942 figures.

Sources: Canadian data, 1871 through 1951, 1961, and 1968 through 1980: Table A.2. 1952 through 1960: Stanislaw Judek, *Medical Manpower in Canada* [Royal Commission on Health Services (Ottawa: Queen's Printer, 1964)]: 26. 1962, 1963: Health Manpower Planning Division, Health and Welfare Canada, *Canada Health Manpower Inventory, 1972* (Ottawa: Health and Welfare Canada, 1972): 63, 64. 1964 through 1967: Health Manpower Directorate, Health and Welfare Canada, *Canada Health Manpower Inventory, 1974* (Ottawa: Health and Welfare Canada, 1974): 115.

American data, 1870 through 1959: Bureau of the Census, *Historical Statistics of the United States* (2 vols.; Washington: Government Printing Office, 1975), II: 75-76 [Series B 275-290]. 1962 through 1980: Bureau of the Census, *Statistical Abstract of the United States* (Washington: Government Printing Office), various issues.

TABLE A.4

MEDICAL SCHOOLS, STUDENTS, GRADUATES, AND
POPULATION PER MEDICAL STUDENT,
1888 TO 1890 AND 1909 TO 1982

Year	Schools	Students	Graduates	Population per Student
1888	13	1,423	319	3,287
1889	13	1,431	277	3,305
1890	13	1,564	351	3,056
1909	8	1,755	327	3,875
1910	8	1,744	308	4,007
1911	8	1,532	342	4,704
1912	8	1,604	263	4,607
1913	8	1,735	305	4,399
1914	8	1,792	321	4,397
1915	8	1,754	318	4,550
1916	8	1,614	206	4,957
1917	8	1,656	315	4,867
1918	8	1,722	270	4,732
1919	8	2,236	296	3,717
1920	8	2,963	251	2,888
1921	8	3,275	406	2,683
1922	8	3,238	434	2,755
1923	8	3,061	492	2,943
1924	8	2,672	645	3,422
1925	9	2,536	473	3,665
1926	9	2,566	517	3,683
1927	9	2,639	417	3,652
1928	9	2,675	444	3,677
1929	9	2,573	406	3,898
1930	9	2,734	448	3,734
1931	9	2,708	484	3,832
1932	9	2,536	495	4,144
1933	9	2,770	475	3,839
1934	9	2,742	476	3,917
1935	9	2,891	457	3,751
1936	9	2,909	473	3,764
1937	9	2,936	508	3,762
1938	9	2,954	594	3,775
1939	9	2,913	486	3,868
1940	9	2,923	606	3,894
1941	9	2,782	562	4,136
1942	9	2,853	539	4,085
1943	9	2,869	496	4,111
1944	9	2,963	523	3,728
1945	9	2,577	769*	4,685
1946	9	2,926	513	4,201
1947	9	3,365	567	3,730
1948	9	3,527	632	3,636
1949	9	3,233	679	4,159

TABLE A.4 — Continued

**MEDICAL SCHOOLS, STUDENTS, GRADUATES, AND
POPULATION PER MEDICAL STUDENT,
1888 TO 1890 AND 1909 TO 1982**

Year	Schools	Students	Graduates	Population per Student
1950	9	3,278	791	4,183
1951	10	3,489	856	4,015
1952	10	3,458	783	4,181
1953	10	3,444	825	4,310
1954	11	3,643	896	4,196
1955	11	3,589	894	4,374
1956	11	3,651	822	4,405
1957	12	3,655	831	4,544
1958	12	3,686	831	4,634
1959	12	3,668	889	4,766
1960	12	3,552	873	5,031
1961	12	3,678	839	4,959
1962	12	3,677	854	5,054
1963	12	3,758	817	5,038
1964	12	3,809	786	5,065
1965	12	4,057	1,032	4,842
1966	12	4,147	887	4,815
1967	12	4,394	921	4,637
1968	12	4,362	1,017	4,746
1969	12	4,832	1,019	4,346
1970	14	5,103	1,108	4,173
1971	16	5,489	1,133	3,929
1972	16	5,933	1,278	3,675
1973	16	6,450	1,328	3,418
1974	16	6,932	1,567	3,226
1975	16	7,029	1,546	3,229
1976	16	7,285	1,710	3,156
1977	16	7,253	1,688	3,211
1978	16	7,306	1,761	3,209
1979	16	7,309	1,756	3,257
1980	16	7,347	1,743	3,278
1981	16	7,387	1,770	3,295
1982	16	7,435	1,749	3,327

Notes: * Includes two graduating classes at the University of Alberta, Dalhousie University, the University of Western Ontario, and the University of Toronto.

Sources: Number of medical schools, students, and graduates, 1888 to 1890: Illinois State Board of Health, *Medical Education, Medical Colleges and the Regulation of the Practice of Medicine in the United States and Canada, 1765-1891* (Springfield, Ill.: Illinois State Board of Health, 1891): 8-20; 1909 through 1982: annual surveys of medical education in the United States and Canada, *Journal of the American Medical Association,* various issues.

TABLE A.5

GRADUATES OF CANADIAN MEDICAL SCHOOLS
PER 100,000 POPULATION, 1885-1982

Year	Graduates	Population ('000)	Graduates per 100,000 Population	Graduates (Three-year Average)	Graduates per 100,000 Population
1885	202[a]	4,537	4.45		
1886	275[a]	4,580	6.00	249	5.43
1887	269[a]	4,626	5.81		
1888	319	4,678	6.82		
1889	277	4,729	5.86	316	6.68
1890	351	4,779	7.34		
1902	320[b]	5,494	5.82		
1903	427	5,651	7.56	363	6.42
1904	341[c]	5,827	5.85		
1909	327	6,800	4.81		
1910	308	6,988	4.41	326	4.67
1911	343	7,207	4.75		
1912	263	7,389	3.56		
1913	305	7,632	4.00	296	3.88
1914	321	7,879	4.07		
1915	318	7,891	3.98		
1916	206	8,001	2.57	280	3.50
1917	315	8,060	3.91		
1918	270	8,148	3.31		
1919	296	8,311	3.56	272	3.27
1920	251	8,556	2.93		
1921	406	8,788	4.62		
1922	434	8,919	4.87	444	4.98
1923	492	9,010	5.46		
1924	645	9,143	7.05		
1925	473	9,294	5.09	545	5.86
1926	517	9,451	5.47		
1927	417	9,637	4.33		
1928	444	9,835	4.51	422	4.29
1929	406	10,029	4.05		
1930	448	10,208	4.39		
1931	484	10,377	4.66	476	4.59
1932	495	10,510	4.71		
1933	475	10,633	4.47		
1934	476	10,741	4.43	469	4.37
1935	457	10,845	4.21		

TABLE A.5 — Continued

GRADUATES OF CANADIAN MEDICAL SCHOOLS
PER 100,000 POPULATION, 1885-1982

Year	Graduates	Population ('000)	Graduates per 100,000 Population	Graduates (Three-year Average)	Graduates per 100,000 Population
1936	473	10,950	4.32		
1937	508	11,045	4.60	525	4.75
1938	594	11,152	5.33		
1939	486	11,267	4.31		
1940	606	11,381	5.32	551	4.84
1941	562	11,507	4.88		
1942	539	11,654	4.62		
1943	496	11,795	4.21	519	4.40
1944	523	11,946	4.38		
1945	769	12,072	6.37		
1946	513	12,292	4.17	616	5.01
1947	567	12,551	4.52		
1948	632	12,823	4.93		
1949	679	13,447	5.05	701	5.21
1950	791	13,712	5.77		
1951	856	14,009	6.11		
1952	783	14,459	5.42	821	5.68
1953	825	14,845	5.56		
1954	896	15,287	5.86		
1955	894	15,698	5.69	871	5.55
1956	822	16,081	5.11		
1957	831	16,610	5.00		
1958	831	17,080	4.87	850	4.98
1959	889	17,483	5.08		
1960	873	17,870	4.89		
1961	839	18,238	4.60	855	4.69
1962	854	18,583	4.60		
1963	817	18,931	4.32		
1964	786	19,291	4.07	878	4.55
1965	1,032	19,644	5.25		
1966	887	20,015	4.43		
1967	921	20,378	4.52	942	4.62
1968	1,017	20,701	4.91		
1969	1,019	21,001	4.85		
1970	1,108	21,297	5.20	1,087	5.10
1971	1,133	21,568	5.25		

TABLE A.5 — Continued

GRADUATES OF CANADIAN MEDICAL SCHOOLS
PER 100,000 POPULATION, 1885-1982

Year	Graduates	Population ('000)	Graduates per 100,000 Population	Graduates (Three-year Average)	Graduates per 100,000 Population
1972	1,278	21,802	5.86		
1973	1,328	22,043	6.02	1,391	6.31
1974	1,567	22,364	7.01		
1975	1,546	22,697	6.81		
1976	1,710	22,993	7.44	1,648	7.17
1977	1,688	23,291	7.25		
1978	1,761	23,445	7.51		
1979	1,756	23,842	7.37	1,753	7.37
1980	1,743	24,086	7.24		
1981	1,770	24,343	7.27		
1982	1,749	24,739	7.07		

Notes: (a) Graduates of the Toronto School of Medicine through the University of Victoria College estimated at 30 per year.

(b) Including the following estimates: Queen's University: 25; Manitoba Medical College (University of Manitoba): 15; Ecole de Médicine: 45.

(c) Including an estimated 45 graduates from the Ecole de Médicine.

Sources: 1885 through 1890: Illinois State Board of Health, *Medical Education, Medical Colleges, and the Regulation of the Practice of Medicine in the United States and Canada, 1765-1891* (Springfield: Ill.: Illinois State Board of Health, 1891): 8-20; 1904 through 1982: annual surveys of medical education in the United States and Canada, *Journal of the American Medical Association,* various issues.

TABLE A.6

INFECTIOUS DISEASES: DATES OF INTRODUCTION OF SPECIFIC MEASURES OF PROPHYLAXIS OR TREATMENT

Disease	Cause Identified*	First Effective Treatment
Cholera, asiatic	1883: *Vibrio cholerae* isolated by Robert Koch	1930s: Use of intravenous therapy
Diphtheria	1883: *Corynebacterium diphtheriae* isolated by Klebs and Loeffler	1894: Antitoxin developed
Dysentery, bacillary	1898: Identification of the *Bacillus dysenteriae* (*Shigella shigae*) by Kiyoshi Shiga	1930s: Use of intravenous therapy
Influenza	1933: Discovery of type A virus by Laidlaw, Andrews, and Wilson Smith	1938: Introduction of sulfapyridine 1946: Civilian use of antibiotics
Measles (rubeola)	1954: Virus first isolated in the laboratory of John Enders	1935: Treatment by sulfonamides, with questionable results 1963: Use of attenuated vaccines
Meningitis, cerebrospinal	1887: Meningococcus identified by Anton Weichselbaum	1938: Introduction of sulfadiazine 1946: Civilian use of antibiotics
Pneumonia (bacterial)	1886: Pneumococcus identified by Albert Fraenkel	1938: Introduction of sulfapyridine 1946: Civilian use of antibiotics
Poliomyelitis	1949: Poliovirus cultivated by Enders, Robbins, and Weller	1955: Introduction of Salk vaccine
Puerperal fever	1933: Lancefield classifies streptococci by antigenic properties, including those causing puerperal fever	1935: Introduction of sulfonamides 1946: Civilian use of penicillin and other antibiotics
Rubella	1962: Isolation of rubella virus	1969: Introduction of attenuated vaccines
Scarlet fever	1924: Linked to toxin-producing streptococci by Dick and Dick	1935: Introduction of prontosil

TABLE A.6 — Continued

INFECTIOUS DISEASES: DATES OF INTRODUCTION OF SPECIFIC MEASURES OF PROPHYLAXIS OR TREATMENT

Disease	Cause Identified*	First Effective Treatment
Smallpox	1915: Isolation of the vaccinia (cowpox) virus by Noguchi	17th century: Early use of variolation 1798: Protective vaccination with cowpox
Syphilis	1905: *Treponema pallidum* identified by Schaudinn and Hoffmann	1910: Introduction of Salvarsan 1946: Civilian use of penicillin
Tetanus	1884: Discovery of *Clostridium tetani* by Arthur Nicolaier	1890: Tetanus antitoxin developed
Tuberculosis	1882: Tubercle bacillus identified by Robert Koch	1947: Introduction of streptomycin 1954: General use of BCG vaccine
Typhoid fever	1880: Discovery of *Salmonella typhi* (*Bacillus typhosus*) by Carl Eberth	1950: Treatment with chloramphenicol
Typhus fever	1916: Discovery of *Dermacentroxenus rickettsi* by Simeon Wolbach	1950: Treatment with chloramphenicol
Whooping cough	1906: Discovery of *Haemophilus pertussis* by Bordet and Gengou	1938: Treatment with sulfonamides, with questionable effect 1952: Wide use of immunization, with variable protective effect

* Earliest significant date, in cases of diseases having multiple causes.

TABLE A.7

DEATH RATES (PER MILLION) FROM DISEASES ATTRIBUTABLE TO MICRO-ORGANISMS, 1871 AND 1921, CANADA*

Cause	Death Rate 1871	Death Rate 1921	Decline (%)	Decline as Percentage of Decline in Death Rate From All Causes (%)
Tuberculosis (respiratory) [a]	1,613.7	606.4	62.2	
Respiratory infections [b]	1,013.0	1,251.4	23.5 Increase	
Sub-Total: respiratory tuberculosis and other respiratory infections	2,626.7	1,859.8	29.2	25.4
Diarrhoeal infections [c]	981.1	553.8	43.6	14.2
Scarlet fever [d]	456.7	63.9	86.0	
Diphtheria	113.6	202.2	78.0 Increase	
Sub-Total: diphtheria and scarlet fever [e]	611.9	266.1	56.5	11.5
Encephalitis and meningitis [f]	456.4	131.8	68.9	10.8
Typhoid fever [g]	362.6	77.8	78.5	9.4
Measles	222.6	46.3	79.2	5.8
Whooping cough	256.5	97.6	61.9	5.3
Puerperal fever [h]	147.5	29.5	80.0	3.9
Smallpox [i]	55.9	6.4	88.6	1.6
Erysipelas	68.0	27.7	59.3	1.3
Tuberculosis (non-respiratory) [j]	146.0	138.1	5.4	.3
Other [k]	1,086.1	533.4	50.9	18.3
TOTAL	7,021.2	3,768.3	46.3	107.8
Total Death Rate from All Causes	13,573.5	10,556.6	22.2	

* Canadian census data for 1871 include Ontario, Quebec, New Brunswick, and Nova Scotia. 1921 data include the entire Dominion except the Territories and Quebec. Since data have not been standardized for age distribution nor area covered, these figures should be regarded as only suggestive.

TABLE A.7 — Continued

DEATH RATES (PER MILLION) FROM DISEASES ATTRIBUTABLE TO MICRO-ORGANISMS, 1871 AND 1921, CANADA*

Notes on Disease Categories

The extremely primitive state of clinical diagnosis in 1871 is reflected in the census categories for cause of death. For the most part, I have followed the analysis of nineteenth-century classifications employed by Dr. Thomas McKeown [*The Role of Medicine* (2d ed.: Princeton: Princeton University Press, 1979)]. The reader would do well to keep in mind that there is a substantial range of error respecting these data on mortality, and that some non-infectious causes of death are inadvertently incorporated in these totals. On the other hand, there is no question that a considerable number of deaths from infectious causes have not been included. Thus, as McKeown points out, mortality from nephritis was almost certainly classified as deaths from dropsy, as were other diseases of infectious origin, but I have not included any deaths in this category. Nor do deaths from "diseases of the heart and blood," which include rheumatic heart disease, appear in the above table. Finally, almost 27% of all deaths in 1871 are listed as "cause not given." By 1921, the percentage of deaths attributed to non-specified causes had dropped to 3%.

The following classifications and their constituent death rates were aggregated to form table A.7:

(a) *Respiratory tuberculosis:* 1871 classifications: consumption (1,613.4); hemoptysis (.3).

(b) *Respiratory infections:* 1871 classifications: bronchitis (113.3); influenza (15.5); diseases of the lungs (499.5); cold (23.8); pleurisy (67.7); croup (293.2). Doubtless a not insignificant proportion of non-tuberculous infections were misdiagnosed as consumption.
1921 classifications: pneumonia (627.3); bronchopneumonia (302.7); bronchitis (141.1); influenza (146.5); pleurisy (33.8).

(c) *Diarrhoeal infections:* 1871 classifications: diarrhoea (403.9); diseases of the bowels (323.9); infantile cholera (115.0); dysentery (106.7); sporadic cholera (30.7); asiatic cholera (0.9).
1921 classifications: diarrhoea and enteritis (501.6); dysentery (44.0); choleriform enteritis (8.3).

(d) *Scarlet fever:* 1871 classification: scarlatina.

(e) Totals include "diseases of the throat" (41.6), the bulk of which were almost certainly the result either of diphtheria or scarlet fever.

TABLE A.7 — Continued

DEATH RATES (PER MILLION) FROM DISEASES ATTRIBUTABLE TO MICRO-ORGANISMS, 1871 AND 1921, CANADA*

(f) *Encephalitis and meningitis:* 1871 classifications: diseases of the brain (423.2); diseases of the spine (33.3), both of which probably included cases of tertiary syphilis and other infectious diseases.

(g) *Typhoid fever:* including paratyphoid fever.

(h) *Puerperal fever:* 1871 classifications: puerperal fever (14.6); childbirth (132.8).

(i) *Smallpox:* 1871 classification: smallpox (55.1); chickenpox (0.6); vaccinia (0.3).

(j) *Non-respiratory tuberculosis:* 1871 classifications: scrofula (16.4); hydrocephalus (128.5); hydrothorax (1.1).

(k) 1871 classifications: convulsions (under four years old) (165.2), and teething (126.5), both almost certainly the result, as McKeown notes, of infectious diseases such as whooping cough, measles, otitis media, meningitis, pneumonia, gastroenteritis, etc.; inflammation (239.5); fever (425.7); intermittent fever (24.4); remittent fever (26.7); abscess (32.4); thrush (13.8); quinsy (7.5); carbuncle (4.9); parotitis (4.9); yellow fever (5.2); chorea (0.6); phlebitis (0.6); leprosy (1.4); rabies (0.3); tetanus (5.4); syphilis (1.1).

1921 classifications: nephritis (318.2); infantile convulsions (95.7); septicemia (54.4); syphilis (30.6); GPI (13.2); tetanus (5.9); chorea (3.7); gonococcal infection (1.6); typhus (0.8); mumps (3.0); malaria (0.6); military fever (0.8); leprosy (0.6); anthrax (0.6); relapsing fever (0.2); mycoses (0.8); "other" (2.8).

TABLE A.8

MEAN INCOME OF SELF-EMPLOYED PHYSICIANS, 1946-1981

Year	Mean Net Income*	Mean Gross Professional Earnings	Mean Net Professional Earnings**	Mean After-Tax Income***
1946	$ 7,446	$	$ 6,884	$ 5,240
1947	7,666		7,120	5,867
1948	8,274		7,821	6,488
1949	9,009		8,532	7,349
1950	9,881		9,182	7,976
1951	9,975		9,257	7,843
1952	10,522		9,935	8,004
1953	11,258		10,441	8,686
1954	11,891		11,113	9,369
1955	12,166		11,363	9,608
1956	13,053		12,300	10,324
1957	13,978	20,804	12,852	11,073
1958	15,264	22,103	13,778	12,032
1959	15,737	22,910	14,590	12,318
1960	16,323	24,288	15,735	12,610
1961	17,006	25,862	16,472	13,109
1962	18,146	26,322	16,970	13,900
1963	19,433	28,690	18,688	14,685
1964	21,474	30,586	20,484	15,979
1965	23,229	32,799	22,064	17,732
1966	24,993	35,223	23,262	18,892
1967	27,343	38,675	26,093	20,023
1968	29,181	42,783	28,615	20,707
1969	32,338	46,328	30,861	24,716
1970	34,757	50,819	34,360	26,186
1971	39,555	56,824	39,203	29,846
1972	41,195	59,324	39,977	31,070
1973	42,730		40,798	32,493
1974	44,585		41,721	34,024
1975	46,661		43,766	35,878
1976	49,310		46,756	37,924
1977	51,718		49,814	41,443
1978	54,668		52,601	44,010
1979	58,393		56,757	47,248
1980	63,411		60,827	50,346
1981	68,377		66,402	53,980

TABLE A.8 — Continued

MEAN INCOME OF SELF-EMPLOYED PHYSICIANS, 1946-1981

Notes: *Taxable returns only.

** Data for 1946 to 1948, 1950 to 1956, and 1973 to 1981 include net professional income and all wages and salaries earned by physicians the major part of whose incomes is derived from professional fees. Data for 1949 include all earned income. Data for 1957 through 1972 are derived from gross professional earnings from professional fee-practice and from wages incidental to medical practice less tax-deductible professional expenses.

*** Federal income tax only: mean net income less aggregate federal tax payments divided by the number of taxable returns.

Sources: Mean net income and mean after-tax income, 1946 through 1981, and mean net professional income for 1946 to 1956 and 1973 to 1981: Taxation Division, Department of National Revenue, *Taxation Statistics,* annual. Mean net and mean gross professional earnings, 1957 through 1965: Research and Statistics Directorate, Department of National Health and Welfare, *Earnings of Physicians in Canada, 1957-1965* [Health Care Series No. 21 (Ottawa: Department of National Health and Welfare, [1967])]; 1966 through 1972: Health Economics and Statistics Division, Health and Welfare Canada, *Earnings of Physicians in Canada, 1962-1972* (Ottawa: Health and Welfare Canada, [1974]).

TABLE A.9

MEAN NET INCOME OF SELF-EMPLOYED PHYSICIANS AND OTHER SELECTED PROFESSIONS, 1946-1981*

Year	Self-Employed Physicians	Self-Employed Dentists	Self-Employed Lawyers	Self-Employed Engineers and Architects	Self-Employed Accountants
1946	$ 7,466	$ 5,289	$ 6,528	$ 5,984	$
1947	7,666	5,713	7,822	7,452	
1948	8,274	5,395	8,309	7,455	
1949	9,009	5,748	9,533	10,428	
1950	9,881	6,202	9,641	10,955	
1951	9,975	6,287	10,214	9,628	8,171
1952	10,522	7,112	9,222	12,266	8,026
1953	11,258	7,485	9,955	10,258	8,096
1954	11,891	7,896	11,925	12,059	8,672
1955	12,166	8,554	12,243	14,007	9,315
1956	13,053	9,230	12,617	13,640	9,940
1957	13,978	10,234	13,244	14,581	10,879
1958	15,264	10,662	13,163	14,260	10,627
1959	15,737	11,605	14,123	14,982	11,033
1960	16,323	12,238	14,597	15,670	11,446
1961	17,006	12,337	15,718	14,692	11,627
1962	18,146	13,707	15,364	14,545	11,183
1963	19,433	13,679	16,283	14,989	10,994
1964	21,474	14,909	17,282	16,801	13,021
1965	23,229	15,693	19,191	19,278	13,447
1966	24,993	17,212	21,045	21,200	13,946
1967	27,347	18,273	22,014	22,111	14,517

TABLE A.9 — Continued

MEAN NET INCOME OF SELF-EMPLOYED PHYSICIANS AND OTHER SELECTED PROFESSIONS, 1946-1981*

Year	Self-Employed Physicians	Self-Employed Dentists	Self-Employed Lawyers	Self-Employed Engineers and Architects	Self-Employed Accountants
1968	$29,181	$20,164	$23,597	$22,707	$17,002
1969	32,338	21,773	25,884	22,612	18,038
1970	34,757	22,794	26,738	22,385	19,303
1971	39,555	25,828	27,862	21,648	18,631
1972	41,195	28,363	30,603	25,477	20,247
1973	42,730	31,160	36,598	33,751	26,993
1974	44,585	35,525	42,751	34,109	30,734
1975	46,661	40,871	42,731	43,409	34,668
1976	49,310	43,336	44,858	40,626	36,616
1977	51,718	43,918	44,098	36,543	37,741
1978	54,668	47,017	44,499	33,977	39,196
1979	58,393	53,027	47,681	36,861	40,599
1980	63,411	56,977	49,481	41,052	44,592
1981	68,377	62,488	56,445	43,682	42,420

* Taxable returns only.

Source: Taxation Division, Department of National Revenue, *Taxation Statistics*, annual.

TABLE A.10

MEAN NET INCOME OF SELF-EMPLOYED PHYSICIANS AS A PERCENTAGE OF MEAN NET INCOME OF OTHER SELECTED SELF-EMPLOYED PROFESSIONALS, 1946–1981

Year	Dentists (%)	Lawyers (%)	Consulting Engineers and Architects (%)	Accountants (%)	Weighted Average* (%)
1946	141.2	119.3	124.8		124.8
1947	134.2	98.0	102.9		111.1
1948	153.4	99.6	111.0		118.3
1949	156.7	94.5	86.4		108.7
1950	159.3	102.5	90.2		115.3
1951	158.7	97.7	103.6	122.1	115.4
1952	147.9	114.1	85.8	128.8	119.6
1953	150.4	113.1	109.7	139.1	126.3
1954	150.6	99.7	98.6	137.1	117.5
1955	142.2	99.4	86.9	130.6	112.2
1956	141.4	103.5	95.7	131.3	115.6
1957	136.6	105.5	95.6	128.5	114.8
1958	143.2	116.0	107.0	143.6	126.1
1959	135.6	111.4	105.0	142.6	121.5
1960	133.4	111.8	104.2	142.6	121.8
1961	137.8	108.2	115.8	146.3	123.7
1962	132.4	118.1	124.8	162.3	130.5
1963	142.1	119.3	129.6	176.8	136.5
1964	144.0	124.3	127.8	164.9	137.1
1965	148.0	121.0	120.5	172.7	136.9
1966	145.2	118.8	117.9	179.2	135.8
1967	149.7	124.2	123.7	188.4	141.5
1968	144.7	123.7	128.5	171.6	137.8
1969	148.5	124.9	143.0	179.3	142.5
1970	152.5	130.0	155.3	180.1	147.1

TABLE A.10 — Continued

MEAN NET INCOME OF SELF-EMPLOYED PHYSICIANS AS A PERCENTAGE OF MEAN NET INCOME OF OTHER SELECTED SELF-EMPLOYED PROFESSIONALS, 1946-1981

Year	Dentists (%)	Lawyers (%)	Consulting Engineers and Architects (%)	Accountants (%)	Weighted Average* (%)
1971	153.1	142.0	182.7	212.3	161.2
1972	145.2	134.6	161.7	203.5	152.1
1973	137.1	116.8	126.6	158.3	130.7
1974	125.5	104.3	130.7	145.1	120.5
1975	114.2	109.2	107.5	134.6	115.8
1976	113.8	109.9	121.4	134.7	117.4
1977	117.8	117.3	141.5	137.0	123.7
1978	116.3	122.9	160.9	139.5	128.0
1979	110.1	122.5	158.4	143.8	127.1
1980	111.3	128.2	154.5	142.2	129.2
1981	109.4	121.1	156.5	161.2	129.8
1946-1950 Average	149.2	101.1	100.0		115.2
1951-1955 Average	149.5	104.2	95.9	132.0	117.9
1956-1960 Average	137.8	109.8	101.7	137.9	120.1
1961-1965 Average	141.2	118.4	123.6	164.7	133.2
1966-1968 Average	146.5	122.3	123.5	179.3	138.4
1969-1973 Average	146.7	129.0	151.4	184.6	145.9
1974-1976 Average	117.4	107.8	119.0	137.8	117.8
1977-1979 Average	114.5	120.9	153.5	140.2	126.3

Notes: * Based on weighted average of net income from all sources of self-employed dentists, lawyers, consulting engineers, architects, and accountants filing taxable returns. From 1946 through 1950, this average does not include data on accountants.

Source: Taxation Division, Department of National Revenue, *Taxation Statistics*, annual.

TABLE A.11

**MEDIAN SALARIES OF SELECTED FULL-TIME UNIVERSITY TEACHERS,
1946–47 TO 1980–81, AND MEAN NET INCOMES OF SELF-EMPLOYED
PHYSICIANS, 1946 TO 1981**

Year**	Median salaries of full professors, all colleges and universities $	Median salaries of all university teachers holding Ph.D.s, all colleges and universities $	Median salaries of full professors, 19 selected universities* $	Mean net incomes of self-employed physicians $
1946–47			5,100e	7,466
1947–48			5,200e	7,666
1948–49			5,400e	8,274
1949–50			5,500e	9,009
1950–51			5,715	9,881
1951–52			6,336	9,975
1952–53			6,431	10,522
1953–54			7,023	11,258
1954–55			7,250	11,891
1955–56			7,670e	12,166
1956–57	7,973	6,285	8,171	13,053
1957–58	9,051	7,165	9,317	13,978
1958–59	10,019	7,869	10,473	15,264
1959–60	...	...	11,591	15,737
1960–61	12,211	9,025	12,304	16,323
1961–62	...	...	12,619	17,006
1962–63	12,848	9,536	12,972	18,146
1963–64	13,401	9,827	13,457	19,433
1964–65	...	...	14,163	21,474
1965–66	14,600	11,000	14,981	23,229
1966–67	...	...	16,201	24,993
1967–68	17,081	12,614	17,743	27,347
1968–69	18,516	13,481	18,982	29,181
1969–70	19,870	14,461	20,162	32,338
1970–71	21,504	15,535	22,136	34,757
1971–72	22,579	...	23,343	39,555
1972–73	23,950	17,150	24,364	41,195
1973–74	25,200	...	25,833	42,730
1974–75	27,400	...	28,070	44,585
1975–76	31,350	23,600	31,835	46,661
1976–77	34,100	26,050	34,486	49,310
1977–78	36,500	28,350	36,583	51,718
1978–79	39,100	30,550	38,788	54,668
1979–80	41,500	33,050	41,194	58,393
1980–81	44,494	35,358	44,800	63,411
1981–82	49,598	40,193	50,300	68,377

290

TABLE A.11 — Continued

MEDIAN SALARIES OF SELECTED FULL-TIME UNIVERSITY TEACHERS, 1946-47 TO 1980-81, AND MEAN NET INCOMES OF SELF-EMPLOYED PHYSICIANS, 1946 TO 1981

Notes: *Comprising the following institutions: University of British Columbia, University of Alberta, University of Saskatchewan, University of Manitoba, University of Western Ontario, McMaster University, University of Toronto, Victoria University (Toronto), University of Trinity College, Queen's University, McGill University, Bishop's University, University of New Brunswick, Mount Allison University, St. Francis Xavier University, Acadia University, and Dalhousie University. In 1965-66, these seventeen universities were augmented by the University of Calgary and the Ontario Institute for Studies in Education.

**Mean incomes of physicians are those for the calendar year ending in December of the first year shown. The bias, therefore, is to underestimate the incomes of physicians as compared to those of university teachers.

ᵉEstimates made by the Dominion Bureau of Statistics and appearing in Dominion Bureau of Statistics, Education Divison, *Salaries and Qualifications of Teachers in Universities and Colleges, 1957-58* (Ottawa: Queen's Printer, 1958): 32 [Table 3].

Sources: Data on salaries of university teachers to 1970-71: Dominion Bureau of Statistics, Education Division, *Salaries and Qualifications of Teachers in Universities and Colleges* [catalogue no. 81-203], annual; data from 1971-72 to 1981-82: Statistics Canada, Education, Science and Culture Division, *Teachers in Universities* [catalogue no. 81-241], annual.

Data on mean net incomes of physicians: table A.8.

Notes

INTRODUCTION

[1] One of the most recent such studies, a history of the Medical Council of Canada, refers to the profession's agitation for protective legislation in the following terms:

"During the nineteenth century, and even into the early part of the twentieth century, there were repeated references in many provinces to the need to curb the activities of unqualified persons who carried out what was considered to be quackery in their so-called medical practice. It was considered essential to create standards, backed by legislation, which would provide for the public the best possible medical care of the time." Robert B. Kerr, *History of the Medical Council of Canada* (Ottawa: The Medical Council of Canada, 1979): 10.

[2] For one of many instances, see Elizabeth MacNab, *A Legal History of Health Professions in Ontario* (A Study for the Committee on the Healing Arts [Toronto: Queen's Printer, 1970]). In discussing the Ontario Medical Council's vigorous campaign to prohibit drugless practitioners from competing with the membership of the provincial College of Physicians and Surgeons in supplying health services to the public, MacNab writes:

"It seems fair to say that Council members generally felt that the purpose of the College was to protect the public by setting the standard to be met by all those who professed to be able to cure their illnesses, and that they had few selfish motives in seeking to eliminate other healing cults. At any rate it was during this period that they made the most determined attempts to ensure that only College members could practise medicine. When it became clear that this end was impossible, they devoted their efforts to preventing the drugless practitioners (as the new cults came to be called) from either abusing or extending their privileges. As well they were concerned that members of the College should not resort to the devices used by the drugless practitioners nor claim the miraculous 'cures' that they did. The Council upheld these policies even in the face of public opinion." (p. 42). Thus, osteopathy, chiropractic, and naturopathy are classified as "cults," whose practitioners were given to claiming "miraculous cures," and to abusing their right to offer their services to the public, while the regular profession's attempts to crush these competing therapies emerged from a concern "to protect the public."

[3] See, for example, Thomas Moore, "The Purpose of Licensing," *Journal of Law and Economics,* IV (1961): 93–117; and, Elton Rayack, *An Economic Analysis of Occupational Licensure* (unpublished report for the United States Department of Labor, September, 1975). One economist has summed up the effects of professional licensing systems in the following way: "Self-regulation in the professions is indeed self-serving. Its ultimate

aim and realized effect is to increase professionals' incomes beyond the levels that would obtain in perfectly competitive professional-service markets. Self-regulation accomplishes this by restricting entry and information and by various market-division schemes, which enhance the individual professional's ability to engage in price discrimination among income groups and which enhance the profession's prospects for achieving superperfect price discrimination within the more narrowly defined submarkets, both service and geographic." Ira Horowitz, "The Economic Foundations of Self-Regulation in the Professions," in Roger D. Blair and Stephen Rubin, eds., *Regulating the Professions* (Lexington, Mass.: Lexington Books, D.C. Heath and Company, 1980): 16. David A. Dodge, in his study of the relation between occupational licensing and returns to investment in education in Canada, concludes that earnings are higher in licensed occupations than would otherwise be the case since incremental costs of entry are imposed on prospective entrants which, in turn, produce a monopoly return for those who practice the profession. "Occupational Wage Differentials, Occupational Licensing, and Returns to Investment in Education: An Exploratory Analysis," in Silvia Ostry, ed., *Canadian Higher Education in the Seventies* (Ottawa: Economic Council of Canada, 1972): 159.

[4] There is virtual unanimity among economists that this has been true in the United States. See Milton Friedman and Simon Kuznets, *Income from Independent Professional Practice* (New York: National Bureau of Economic Research, 1945); Reuben A. Kessel, "Price Discrimination in Medicine," *Journal of Law and Economics,* I (1958): 20–54; *idem,* "The AMA and the Supply of Physicians," *Law and Contemporary Problems,* XXXV (1970): 267–283; and, Elton Rayack, *Professional Power and American Medicine: The Economics of the American Medical Associaton* (Cleveland: World Publishing Co., 1967). A survey of the more significant literature in the area appears in Frank Sloan and Roger Feldman, "Competition Among Physicians," in Warren Greenberg, ed., *Competition in the Health Care Sector: Past, Present and Future* (Germantown, Md.: Aspen Systems Corporation, 1978): 45–102.

There is little doubt that similar monopoly returns accrue to physicians in Canada. See Dodge, "Occupational Wage Differentials."

[5] In writing of the British guilds, one noted historian observed: "It is very likely that at first the terms of admission were easy.... But, before the middle of the fourteenth century, there are unmistakable traces of the desire to limit competition by diminishing the influx of new-comers.... A century later all pretense of unconsciousness was abandoned, and the members of the crafts frankly avowed that they sought (such) protection." William J. Ashley, *Introduction to English Economic History and Theory* (4th ed.; 2 vols.; New York: G. P. Putnam, 1906), I: 75–77, fn. 2; quoted in J. A. C. Grant, "The Guild Returns to America," *Journal of Politics,* IV (August, 1942): 305.

[6] Dodge, "Occupational Wage Differentials," 145.

[7] *Ibid.* Dodge concludes that "very high social returns are to be gained from improvement of the allocation of human resources by the removal of these restrictions on entry to trades and professions." *Ibid., 159.*

[8] Simon Rottenberg, "The Economics of Occupational Licensing," in *Aspects of Labor Economics* (Princeton, N.J.: National Bureau of Economic Research, Princeton University Press, 1962): 19.

[9] Kessel, "The AMA and the Supply of Physicians," 272-273. A similar point is made by H. E. Frech, "Occupational Licensure and Health Care Productivity: The Issues and the Literature," in John Rafferty, ed., *Health Manpower and Productivity* (Lexington, Mass.: Lexington Books, D. C. Heath and Company, 1974): 121-122.

Sloan and Feldman, among others, contend that licensure in fact reduces the quality of medical care administered to consumers. "Competition Among Physicians," 46.

[10] Stephen J. Kunitz, "Professionalism and Social Control in the Progressive Era: The Case of the Flexner Report," *Social Problems, XXII* (1974): 24; and, Marie Haug, "The Sociological Approach to Self-Regulation," in Roger D. Blair and Stephen Rubin, eds., *Regulating the Professions* (Lexington, Mass.: Lexington Books, D. C. Heath and Company, 1980): 62. Also see, Magali Sarfatti Larson, *The Rise of Professionalism: A Sociological Analysis* (Berkeley: University of California Press, 1977).

The conclusions of one Canadian historian of medicine that in Canada "the process of professionalization ultimately rested on the pressures and expectations of a society increasingly concerned with matters of health" has no foundation in fact. Indeed, both sociological theory and the historical data themselves directly contravene the following observation: "Far from being a group which consciously determined the course of their own development, it is clear that the character of medical practice [in Canada] was largely dependent on external influences." Samuel Shortt, "The New Social History of Medicine: Some Implications for Research," *Archivaria,* No. 10 (Summer, 1980): 12-13.

Shortt similarly misconstrues the process by which medical practice became professionalized in the United States and misplaces the period in which this occurred. "This process of professionalization, well-established by 1870," he writes, "antedated significant interest in or contributions by medical science; rather it represented a series of responses to shifts in the popular perceptions of legitimate sources of health care. The structure of the American medical profession at the end of the nineteenth century, then, reflected demands made by the public with which the practitioners attempted to harmonize their own views of appropriate professional standards of behavior." *Ibid.,* 14. Rather than reacting to forces exogenous to medicine, both American and Canadian physicians were directly responsible for the changes that raised their status to that of a profession, with all the economic and social benefits that followed this shift. The methods used were, of course, identical: enactment of legislation that restricted entry into medical practice. Although it is true that advances in medical therapeutics played no role in professionalizing medicine in either country, the process did not approach success in the United States until well after the turn of the century. The following studies deal extensively with the American experience: James G. Burrow, *AMA: Voice of American Medicine* (Baltimore: The Johns Hopkins University Press, 1963); *idem, Organized Medicine in the Progressive Era: The Move Toward Monopoly* (Baltimore: The Johns Hopkins University Press, 1977); Ronald Hamowy, "The Early Development of Medical Licensing Laws in the United States, 1875-1900," *Journal of Libertarian Studies,* III (1979): 73-119; and, Rayack, *Professional Power and American Medicine.*

11 Haug, "Sociological Approach to Self-Regulation," 63-64.

12 There are, of course, exceptions, the most notable being Charles M. Godfrey's *Medicine for Ontario: A History* (Belleville, Ont.: Mika Publishing Co., 1979). Godfrey's history is not, nor does it pretend to be, a thorough study of the profession in Ontario during the nineteenth century. It does, however, contain much valuable information and data on the history of medical education in the province and recounts the struggle between orthodox and irregular practitioners with a fair measure of objectivity.

13 The following reference to the legal recognition of homeopathic and eclectic practice in Ontario is typical: "Disturbing legislation had been enacted in 1859, in the form of a Bill incorporating a homoeopathic board, with the power to grant licenses to practise physic, surgery and midwifery 'on homoeopathic principles.' This had been the thin edge of a wedge which was soon fully driven in by the cult of eclectics, who before long obtained similar legal recognition." H. E. MacDermot, *History of the Canadian Medical Association* (2 vols.; Toronto: Murray Printing Co., 1935-1958), I:11.

14 Histories of the Canadian profession have, on the whole, been so biased in advancing the profession's public image that they read more like propaganda tracts than historical essays. In addition, these studies tend to be so poorly researched that errors appearing in earlier accounts are often perpetuated by later writers and have eventually taken on the status of incontrovertible fact. In light of these and a host of other failings, it is difficult to share Shortt's sentiment respecting these works that "it is unfair to make demands of past historians from the perspective of present historiographic sophistication." S. E. D. Shortt, "Antiquarians and Amateurs: Reflections on the Writing of Medical History in Canada," in S. E. D. Shortt, ed., *Medicine in Canadian Society: Historical Perspectives* (Montreal: McGill-Queen's University Press, 1981): 6.

15 *Ibid.,* 3.

16 College of Physicians and Surgeons of Ontario, *Brief of the College to the Ontario Committee on the Healing Arts* (Toronto: College of Physicians and Surgeons of Ontario, July, 1967): x.

CHAPTER 1
MEDICAL LICENSING IN CANADA IN THE PERIOD TO 1840

1 Strictly speaking, medical practitioners in New France were not "physicians" but, rather, "surgeons" or, in a few cases, "apothecaries." Surgery had been entirely divorced from and made inferior to medicine in the Middle Ages, and both surgeons and apothecaries, who also attended patients, were nominally subordinate to physicians, although all three had their own guilds. This situation persisted in Europe until the French Revolution finally brought about the equality of physicians and surgeons. Although the distinction remains important in British law until the late nineteenth century, it was never of great significance in Canada and, in this monograph, is disregarded unless otherwise indicated.

For an overview of the history of the medical profession in Europe from its beginnings through the eighteenth century, see Joh. Hermann Baas, *Outlines of the History of Medicine and the Medical Profession,* rev. and trans. H. E. Handerson (New York: J. H. Vail & Co., 1889), *passim.*

2 The bill is quoted in full in John J. Heagerty, *Four Centuries of Medical History in Canada* (2 vols.; Toronto: The Macmillan Company of Canada Ltd., 1928), I:315–316. Heagerty refers to the ordinance as "the code of the medical profession in Canada."

3 *Ibid.,* 315.

4 *Ibid.*

5 When assessing arguments respecting the necessity of protecting the public from poorly trained and comparatively incompetent medical practitioners, the reader would do well to keep in mind the extremely primitive state of orthodox medicine, even at its best, throughout the eighteenth and well into the nineteenth centuries. David M. Vess, in his brief discussion of French medicine before the Revolution, notes that even the most elementary principles of sanitation were unknown, that diagnosis of the most common diseases such as diphtheria, measles, smallpox, and scarlet fever, was faulty, that lice and itches were endemic, that venereal disease was common but syphilis and gonorrhea could not be distinguished, and that physicians routinely prescribed a host of "remedies" comprising large doses of mineral poisons. Finally, bleeding was employed for almost all ailments. *Medical Revolution in France, 1789–1796* (Gainesville, Fla.: University Presses of Florida, 1975): 10–18. There was, in fact, little to choose between the highly educated physician and the "quack" before the end of the nineteenth century.

6 Heagerty, *Four Centuries of Medical History,* I:237.

7 *Ibid.,* 223–224.

8 *Ibid.,* 315.

9 *Ibid.,* 238. Statistics for the year 1655 are perhaps indicative. In that year, the population of New France is estimated to have been approximately 2,000, while there were about ten physicians practicing in the colony. This

provides a startlingly high ratio of one physician to each 200 permanent residents. (For contrast, see footnotes 71 and 135, below; chapter 3, footnote 154; and, tables A.1 and A.2.)

Population data are contained in Warren E. Kalbach and Wayne W. McVey, *The Demographic Bases of Canadian Society* (2d ed.; Toronto: McGraw-Hill Ryerson Ltd., 1979): 21. The physician population is estimated by taking the names of those physicians listed on the Quebec register for the ten years prior to 1655, as shown in Heagerty, *Four Centuries of Medical History,* I:224.

10 The legal and governmental arrangements of Canada after Wolfe's conquest are discussed in W. P. M. Kennedy, *The Constitution of Canada: An Introduction to Its Development and Law* (London: Oxford University Press, 1922): 25–49. It is rare to find a work so unrelievedly adulatory of every governmental depredation either conceived or executed by the British authorities in their conquest and occupation of Quebec. To accept Kennedy's conclusions is to believe—especially after the passage of the Quebec Act of 1774—that the inhabitants of New France were transferred from a state of abject misery into citizens of the New Jerusalem through the intercession of the more despotic elements of the British military and civil administration. Despite this somewhat repellent shortcoming, Kennedy's work is occasionally useful in tracing the evolution of Canada's legal and governmental structure from the earliest colonization of the area through World War I.

11 William Canniff, *The Medical Profession in Upper Canada, 1783–1850* (Toronto: William Briggs, 1894): 12. Canniff notes that a census of those living in the eastern part of Upper Canada in 1784 shows a population of 3,776. *Ibid.,* 12–13.

12 *Ibid.,* 12.

13 Canniff, who, with Heagerty, offers a slavish apologia for every piece of restrictive legislation respecting the medical profession, provides the following account of the profession in Upper Canada before passage of the medical bill of 1788:

"Among the non-combatant refugees there were few, if any, possessing skill in the practice of medicine, and the further the settlements extended from the garrisons, the greater was the want of a physician. At first anyone offering his services as a doctor among the English-speaking people of Canada was able to show some evidence of qualification from the parent country. But after a time, in Upper Canada, there came, now and then, persons from the United States professing to possess medical skill. They came generally, not for attachment to the British flag, but to turn a penny. Sometimes they had a degree of medical education which had been acquired in the United States medical schools; sometimes they knew a little about the use of drugs; but too frequently they only knew how to deceive the people by arrant quackery. This class of doctors, being natives of the United States, managed to make themselves agreeable to the U. E. Loyalist settler, who was also generally a native of America. For many years only a few with qualifications from British colleges settled in Upper Canada, and only in places where there was an aggregation of settlers. As villages were formed and grew into towns, the number of doubtful practitioners increased, and as a natural result of this state of affairs, it became necessary to protect the settlers from imposters." *Ibid.,* 15–16.

¹⁴ 28 Geo. III, c. 8 (Quebec).

¹⁵ It was claimed that the epidemic originated at Mal Baie (Baie St.-Paul), having been imported there by a detachment of Scottish troops. Hence its appellation of Mal de la Baie St.-Paul. Heagerty, *Four Centuries of Medical History,* I:131.

¹⁶ *Ibid.,* 142–143.

¹⁷ Quoted in Heagerty, *ibid.,* 135.

¹⁸ *Ibid.*

¹⁹ Quoted in Heagerty, *ibid.,* 137.

²⁰ Quoted in Heagerty, *ibid.,* 152.

²¹ Heagerty, *ibid.,* 317.

²² 31 Geo. III, c. 31 (1791). The population of Upper Canada at this time is estimated to have been 20,000. Canniff, *Profession in Upper Canada,* 19.

²³ Kennedy, *Constitution of Canada,* 117.

²⁴ Elizabeth MacNab, *A Legal History of Health Professions in Ontario* (A Study for the Committee on the Healing Arts [Toronto: Queen's Printer, 1970]): 4. This study has been consulted frequently in the following discussion of early legislative attempts to enact medical licensing laws in the province. MacNab's history, although extremely valuable in providing the broad outlines of legislation in Ontario, suffers from a number of factual errors respecting the details of specific medical statutes. This has made it necessary to consult the acts themselves, rather than her summaries.

²⁵ *Ibid.,* 4.

²⁶ This act was the first statute passed at the 1795 session of the provincial parliament.

²⁷ 35 Geo. III, c. 1 (Upper Canada).

²⁸ Canniff, *Profession in Upper Canada,* 22.

²⁹ McNab is in error when she writes that female midwives were exempt from the provisions of the act. *Legal History of Health Professions,* 5.

³⁰ At least this is the opinion of Heagerty. *Four Centuries of Medical History,* I:320.

³¹ W. P. M. Kennedy dismisses Gourlay with these words: "Gourlay's history, taken by itself, proves that he was foolish and impulsive, and that he lost excellent opportunities for constructive reform by flying too much in the face of unfavourable conditions and by allowing his pen to conquer his sanity." *Constitution of Canada,* 135.

Gourlay had been indiscreet enough to criticize the huge land reserves set aside for the Crown and the protestant clergy in each township, which continued to remain undeveloped despite colonization in the area. The result was that each settler was isolated from his neighbors by uncleared land and communications and transportation were, at best, exceedingly difficult. Gourlay organized a series of meetings of settlers—the largest of which was at York—to air their grievances and this drew the ire of the authorities, who regarded Gourlay as a fomenter of sedition in the province. Kennedy writes of the treatment accorded him by the government of Upper Canada:

"Gourlay's convention at York 'for the purpose of deliberating upon matters of public concern,' was pronounced 'highly derogatory and repugnant to the spirit of the constitution of this province' and tending 'greatly to disturb the public tranquility'. His supporters were treated to some sound advice on the folly of good citizens endangering the security and the good name of Upper Canada both in the United States and in England by 'lending their countenance to measures so disgraceful'. A statute was passed constituting such meetings unlawful assemblies and making those in any way connected with them guilty of high misdemeanour. Gourlay attacked this bill in the public press. His article was promptly pronounced a gross libel by the assembly and the editor was severely punished. Proceedings were taken against Gourlay under the old Alien Act of 1804. An ignorant and uneducated member of the assembly, Isaac Swayzie, actually swore against common knowledge that Gourlay had not resided in the province for the statutory six months, and that he was a seditious character. It was little wonder, when ordered to leave the province within ten days, that Gourlay ignored the verdict. He was arrested and imprisoned. He established the falsity of the charges against himself on a writ of *habeas corpus* before the chief justice, who, however, refused bail on a technicality. For months he lay in Niagara jail, and when finally he was tried he was no longer capable of self-control. He was condemned on a mere quibble—that he had not left the country when ordered—and sentenced to death without benefit of clergy unless he departed from Upper Canada within twenty-four hours. Gourlay lived to be an old man. His sufferings were pronounced illegal and unconstitutional by the Canadian parliament in 1842." *Ibid.*, 134–135.

From this narrative it is apparent that the civil authorities of Upper Canada did not take kindly to men who behaved foolishly and impulsively by allowing their pens to conquer their sanity!

[32] Quoted in Canniff, *Profession in Upper Canada,* 22.

[33] Canniff, *ibid.,* 24.

[34] *Ibid.,* 24–25, and MacNab, *Legal History of Health Professions,* 5.

[35] 55 Geo. III, c. 10 (Upper Canada).

[36] MacNab, *Legal History of Health Professions,* 5.

[37] Canniff, *Profession in Upper Canada,* 32.

[38] Kalbach and McVey, *Demographic Bases,* 24.

[39] William Perkins Bull, *From Medicine Man to Medical Man* (Toronto: [The Perkins Bull Foundation] George J. McLeod Ltd., 1934): 43.

One historian of Canadian medicine describes the professional life of a physician in Upper Canada in the following terms: "The medical practitioner in Upper Canada had no sinecure. His patients were far apart and often to be reached only after hours of riding or walking along corduroy roads or forest trails. If he had several patients to see, his rounds might keep him away from home for days. There was little driving; progress along the roads was too slow and uncertain. Sometimes he went by water; a method of travelling which might be pleasant enough in summer, but which in spring and autumn was often dangerous and uncomfortable. At least one of these pioneer doctors, in a hurry to reach a patient dangerously ill, is known to have swum his horse across a river when the melting snow had raised its icy waters to flood level. There was always the chance of being lost in the woods, a misadventure that might cost a man his life. In the summer the traveller was tormented in his journeys by mosquitoes and black flies." William Boyman Howell, *Medicine in Canada* (New York: Paul B. Hoeber, Inc., 1933): 91.

[40] Quoted in Canniff, *Profession in Upper Canada,* 35.

[41] Quoted in Canniff, *ibid.,* 29. "Empirics" were practitioners who, for the most part, lacked professional training but had usually undergone an informal apprenticeship to a botanical physician. They confined their practice to prescribing botanical remedies and were often far more knowledgeable in the therapeutic properties of herbs and roots than were regular physicians, who relied heavily on the administration of mineral poisons, and bleeding and blistering. William G. Rothstein, *American Physicians in the Nineteenth Century: From Sects to Science* (Baltimore: The Johns Hopkins University Press, 1972): 35. Orthodox physicians regarded all empirics as quacks and the terms were commonly used interchangeably. Indeed, an orthodox practitioner traveling in Georgia, struck by the "numerous train of empirics" operating there, proposed the following coat of arms: "a coat ornamented with three Ducks heads, and the motto Quack, Quack, Quack." Quoted in Wyndham B. Blanton, *Medicine in Virginia in the Eighteenth Century* (Richmond: Garrett & Massie, Inc., 1931): 209.

[42] Edwin Seaborn, *The March of Medicine in Western Ontario* (Toronto: The Ryerson Press, 1944): 36.

[43] Bull, *From Medicine Man,* 52. This technique of catering to the public's anti-Americanism as a method of garnering support for limiting competition has, of course, been a recurring theme throughout Canadian history and appears as effective a device today as it was 170 years ago.

[44] Quoted in Canniff, *Profession in Upper Canada,* 34–35.

[45] *Ibid.,* 34.

46 The term is Bull's. *From Medicine Man,* 43.

47 59 Geo. III, c. 13 (Upper Canada).

48 Due to administrative difficulties, the act was amended in 1819 to provide for four sittings a year and for the appointment of a permanent secretary to the Board to whom all applications were to be directed [59 Geo. III (2d), c. 2 (Upper Canada)].

49 Canniff, *Profession in Upper Canada,* 39–41. Canniff's work contains session-by-session extracts from the proceedings of the Board to 1850.

50 *Ibid.,* 42–43.

51 *Ibid.,* 43–47.

52 The population of Upper Canada grew from approximately 95,000 in 1811 to over 150,000 in 1824. Kalbach and McVey, *Demographic Bases,* 24.

53 Bull, *From Medicine Man,* 46. Bull writes of the Board's early years, "exulting in its prerogatives, the Medical Board dealt almost ruthlessly with applicants seeking the right to minister to suffering humanity. It set its own standards, and took no cognizance of beribboned parchments flourished by aspiring candidates. It resolved 'that in every case the examination of a candidate shall be rigidly entered upon and pursued, let his testimonials be of whatever nature they may.'" *Ibid.,* 44.

54 Canniff, *Profession in Upper Canada,* 52.

55 *Ibid.,* 47–53.

56 8 Geo. IV, c. 63 (Upper Canada).

57 Canniff, *Profession in Upper Canada,* 59.

58 *Ibid.*

59 *Ibid.,* 60.

60 *Ibid.*

61 *Ibid.,* 62.

62 *Ibid.,* 61, 63, 75, 76, 77–78, 85. It should perhaps be pointed out that, by the beginning of the nineteenth century, no medical text or reference work used by any medical faculty in either the United States or Great Britain was unavailable in English. Mastery of Latin or Greek would have added nothing to the competence of a physician, either in his capacity as a diagnostician or as a therapist. Indeed, in Great Britain, to the extent that a knowledge of Latin was a qualification for being awarded the title of physician after the beginning of the eighteenth century, this knowledge was solely indicative of the requirement that one's educational background had reached a certain level of scholarship, and in no sense constituted a test of one's medical knowledge or expertise. A classical education, of course, was not an aspect of the training needed to qualify for membership in the Royal College of Surgeons. Nor were apothecaries, who, at the beginning of the nineteenth century, most closely approximated what later became general practitioners, required to know Latin except to the extent that they

were capable of readily dealing with physicians' prescriptions. For a detailed discussion of medical education in Great Britain over the course of the nineteenth century, see Charles Newman, *The Evolution of Medical Education in the Nineteenth Century* (London: Oxford University Press, 1957), and F. N. L. Poynter, ed., *The Evolution of Medical Education in Britain* (London: Pitman Medical Publishing Co. Ltd., 1966).

In the United States the requirement of a liberal academic background — including the requisite knowledge of Latin — preparatory to the study of medicine had effectively disappeared by the beginning of the nineteenth century at even the best schools. The history of American medical education is covered in Martin Kaufman, *American Medical Education: The Formative Years, 1765-1910* (Westport, Conn.: Greenwood Press, 1976), and Ronald L. Numbers, ed. *The Education of American Physicians: Historical Essays* (Berkeley: University of California Press, 1980). See also the essays on England, Scotland, and the United States in C. D. O'Malley, ed. *The History of Medical Education* (An International Symposium held February 5-9, 1968) (Berkeley: University of California Press, 1970).

The transmutation of medical education during the early part of the nineteenth century from what was primarily a philosophical discipline, in which physicians were steeped in the classics and in which empirical data played a negligible role (and from which the requirement that physicians be conversant with Latin remained a vestige) to a clinical science, based squarely on observation, is recounted in Arturo Castiglioni, *A History of Medicine,* E. B. Krumbhaar, trans. (New York: Alfred A. Knopf, 1947): 650-666, 756-761.

63 Canniff, *Profession in Upper Canada,* 77.

64 *Ibid.,* 85.

65 *Ibid.,* 78.

66 *Ibid.,* 78, 83.

67 *Ibid.,* 79.

68 *Ibid.,* 83.

69 *Ibid.,* 103.

70 Kalbach and McVey, *Demographic Bases,* 24.

71 The ratio of 1:2,400 assumes, of course, that all those candidates passed by the Board remained in practice in the province, and that no deaths or retirements reduced their numbers over the course of nineteen years, an unrealistic assumption at best.

72 Edwin Seaborn, whose history of the profession in the province tends to focus on biographical detail, characterizes the Board's requirements during this period as "far from exacting," but all available evidence runs contrary to this description. *March of Medicine,* 36.

73 Bull, *From Medicine Man,* 52.

74 McNab, *Legal History of Health Professions,* 6.

[75] *Ibid.*

[76] Charles M. Godfrey, *Medicine for Ontario: A History* (Belleville, Ont.: Mika Publishing Co., 1979): 18.

[77] Quoted in Canniff, *Profession in Upper Canada,* 68–69.

[78] Letter from Drs. James Muirhead, Walter Telfer, and F. W. Porter to Attorney-General Henry T. Boulton, dated October 22, 1832, quoted in Canniff, *ibid.,* 64.

[79] From the context of the letter, together with the replies of both the Attorney-General and the Upper Canada Medical Board—to whom a copy of the letter was directed—it appears that the authors had in mind as one of the functions of the proposed College the disciplining of licentiates who engaged in unorthodox treatment, such as botanical medicine. See Canniff, *Profession in Upper Canada,* 61–67.

[80] "A regular physician would no sooner go to see his patient without his bleeding lancet than he would go to church without his common prayer book." Godfrey, *Medicine for Ontario,* 23.

[81] "Many children died from over-dosing with calomel, a standard pediatric medicine." *Ibid.,* 22.

 Properly speaking, calomel is not, in small doses, poisonous; in fact, together with the other mercury salts, particularly its more toxic relative, mercuric chloride (corrosive sublimate), it was effectively used as a specific for syphilis since the sixteenth century. However, largely because of its cathartic properties, by the eighteenth century it was regarded by physicians as the drug of choice for virtually every disease, venereal or otherwise, including rheumatism, cholera, diarrhoea, tetanus, yellow fever, typhus, smallpox, and a long list of other ailments. More importantly, the doses prescribed were massive and, far more often than not, resulted in mercury poisoning. Thus, an 1861 text on therapeutics refers to doses of 60 grains (4,000 mg.) of calomel every hour in cases of Asiatic cholera, certainly sufficient to kill. (For purposes of comparison, the cathartic dose recommended in 1960 was between 120 to 300 mg. daily.) Indeed, mercurial salivation, which precedes death by mercury poisoning by some ten to twenty hours, was regarded by physicians as an essential part of any mercurial cure. For an informative discussion of the central role of calomel in the armamentarium of the nineteenth century physician, see Harris L. Coulter, *Divided Legacy: The Conflict Between Homoeopathy and the American Medical Association* (2d edition; Richmond, Calif.: North Atlantic Books, 1982): 61–67.

[82] For a discussion of the therapeutic principles of regular medicine and those of homeopathy and eclecticism, see Rothstein, *American Physicians,* 41–62 and 125–197, and Harris Livermore Coulter, *Political and Social Aspects of Nineteenth-Century Medicine in the United States: The Formation of the American Medical Association and its Struggle with Homeopathic and Eclectic Physicians* (unpublished Ph.D. dissertation, Columbia University, New York, 1969): 23–33, 92–118, and 195–231. For

a brief overview of the more popular remedies recommended in the 1830s by both orthodox and Thomsonian practitioners in Canada, see William Renwick Riddell, "Popular Medicine in Upper Canada a Century Ago." *Ontario Historical Society Papers and Records,* XXV (1929): 398-404.

[83] Woolverton studied medicine at both McGill and at the University of Pennsylvania, from which school he graduated in 1834. The medical faculty at Pennsylvania was considered one of the best in North America and a rival of the better schools in Britain at that time.

[84] Charles G. Roland, "Diary of a Canadian Country Physician: Jonathan Woolverton (1811-1883)," *Medical History,* XV (1971): 173.

[85] *Ibid.*

[86] Rothstein's observations on the effect the multiplication of orthodox medical schools in the United States had on the progress of medical therapeutics is equally applicable to the effect of licensing laws on the practice of medicine in Canada. Rothstein notes:

"The proliferation of medical schools brought about the standardization of regular medical therapeutics as a few dozen medical schools, using a small number of textbooks, replaced thousands of preceptors, each of whom taught his own idiosyncratic practices. The schools inculcated in their students the regimen of bloodletting, cathartics, blistering, and all the other therapies characteristic of heroic medicine. Eventually, an aroused public rebelled against this form of medical practice." *American Physicians,* 125.

There is little doubt that medical therapy in Canada would have been far more open to innovation and advancement in the absence of the stultifying effects of licensing boards, which had every incentive to demand of their applicants adherence to the strictest orthodoxy of the day.

[87] Canniff, *Profession in Upper Canada,* 71.

[88] *Ibid.,* 74. A fairer treatment is that offered by Godfrey, *Medicine for Ontario,* 20-23.

Canniff penned a book of close on 700 pages, 450 pages of which are devoted to detailed biographies of the early physicians of Upper Canada who possessed few attainments and are of little note. It is inexplicable that he should have neither known the correct spelling of Thomson's name nor whether or not he was a "subject" of the United States. There is perhaps no better example of the parochialism of nineteenth-century Canadian medicine than that an eminent physician and historian of medicine should appear to be unaware of a sect that was to become strong enough to be granted its own licensing board in Upper Canada only eleven years after the close of Canniff's narrative.

Dr. Heagerty's work, the full title of which is *Four Centuries of Medical History in Canada, and a Sketch of the Medical History of Newfoundland,* comprises almost 800 pages of text in two volumes, yet not once mentions either eclecticism or Samuel Thomson (nor homeopathy, for that matter), despite devoting countless pages to the minutiae of Canadian medicine and the medical profession in the nineteenth century.

[89] The brief summary of homeopathy which follows is taken from my essay on "The Early Development of Medical Licensing Laws in the United States, 1875–1900," *Journal of Libertarian Studies,* III (1979): 74.

[90] "Of all those medicines, that one whose symptoms bear the greatest resemblance to the totality of those which characterize any particular natural disease, ought to be the most appropriate and certain homoeopathic remedy that can be employed; it is the specific remedy in this case of disease." Samuel Hahnemann, *Organon of Homoeopathic Medicine* (3d American ed., New York: William Radde, 1849): 171.

[91] Rothstein, *American Physicians,* 157.

[92] *Ibid.,* 158.

[93] Godfrey, *Medicine for Ontario,* 193; Seaborn, *March of Medicine,* 194.

[94] Seaborn, *March of Medicine,* 197–199; Bull, *From Medicine Man,* 133.

[95] *Ontario*

A separate homeopathic board of examiners, empowered to license homeopathic practitioners in Canada West, was established in 1859 [22 Vic., c. 47 (Canada)]. The law was repealed in 1869, upon passage of a new medical act [32 Vic., c. 45 (Ontario)], and homeopaths were given representation on the Council of the newly-created College of Physicians and Surgeons of Ontario. By amendment in 1874 [37 Vic., c. 30 (Ontario)], homeopathic applicants were granted the right to be examined in the theory of materia medica and of physic, and the theory of surgery and midwifery, by homeopathic examiners. In 1932 [22 Geo. V, c. 22 (Ontario)], homeopathic representation on the Council was reduced from five members to one, and in 1960 [8 & 9 Eliz. II, c. 66 (Ontario)], was abolished altogether, although the other special provisions concerning homeopathic applicants remained in force. Finally, in 1974 [23 & 24 Eliz. II, c. 47 (Ontario)], the laws respecting licensing in the health field were completely revised with passage of the Health Disciplines Act, and all provisions respecting homeopathy were deleted.

Quebec

In 1865, the provincial parliament created the Montreal Homeopathic Association, with authority to establish a board of examiners for the purpose of examining homeopathic candidates throughout Canada East in specific fields [28 Vic., c. 59 (Canada)]. The act was amended in 1883 [46 Vic., c. 31 (Quebec)], and the homeopathic board's powers were broadened to include authority to determine the curriculum of study of its applicants. This act appears among the statutes of the province as late as 1941, but is omitted from the Revised Statutes of Quebec, 1964. The laws governing all the professions in Quebec were totally restructured in 1973 [22 Eliz. II, c. 43 (Quebec)], with the enactment of the Professional Code, and the statute creating a homeopathic board was formally repealed at that time [22 Eliz. II, c. 46 sec. 54 (Quebec)].

96 Godfrey, *Medicine for Ontario,* 195. Dr. Lancaster's torments at the hands of allopathic practitioners were apparently unending, according to Seaborn. He recounts that "once and probably often he [Lancaster] successfully defended himself against unjust charges of malpractice and once for homicide." *March of Medicine,* 200.

97 Godfrey, *Medicine for Ontario,* 193. Homeopathic practitioners apparently were extremely effective in competing with orthodox physicians in the United States and this doubtless contributed substantially to the antagonism between the two groups. See Coulter, *Divided Legacy,* 119-124.

98 The Rev. Isaac Fidler, in his *Observations,* published in 1832, has this to say about Americans practicing in Canada: "Some medical gentlemen emigrate from the States into Canada; but I believe they are never employed where one from Great Britain or Ireland can be procured. American physicians do not commonly place themselves in any situation in which competition with Europeans is hazarded. If any professional gentleman from the States be found in such neighbourhood, he forms an exception from the general rule. There was one such at Thornhill, but his skill was not considered as entitling him to much patronage. His practice was very limited, chiefly to the lower orders." Quoted in Canniff, *Profession in Upper Canada,* 69-70. If Fidler is correct in his claim that Americans tended to confine their practice to the rural areas, it is unlikely that they would have gone through the difficulties of acquiring a license.

99 The following table appears in Rothstein, *American Physicians,* 93:

Regular Medical Schools Providing Instruction on a Degree-Granting Basis, by Year, 1770-1860

Year	All Schools	Schools in New England, New York State, and Philadelphia
1770	2	2
1780	2	2
1790	3	3
1800	4	4
1810	6	5
1820	13	10
1830	22	14
1840	30	16
1850	42	17
1860	47	16

100 See Hamowy, "Medical Licensing Laws," 73.

101 Among the applicants rejected by the Upper Canada Medical Board were a number of Canadians who had undergone their medical training at schools in the United States. Doubtless these unsuccessful candidates felt

particular resentment at the existence of a licensing authority that could prevent them from entering practice in their home country, especially since they would have been able to practice freely in the United States.

[102] This attitude has been summarized by one American historian of medicine: "Canadian nationalism then as now contained a dose of anti-Americanism. Especially in the politically troubled 1830s there were widespread and not unjustified fears that lax enforcement of licensing laws would invite a descent on Canada by battalions of American quacks armed with republicanism as well as charlatanism. Regulations, then, always had a political as well as a purely professional goal. It meant not only safeguards for health but guarantees of stability. Here the reverse was true in the United States. Amidst the democratic agitation of the 1830s attempts by the profession to secure enforcement of licensing laws had the rubric of monopoly and were given the kiss of death, a comparison to the Bank of the United States. Medical institutions in America seemed out of step with triumphant egalitarianism; in Canada they appeared to be guarantors of triumphant paternalism." Joseph F. Kett, "American and Canadian Medical Institutions, 1800–1870," *Journal of the History of Medicine and Allied Sciences,* XXII (1967): 348.

[103] Letter to Sir Peregrine Maitland, dated March, 1826, quoted in Canniff, *Profession in Upper Canada,* 53. G. M. Craig writes of Strachan during this period that "his offices do not begin to suggest the real influence he exercised for a fairly limited time, roughly the regime of Sir Peregrine Maitland (1818–1828), when in many respects he dominated the government, either directly or through his former pupils, particularly John Beverley Robinson." "Two Contrasting Upper Canadian Figures: John Rolph and John Strachan," *Transactions of the Royal Society of Canada,* series 4, XII (1974): 240.

Strachan had earlier deplored the large number of poorly trained practitioners operating in the province during the hiatus between the repeal of the 1795 act in 1806 and the enactment of the 1815 medical statute. In 1812, under the pseudonym "Reckoner," he wrote in the Kingston *Gazette* that "the Province is overrun with self-made physicians who have no pretensions to knowledge of any kind and yet there is no profession that requires more extensive information.

"They comprehend not the causes or nature of diseases, are totally ignorant of anatomy, chemistry, and botany; many know nothing of classical learning or general science.... The welfare of the people calls aloud for some legislative provision that shall remedy this increasing evil; any examination, however slight, would terrify nine-tenth of the present race." Quoted in Canniff, *Profession in Upper Canada,* 26–27.

[104] Quoted in Caniff, *ibid.,* 175–176.

[105] Efforts to strengthen the 1827 act began almost immediately after its passage. Between 1828 and 1835, at least six bills aimed at amending the 1827

statute were proposed in the Upper Canada legislature. MacNab, *Legal History of Health Professions,* 7.

[106] Quoted in Canniff, *Profession in Upper Canada,* 110.

[107] *Ibid.,* 109–110.

[108] Quoted in Caniff, *ibid.,* 111.

[109] The preamble to the 1839 act makes explicit reference to the petition of the Medical Board:

"Whereas [there follows a list of signers of the petition] have by their petition amongst other things represented, that the Laws now in force in this Province, regulating the practice of the Medical profession, and for the prevention of persons practising without License, have been found very inadequate, and have prayed that such alterations and amendments may be made in the existing Laws, as may be most conducive to the interests of the Medical profession and the public at large: *And whereas* it is highly desirable that the profession of Medicine in this Province should be placed upon a more respectable and efficient footing, and that a more summary mode should be provided for the conviction and punishment of persons practising without a License: ... " 2 Vic., c. 38 (Upper Canada).

[110] There is evidence that the medical boards' actions were often arbitrary and reflected the animosity that existed between the English-speaking physicians of the province, who controlled the boards, and the French-speaking profession. The Laterrière case is an example. In 1789, Pierre de Sales Laterrière became the first person examined for a physician's license by the Quebec board. Despite the fact that the 1788 statute explicitly exempted from examination all holders of medical degrees, and despite his having been earlier assured by the provincial board that a degree would prove sufficient for licensure, Laterrière's degree from the medical faculty at Harvard was not regarded as grounds for exemption, and he was forced to sit a lengthy and difficult examination. See Donald Jack, *Rogues, Rebels, and Geniuses: The Story of Canadian Medicine* (Doubleday Canada Ltd., 1981): 53–54, and Charles-Marie Boissonnault, *Histoire de la Faculté de Médecine de Laval* (Quebec: Les Presses Universitaires Laval, 1953): 62, for a discussion of Laterrière's treatment by the Quebec licensing authorities. See also Maude E. Abbott's jejune account of the episode in her *History of Medicine in the Province of Quebec* (Montreal: McGill University, 1931): 48, where the incident is described as "colourful."

Control of the province's medical boards by the civil authorities and, through them, by the English-speaking profession, led one francophone historian to comment of the 1788 law: "It placed the study and practice of medicine completely in the hands of the executive authority [and thus] opened the door to favoritism, injustice, and administrative tyranny. Licenses were to be granted by the governor, who, in addition, appointed the examiners, thus making of them simply officers of the executive power. In a period when so much prejudice and narrow-mindedness dominated official circles, such control over the profession permitted serious injustices." Joseph-Edmond Roy, *Histoire du notariat du Canada,* quoted in Boissonnault, *Histoire de la Faculté,* 62.

111 A[nthony] von Iffland, "Sheets from my Portfolio," *British American Journal of Medical & Physical Science,* IV (May, 1848): 24.

112 *Ibid.*

113 H. E. MacDermot, *History of the Canadian Medical Association* (2 vols.; Toronto: Murray Printing Co., 1935–1958), I:3.

114 In August, 1822, Dr. John Stephenson received permission to advertise lectures on anatomy, surgery, and physiology to be held at the Montreal General Hospital during the following winter and Dr. Andrew Holmes soon followed with a series of lectures in experimental chemistry. In October of that year, at the instigation of the medical officers of the hospital, these two physicians drew up a statement outlining the need for a medical school in Canada, suggesting its affiliation with the Montreal General Hospital, and listing its proposed faculty, comprising the authors of the statement, together with Drs. William Caldwell, Henry P. Loedel, and William Robertson. This statement was appended to Dr. Robertson's letter to Lord Dalhousie recommending a restructuring of the board of medical examiners in Montreal. The school was opened in November, 1824, and on June 29, 1829, the officers of the Montreal Medical Institution were constituted the medical faculty of McGill University. Heagerty, *Four Centuries of Medical History,* II:59–64. Thus was established the first degree-granting medical school in Canada, "to meet a pressing educational demand [since] quacks abounded everywhere and the need for medical training was acute." *Ibid.,* 59.

In fact, it appears that the residents of Quebec had ample opportunity to formally pursue the study of medicine without great difficulty even before the establishment of the Montreal Medical Institution. The Castleton Medical Academy, located near the Canadian border in Castleton, Vermont, was founded in 1818, and its student body included a large number of Canadians. See Sylvio Leblond, "La médecine dans la province de Québec avant 1847," *Les Cahiers des Dix,* No. 35 (1970): 69–95. During its first decade the school grew into one of the outstanding medical colleges in the United States, but it quickly declined after 1828, in great part because of the establishment of a medical school in Montreal and the increased competition generated by other new medical colleges in the area. For a brief history of the college, see M. Therese Southgate, "Castleton Medical College, 1818–1862," *Journal of the American Medical Association,* CCIV (May 20, 1968): 698–701.

115 The profession again submitted petitions to the legislature requesting improvements in the medical law in 1823, 1827, and 1828. Boissonnault, *Histoire de la Faculté,* 63.

116 Leblond, "La médecine dans Québec," 78, and Barbara R. Tunis, "Medical Licensing in Lower Canada: The Dispute Over Canada's First Medical

Degree," *Canadian Historical Review,* LV (1974): 491. The *Free Press* strongly criticized the appointment of the medical officers of the Montreal General Hospital "as the sole examiners of all those who wish to be admitted to practise the medical profession in Canada. This accomplished, no young man, however superior his natural and acquired abilities might be, who had not walked the Montreal General Hospital, and attended the lectures of the learned officers of this enlightened medical school, would pass this Board; in fact, none who had not been reared by these *soi-disant* lecturers would be admitted to the practice of the profession here." The *Free Press,* March 27, 1823, quoted in Tunis, "Medical Licensing in Lower Canada," 491.

There is little doubt that the reconstitution of the membership of the Montreal medical board was deliberately designed to consolidate the position of the English-speaking and British-educated physicians in Quebec. On February 11, 1823, Lord Dalhousie, in a letter to two physicians whose names had been omitted from the new membership list, noted that they were not included because of "considerations of a Public nature on new modelling the Board of Medical Examiners of Montreal so that it shall in future consist of persons holding diplomas or testimonials from Medical Institutions in Great Britain, of those who are at present Medical Officers of the Montreal General Hospital now about to be incorporated." Quoted in Abbott, *History of Medicine,* 59.

117 Heagerty, *Four Centuries of Medical History,* I:283. Its opening resolution was typically self-laudatory: "That of all the various classes of society which have a direct influence on the prosperity of the State, the Medical Profession, having for its object to ensure comfort and happiness to every individual, must be considered as the most beneficial to mankind. . . .

"That the improvements which have lately taken place in the Profession of Medicine in this country, enforce on its members the necessity of adopting such measures as may ensure the further support and protection which the interest of Medical Science imperiously requires." And so on. The resolution is quoted in full in Heagerty, *ibid.*, 282.

118 *Ibid.,* 283, and Boissonnault, *Histoire de la Faculté,* 62.

119 Quoted in Heagerty, *Four Centuries of Medical History,* I:283.

120 1 William IV, c. 27 (Lower Canada). Several representatives of the Assembly were elected to membership of the newly created medical boards, including two physicians who had served on the Assembly's committee to review and recommend changes to the 1788 statute. Tunis, "Medical Licensing in Lower Canada," 493.

121 Thus meeting the demands of French-speaking physicians that they be granted a role in controlling the profession in Lower Canada.

122 Tunis, "Medical Licensing in Lower Canada," 495.

123 *Ibid.,* 494. Tunis notes that "a second provision of Article VI required that the diploma or license conferring the degree be produced and verified 'to

the satisfaction of the Board.' This latter clause gave almost unlimited power for the board to reject a diploma, since it did not say what criteria for this 'satisfaction' should be." *Ibid.,* 494-495.

[124] *Ibid.,* 495.

[125] The case is covered in great detail in Tunis, *ibid.,* 497-504.

[126] Memorial of the Medical Faculty of McGill College to Lord Aylmer, 29 October 1831, quoted in Tunis, *ibid.,* 492.

[127] Tunis, *ibid.,* 493.

[128] *Ibid.,* 503. Logie, it appears, never reapplied to the board. Ms. Tunis notes: "Although the dispute over Canada's first medical degree was settled, it is perhaps ironic that the man who precipitated the controversy never claimed his license to practise in Lower Canada.... William Logie, for reasons unknown, had left Lower Canada before the end of 1833. He applied for and received a license to practise medicine in New Orleans, Louisiana, in January, 1834, and spent his entire professional career in the United States. He died in 1879, and is buried in Geneva, New York." *Ibid.,* 504.

Logie would have found no difficulty in setting up practice in Louisiana. Although an act had been passed in 1816 setting up medical licensing boards in the state and providing penalties for its violation, the law exempted any inhabitant who could produce the testimonial of a neighbor that he had furnished him relief at any time or that the practitioner was capable of ministering to any ailment. The statute was a dead letter from the date of its passage and was eventually repealed. Rothstein, *American Physicians,* 335-336.

[129] During its six years of operation under the 1831 act, the medical board at Quebec licensed sixty-nine applicants to practice medicine in the province. Leblond, "La médecine dans Québec," 86.

[130] "Sheets from my Portfolio," 25.

[131] 56 Geo. III, c. 16 (New Brunswick). Under the terms of the statute, physicians possessing a diploma or "other authentic and sufficient testimonial of ... skill and ability" from some college or other public institution in Great Britain or Ireland were to be granted a license to practice medicine and surgery in the colony. Practitioners not possessing the requisite medical qualification were required to undergo an examination by judges appointed for that purpose by the governor, and, if found qualified, were entitled to a license, as were all physicians who had been in practice in the colony for at least seven years. Military doctors were exempt from the provisions of the act.

[132] 9 Geo. IV, c. 5 (Nova Scotia). The act provided that all physicians not holding diplomas or "other sufficient testimonial" from a medical college or other public institution were to be examined by judges appointed by the governor and, if found qualified, granted a license to practice. The act

exempted military physicians and, by amendment in 1829 [10 Geo. IV, c. 10 (Nova Scotia)], all physicians who had been in practice in the colony for at least seven years.

¹³³ Unlike her sister colonies, Prince Edward Island did not enact a law regulating the practice of medicine until 1871.

¹³⁴ W. Brenton Stewart, *Medicine in New Brunswick* (Moncton, N.B.: New Brunswick Medical Society, 1974): 41.

¹³⁵ "After the founding of Halifax [in 1749], about nine-tenths of the physicians who came to Nova Scotia, came from New England, and of the thirty-five practitioners in 1790 fully three-fourths were Loyalists." D. A. Campbell, "The Growth and Organization of the Medical Profession in Nova Scotia," quoted in M. Charlton, "Outlines of the History of Medicine in Lower Canada," *Annals of Medical History,* 1st series, VI (1924): 223. Dr. Charlton's article appeared in the *Annals* in four parts: V (1923): 150–174; V (1923): 263–278; VI (1924): 222–235; and, VI (1924): 312–354. At least a half of his commentary concerns itself with events outside Lower Canada.

Nova Scotia appears to have been well supplied with physicians at the close of the eighteenth century. Campbell estimates the population of the colony in 1790 to be about 35,000. D. A. Campbell, "Medical Legislation in Nova Scotia; Past, Present and Future," *Maritime Medical News,* I (July, 1889): 96. If he is correct in concluding that thirty-five physicians were then practicing there, the physician-population ratio would have been 1:1,000.

¹³⁶ The population of Nova Scotia in 1827 was slightly under 124,000, and that of New Brunswick in 1824, less than 75,000. Prince Edward Island's population did not exceed 47,000 until 1841. Kalbach and McVey, *Demographic Bases,* 24–25.

¹³⁷ Norman MacDonald, *Canada, 1783–1841, Immigration and Settlement* (London: Longmans, Green and Co., 1939): 466.

¹³⁸ Campbell, "Medical Legislation in Nova Scotia," 96.

¹³⁹ S. F. Wise, "Colonial Attitudes from the Era of the War of 1812 to the Rebellions of 1837," in S. F. Wise and Robert Craig Brown, eds., *Canada Views the United States: Nineteenth-Century Political Attitudes* (Seattle: University of Washington Press, 1967): 28–29.

¹⁴⁰ A detailed tabulation of early American medical licensing legislation is contained in Joseph F. Kett, *The Formation of the American Medical Association: The Role of Institutions, 1780–1860* (New Haven: Yale University Press, 1968): 181–184, and Rothstein, *American Physicians,* 332–339.

¹⁴¹ The introduction of restrictive legislation in the United States is discussed at some length in Hamowy, "Medical Licensing Laws," 73–119.

¹⁴² Sir William Osler, "The Growth of a Profession," *Canada Medical and*

Surgical Journal, XIV (October, 1885): 131. Osler has considerably over-simplified the licensing system operating in Great Britain before passage of the Medical Act of 1858. Before that time, there were no less than twenty-one corporations throughout the British Isles empowered to examine and license medical practitioners of various sorts, most operating within distinct geographic limits. Unlicensed practice was common and, in most cases, legal. The standard histories of the most prestigious of these licensing bodies are, Sir George Clark, *A History of the Royal College of Physicians of London* (3 vols.; Oxford: Clarendon Press, for the Royal College of Physicians, 1964–1972) [The third and final volume, carrying the narrative of the College from 1858 through 1948 is authored by A. M. Cooke] and, Zachary Cope, *The Royal College of Surgeons of England: A History* (London: Anthony Blond, 1959). A brief summary of the history of medical legislation in England is contained in the *Encyclopedia of the Laws of England* (2d ed.; London: Sweet & Maxwell, Ltd., 1908): IX: 171–178, *s.v.* "Medicine; Medical Practitioners." See also the discussion of the medical profession in early nineteenth-century England in M. Jeanne Peterson, *The Medical Profession in Mid-Victorian London* (Berkeley: University of California Press, 1978): 5–39.

¹⁴³ 2 Vic., c. 38 (Upper Canada).

¹⁴⁴ The provision allowing for the licensing without examination of licentiates of the various medical faculties in the United Kingdom does not appear in Upper Canada's medical act of 1818. It was only after strong opposition to the provisions of the act by licentiates of the Royal College of Physicians, London, and the Royal College of Surgeons, London, that the medical act of 1827 exempted these two groups from examination, thus granting them the same status the law had accorded holders of medical degrees from British universities. One historian notes that, immediately after passage of the 1827 act, "other independent medical colleges, including the Colleges of Surgeons of Edinburgh and Dublin, and the Faculty of Physicians and Surgeons of Glasgow, also claimed exemption from examination by the Medical Board, and pressed their claims energetically until their grievances were removed in 1839." Bull, *From Medicine Man,* 46. Goldwin Smith is thus correct in his observation that the Family Compact "showed its exclusiveness even towards British immigrants, excluding them by jealous restrictions from free practice in the legal and medical professions." *Canada and the Canadian Question* (London: Macmillan and Co., 1891): 110.

¹⁴⁵ Canniff, *Profession in Upper Canada,* 132. In reply to a query from the College respecting these two points, which had been brought to its attention by a letter of complaint, the College's solicitor, Henry Sherwood, wrote: "I cannot discover any ground upon which it can be urged that the College of Physicians and Surgeons can not legally take upon themselves the prevention of those who, offending against the law by practising

physic, surgery and midwifery without lawful authority, are subjected by the law to certain fines. Nor can I see upon what principle it can be contended, that they cannot lawfully appropriate any portion of those fines, as of their other funds, to bring such offenders to justice. I consider the College as a body incorporated for the purpose of placing the medical profession upon a more respectable and efficient footing. It is the only body which now legally has any control over the members of the profession. From the College the right to practise the various branches of the profession can now only be obtained, and it does appear to me there would be great reason for complaint against the Fellows of the College, not only by its members but by the community generally, if knowingly they suffered unauthorized persons openly to practise the various branches of the profession, without any exertion on their part to stop the evil of barretry. What is termed a common barretor is a common quarreler, a common exciter or maintainer of quarrels and suits in courts – a person who invents or disperses false rumours whereby discord arises – but to insist that an incorporated body established by law to regulate and control one of the learned professions, would be guilty of barretry by appointing a person to prosecute before a proper tribunal persons who are practising contrary to law, who are, in fact, guilty of misdemeanours, would, in my humble judgment, be extending the meaning of the term beyond any reasonable limit." Quoted in Canniff, *ibid.,* 132–133.

146 "*Resolved* unanimously – That the Fellows of the College of Physicians and Surgeons avail themselves of the earliest opportunity of tendering to Henry Sherwood, Q.C., and M.P.P., their unanimous thanks for the persevering efforts he has made in procuring the passage through the Legislature of the Act of Incorporation, a measure so well calculated to raise the character of the profession and benefit the public at large." Minutes of the College of Physicians and Surgeons of Upper Canada, Toronto, May 13, 1839, quoted in Canniff, *ibid.,* 113.

147 Minutes of the College of Physicians and Surgeons of Upper Canada, Toronto, August 29, 1839, quoted in Canniff, *ibid.,* 128.

148 There had been earlier attempts to establish a medical school in the province, although not one empowered to grant degrees. In 1824, Drs. John Rolph and Charles Duncombe attempted to organize a private medical school at the St. Thomas Dispensatory at York, but they were forced to abandon the project after two sessions. The continuing absence of any organized medical school in the province encouraged Rolph to once again offer private classes in medicine in the city in 1832, and his school appears to have been successful in attracting a large number of students. Because of his sympathies with the reform movement, however, the government brought charges of treason against Rolph in 1837, and he was forced to escape to Rochester. He did not return to Toronto until after the general pardon of 1843, at which time he re-established his school, which was

incorporated as the Toronto School of Medicine in 1853. Hence, between 1837 and 1843, no medical school, proprietary or otherwise, existed in Upper Canada. Heagerty, *Four Centuries of Medical History*, II: 72–80.

[149] The petition, in part, reads: "The establishment at once of an efficient school of medicine with an ample library and museum is intended by us, as the first step towards the accomplishment of this desirable object; this will, by affording within the Province the means of instruction in medical science, prevent hundreds of our youths resorting to the neighbouring States for their education, from whence they too often return with little addition to their information, and most commonly with principles at variance with the allegiance due to their Sovereign.

"His Excellency Sir John Colborne was so deeply impressed with the baneful effects of an education acquired in the United States upon the morals of our youths intended for the profession of medicine, that he upon many occasions stated that he saw that 'a medical school could no longer be delayed without manifest injury to the best interests of the Province.'" Quoted in Canniff, *Profession in Upper Canada*, 116.

[150] Minutes of the College of Physicians and Surgeons of Upper Canada, Toronto, September 3, 1839, quoted in Canniff, *ibid.*, 130.

[151] "It being obvious that the College of Physicians and Surgeons have not at their disposal means to defray the expenses of an efficient school of medicine, and it being evident that the Council of King's College are not prepared to set on foot an establishment equal to the wishes or wants of the medical community, this College therefore propose to the Council the propriety of meeting the wants of the medical youth of the Province, by conjointly establishing a school of medicine.

"Such a course was adopted with success, when the School of Physics in Ireland was perfected conjointly by the University of Dublin and the King and Queen's College of Physicians in Ireland; ...

"The medical profession of both Institutions form conjointly the faculty of medicine of the University; and the examinations of all matters connected with the medical department, as well as that of candidates for degrees in medicine, are conducted by them." Report upon a communication from the President of King's College, to the President of the College of Physicians and Surgeons of Upper Canada, contained in the Minutes of the College, May 30, 1839, quoted in Canniff, *ibid.*, 121.

[152] Minutes of the College of Physicians and Surgeons of Upper Canada, Toronto, November 28, 1839, quoted in Canniff, *ibid.*, 136. The College further resolved:

"That Mr. William Higgins, High Constable of the Home District, be appointed collector," and,

"That a notice be inserted in the Toronto *Patriot, Commercial Herald,* Kingston *Chronicle,* Hamilton *Gazette,* Cobourg *Star* and Niagara *Chronicle* newspapers, requesting all magistrates convicting any offenders against the Act incorporating the College of Physicians and Surgeons of

Upper Canada, to remit the amount of all fines to the collector of the College. . . . " *Ibid.*

153 Minutes of the College of Physicians and Surgeons of Upper Canada, Toronto, July 5, 1839, quoted in Canniff, *ibid.,* 125.

154 *Ibid.*

155 The figure does not include seven applicants who held licenses granted by the Medical Board of Upper Canada, the College's predecessor.

156 Despite the provisions of the law exempting from examination all members and licentiates of any college or faculty of medicine or surgery within the United Kingdom, the College regularly required such applicants to undergo an examination in that area of medicine not embraced by the candidate's faculty—that is, in either medicine or surgery—and, in some cases, in direct contravention of the act, in both fields.

157 Minutes of the College, quoted in Canniff, *ibid.,* 113–166. The College also refused to consider the applications of three candidates, including two diplomates of the Royal College of Surgeons, Edinburgh, because they refused to appear personally before the College in Toronto. A motion that "no application for license be entertained unless on the personal appearance of the applicant, and that a 'statute' to that effect be adopted" was put before the Fellows of the College at their meeting of January 6, 1840, but the motion was never voted upon. Cited in Canniff, *ibid.,* 140.

 Given the difficulties of travel and the distances and costs involved, especially in the case of an applicant living in the outlying regions of the province, the demand that all candidates personally appear before the College underscores the petty and arbitrary behavior consistently displayed by the College's fellows in its dealings with prospective practitioners.

158 Kalbach and McVey, *Demographic Bases,* 24.

159 It is interesting that the province's attorneys, themselves protected from unwelcome competition, joined in condemning the 1839 statute. "The lawyers of Upper Canada, secure within the Law Society which was one of the first institutions created in the province, agreed that medicine should be a trade open to all with the law as the remedy against error." Geoffrey Bilson, *A Darkened House: Cholera in Nineteenth-Century Canada* (Toronto: University of Toronto Press, 1980):145.

160 Minutes of the Special Meeting of the College of Physicians and Surgeons of Upper Canada, Toronto, August 24, 1840, quoted in Canniff, *Profession in Upper Canada,* 151–152.

161 *Ibid.,* 155–156 (italics mine).

162 Letter from S. B. Harrison, secretary to the Lieutenant-Governor, to the College of Physicians and Surgeons of Upper Canada, dated December 28, 1840, quoted in Canniff, *ibid.,* 161–162.

163 Indeed, it appears to have been the policy of the Colonial Office to let stand colonial acts repugnant to imperial statutes if the colonial legislation were judged reasonable. Thus, unlike the treatment accorded the

Upper Canada act of 1839, a Queensland act of 1862 requiring doctors duly qualified in England to register before being permitted to practice in the colony was allowed to stand, despite its being in direct conflict with the Imperial Medical Act of 1858, which authorized its registrants to practice throughout the Empire. Conceding the repugnancy of the Queensland law, Sir Frederic Rogers, then Permanent Under-Secretary of State for the Colonies, argued that since the act was a reasonable one it should be permitted to come into operation, where it would lay open to challenge in a court of law. D. B. Swinfen, *Imperial Control of Colonial Legislation, 1813–1865* (Oxford: Clarendon Press, 1970): 61.

[164] 28 & 29 Vic., c. 63 (1865). The notion of repugnancy contained in the Colonial Laws Validity Act had been anticipated in the language of the Canada Act of Union [3 & 4 Vic., c. 35 (1840)].

[165] 30 Vic., no. 31 (British Columbia).

[166] 21 & 22 Vic., c. 90 (1858).

[167] The Colonial Laws Validity Act was made inoperative respecting the colonies achieving dominion status under the Statute of Westminster [22 Geo. V, c. 4, sec. 2 (1931)].

CHAPTER 2
THE PERIOD FROM 1840 TO CONFEDERATION

[1] 3 & 4 Vic., c. 35 (1840).

[2] 4 & 5 Vic., c. 41 (Canada).

[3] W. P. M. Kennedy, *The Constitution of Canada: An Introduction to its Development and Law* (London: Oxford University Press, 1922): 281.

[4] Elizabeth MacNab, *A Legal History of Health Professions in Ontario* (A Study for the Committee on the Healing Arts [Toronto: Queen's Printer, 1970]): 8, fn. 30.

[5] In January, 1842, a memorial — similar in wording and identical in substance to that sent in 1839 by the College of Physicians and Surgeons of Upper Canada to the then Lieutenant-Governor, Sir George Arthur, requesting his intercession in the establishment of a medical school at King's College — was forwarded by the medical board of Canada West to Sir Charles Bagot. The memorial is quoted in full in William Canniff, *The Medical Profession in Upper Canada, 1783–1850* (Toronto: William Briggs, 1894): 175–176.

[6] John J. Heagerty, *Four Centuries of Medical History in Canada* (2 vols.; Toronto: The Macmillan Company of Canada Ltd., 1928), II:77–80.

It is fortuitous that, with the return of John Rolph from exile in the United States, a second medical school was established in Toronto in 1843.

Rolph's school, later incorporated as the Toronto School of Medicine, was joined by yet a third, in 1850. In that year, Drs. James Bovell and Edward Hodder established the Upper Canada School of Medicine, which became the medical faculty of the University of Trinity College in 1852. See Charles M. Godfrey, *Medicine for Ontario: A History* (Belleville, Ont.: Mika Publishing Co., 1979): 46-58.

With the establishment of several schools of medicine in Canada West, some of which were proprietary, it is predictable, as MacNab observes, that "after 1844, the Bills presented to the Legislature sought to control the *study* and practice of medicine." *Legal History of Health Professions,* 9. A summary of medical schools established in Canada prior to 1920 is contained in table 2.1.

[7] Report of the medical committee of King's College, October, 1843, quoted in Canniff, *Profession in Upper Canada,* 184-185.

[8] William G. Rothstein, *American Physicians in the Nineteenth Century: From Sects to Science* (Baltimore: The Johns Hopkins University Press, 1972): 92.

[9] *Ibid.,* 97.

[10] *Ibid.*

[11] Letter from the Medical Board of Canada West to the Medical Board of Montreal, dated April 26, 1847, quoted in Canniff, *Profession in Upper Canada,* 197.

[12] Minutes of the Medical Board of Canada West, Toronto, April, 1847, quoted in Canniff, *ibid.,* 196. The Montreal medical board responded that its requirements were—in the main—the same as those of the Medical Board of Canada West, but that the Quebec board, on the advice of its attorney, had enforced a period of four years' study only. Letter from the Montreal Board to the Medical Board of Canada West, dated May 7, 1847, quoted in Canniff, *ibid.,* 198.

[13] Minutes of the Medical Board of Canada West, Toronto, July 7, 1845, quoted in Canniff, *ibid.,* 192.

[14] Minutes of the Medical Board of Canada West, Toronto, October, 1845, quoted in Canniff, *ibid.*

[15] Warren E. Kalbach and Wayne W. McVey, *The Demographic Bases of Canadian Society* (2d ed.; Toronto: McGraw-Hill Ryerson Ltd., 1979): 25.

[16] Charles-Marie Boissonnault, *Histoire de la Faculté de Médecine de Laval* (Quebec: Les Presses Universitaires Laval, 1953): 137-141, and, Heagerty, *Four Centuries of Medical History,* II:113-116. Professors at the Ecole de Médecine were originally required to deliver their lectures in both French and English, one in the morning in one language, and again in the afternoon in the other. Heagerty, *ibid.,* 94.

[17] A draft of the 1845 bill is contained in "The Medical Bill," *British Ameri-*

can Journal of Medical & Physical Science, I (May, 1845): 56-57. The proposed law is examined in some detail in the following issues of the *Journal:* I (June, 1845): 81-83; I (July, 1845): 110-112; and, I (October, 1845): 195-196.

[18] "The Medical Bill," *British American Journal of Medical & Physical Science,* I (June, 1845): 82.

The *Journal,* one of the first English-language medical periodicals published in Canada, had, in its first number, argued the need for a strong medical licensing law in the following terms:

"The propriety of making an Act of this kind of Government measure, cannot be doubted. Governments are bound, by every principle of justice, to place within the reach of their subjects, without any restriction, or with as little as possible, those articles which may be deemed to be among the actual necessities of life; and among such a list, without the slightest fear of contradiction, may be indubitably placed proper medical remedial assistance, as affecting in the most immediate and direct manner their happiness, their health, nay, their very lives. Proper remedial assistance cannot be viewed as, nor is it in reality, one of the luxuries of life, (although we doubt not it would be esteemed so in many sections of this Province,) of which those who have the longest and best filled purses can have the best quality. The poor man should be equally as well provided for in this respect as the rich. His life is equally as valuable, and its sacrifice awakens equally as keen an expression of anguish and sorrow among surviving relatives and friends, while it is not unfrequently attended with much more distressing consequences. To secure, then, an object of such paramount importance, should be the anxious solicitude of every government, and there are no means of effecting it, but by the entailment of a thorough education on the part of all who aspire to such duties, thus fitting them for their due and faithful discharge, with their subsequent protection in their avocation, from the inroads and incursions of unlicensed and unlettered pretenders." "The Medical Bill," *ibid.,* I (April, 1845): 27.

[19] H. E. MacDermot, *History of the Canadian Medical Association* (2 vols.; Toronto: Murray Printing Co., 1935-1958), I:4. Dr. Hall was at that time both a member of the Board of Medical Examiners in Montreal and lecturer in chemistry at the University of McGill College. Heagerty, *Four Centuries of Medical History,* I:277.

[20] "The Medical Bill and the School of Medicine of Montreal," *British American Journal of Medical & Physical Science,* II (May, 1846): 22-25.

[21] "Three months have now elapsed since our remarks against an augmentation of licensing boards for the Province were submitted to the profession. At that period the Provincial Legislature was in session, and we have some good grounds for believing that our observations tended, in no small degree, to that result which ended in the arrest of the bill until the

deliberate opinion of the profession at large was heard on a matter of such vital importance to their interests. With the simple exception of an anonymous scribbler in one of the French Canadian newspapers, who, from *interested motives,* made a miserable attempt to pervert the plain meaning and spirit of our remarks to subserve his own ends, not one sentence condemnatory of the position which we assumed and upheld has been publicly expressed." "Augmentation of Licensing Boards for the Province," *ibid.,* II (August, 1846): 111.

22 MacDermot, *Canadian Medical Association,* I:21–22.

23 "The Adjourned Convention of Medical Delegates," *British American Journal of Medical & Physical Science,* II (October, 1846): 164. English physicians were quick to see in the proposals as first drafted an attempt to subvert their influence in the profession to the benefit of the French party. The offending clauses had reference to the original composition of the proposed College, which was to comprise all physicians legally practicing in Canada East for at least twenty years, and to the membership of its Board of Governors, which was to be elected by the general membership. Additionally, provincial licentiates of more than seven but less than fifteen years were eligible for election to the Board only after having passed an examination. As the *British American Journal* remarked, had these provisions remained, "French Canadian interests should then prevail," since "composed, as the Profession is in this part of the Province, mainly of French Canadian members, the power would become lodged in the majority." Finally, all applicants for a license to practice were required, under the proposal, to sit the examination of the Board unless their curriculum of study was that prescribed for medical schools in Canada East. English physicians objected that this requirement would have made it obligatory for graduates and licentiates of the various universities and faculties in Great Britain to submit to "the degradation of an examination" to practice in the area. See "Proposal for a College of Physicians and Surgeons for Canada East," *ibid.,* II (October, 1846): 164–166, and "Medical Meeting at Three-Rivers," *ibid.,* II (November, 1846): 190–191.

24 Minutes of the meeting of the medical profession resident in Canada East, held at Three Rivers, October 14, 1846, quoted in *ibid.,* II (November, 1846): 191.

25 *Ibid.,* 191–192.

26 The medical boards in Quebec and Montreal had, in fact, arrogated to themselves the power to assess the educational qualifications of nondegree holders under the powers granted them by the 1788 act to both examine and "approve" applicants.

27 "Summary Punishment of Illegal Practitioners of Medicine," *ibid.,* II (April, 1847): 335–336, quoting the *Morning Courier* of February 4, 1847. The "Yankee quack" to which the editorial alluded, refers to a Dr. F. A. Caldwell of the "American Eye and Ear Institute of New York," who

offered his services in the treatment of diseases of the eye and ear to the residents of Montreal in late 1846 and advertised his presence in the local press. The profession in Montreal was extremely exercised by this innocuous bit of competition, especially after finding no record of the "American Eye and Ear Institute" in New York, and the incident was constantly used as an example of the rampant charlatanism in Canada East and of the need for stricter legislation. The episode is recounted in "Quackery in Montreal," *ibid.,* II (October, 1846): 166–167.

The editorial is totally misleading in suggesting that foreigners were immune from prosecution if they practiced in Canada East without a license granted by one of the provincial medical boards. The 1788 law made no provision for treating visiting physicians any differently than residents and all instances of unlicensed practice were punishable under the act.

28   10 & 11 Vic., c. 26 (Canada).

29   The Medical Board was to take the requirement that all applicants proposing to study medicine be bilingual quite literally. In 1851, two candidates were failed solely on the grounds that one did not know English, while the other was ignorant of French. Boissonnault, *Histoire de la Faculté,* 127.

30   There was some dissatisfaction with the act during the period immediately following its passage, centering on the powers accorded the Board of Governors of the College and their possible abuse, and the fact that graduates of the Ecole de Médecine — unlike those of McGill — were required to sit the licensing examination after having completed their studies. These discontents gave rise to the formation of a Repeal Association, which sought repeal of the 1847 statute and its replacement with a new law. The dispute within the profession — as was commonly the case in Lower Canada — tended to fall along ethnic and linguistic lines, French-speaking physicians comprising the preponderance of signatories to the Association's petitions. A summary of the activities and goals of the Association is contained in a lengthy letter by Dr. J. E. Coderre, published in French, in "Past Proceedings of the Governors of the College of Physicians and Surgeons," *British American Journal of Medical & Physical Science,* IV (August, 1848): 104–109. Unfriendly accounts of the Repeal Association appear in "The Doings of the 'Repeal Association,'" *ibid.,* III (February, 1848): 276–278; "The Repeal Association Again," *ibid.,* III (March, 1848): 311–313; and, "Dr. Coderre's Letter and the Repeal Association," *ibid.,* IV (September, 1848): 134–136. Also see the Proceedings of the Board of Governors of the College of Physicians and Surgeons of Lower Canada, held at Quebec on May 9 and 10, 1848, containing a protest against the activities of the Board of Governors, which the Association accused of certain irregularities tending "à détruire l'ordre et l'harmonie et les pouvoirs que le dit Acte d'incorporation avait en vue d'établir pour le corps social des Médecins." The proceedings are reprinted in the *British American Journal,* IV (June, 1848): 49–51.

[31] "College of Physicians and Surgeons of Canada East," *ibid.*, III (July, 1847): 76. One practitioner observed soon after passage of the measure that "I really cannot perceive why the numerous quacks, who so long have infested the country, should continue to exist in that capacity, provided the medical profession be only true to itself, and will combine for the purpose of protecting its own and the public interest." Letter from F. D. Gilbert, dated September 11, 1847, *ibid.*, III (November, 1847): 193.

[32] Letter from "Rusticus," dated June 7, 1847, *ibid.*, III (July, 1847): 81–82.

[33] 12 Vic., c. 52 (Canada).

[34] The society was formed in July, 1844, to replace the Medico-Chirurgical Society of Upper Canada, which had been founded at York in 1833 and had apparently ceased to function after the dissolution of the College of Physicians and Surgeons of Upper Canada in 1841. MacDermot, *Canadian Medical Association,* I:139. The successor organization, "the sole object of which is, and shall always be, the dissemination and improvement of the various branches of medicine and the collateral sciences," almost immediately began to agitate for new restrictive legislation.

[35] A draft of the original measure is reprinted in "Bill: An Act to Incorporate a College of Physicians and Surgeons in Upper Canada," *British American Journal of Medical & Physical Science,* II (June, 1846): 56–58. The original draft contains the somewhat curious provision whereby the first fellows of the College would consist of the members of the Toronto Medico-Chirurgical Society! A later draft, more acceptable to the profession in western Canada, appears in "Rough Draft of a Proposed Bill to Incorporate the Profession in Upper Canada," *ibid.*, II (November, 1846): 192–193.

[36] The petition is reprinted in the *British American Journal*, I (March, 1846): 335. The petitioners' contention that unlicensed practitioners commonly escaped the law by not billing their patients until one year after treatment is, needless to say, absurd. Nor is there any more sense to the claim that the public expected regular physicians to take on the duty of initiating prosecutions against unauthorized doctors. In fact, the public was strongly opposed to such prosecutions.

[37] Anonymous letter, dated August 20, 1846, *ibid.*, II (September, 1846): 141.

[38] Anonymous letter, dated May 25, 1846, *ibid.*, II (June, 1846): 55–56. In a second letter authored by the same physician, and which appeared in the next issue of the *Journal,* the writer undertakes an elaborate and detailed defense of the bill against a few of its detractors within the profession and, in the course of his argument, admits to having taken part in drafting the original petition. Anonymous letter, dated June 26, 1846, *ibid.*, II (July, 1846): 85–86.

[39] "In Lower Canada, a difference of race, and a difference in habits, and to some extent, of practice, between the members of our profession, will

account for the want of concord sometimes displayed amongst us, but when the interests of the profession demanded removal of the feelings originating from the above causes, we did overcome them and acted in unison for our common good, and as a reward, have obtained our act of incorporation, which has already, in many instances, afforded redress to the aggrieved practitioner." *Canada Medical Journal,* I (August, 1852): 381.

The periodical, whose full title was the *Canada Medical Journal and Monthly Record of Medical and Surgical Science,* was published in Montreal from March, 1852, to February, 1853, under the editorship of Robert L. MacDonnell and Aaron H. David. A second medical journal with the identical title began publication in Montreal in July, 1864, with George E. Fenwick and Francis W. Campbell as editors. It continued to publish through June, 1872. Both journals began their series with volume I. A thorough examination of Canadian medical journals is contained in Charles G.Roland and Paul Potter, *An Annotated Bibliography of Canadian Medical Periodicals, 1826–1975* ([Toronto]: Hannah Institute for the History of Medicine, 1979).

40 *Upper Canada Journal of Medical, Surgical and Physical Science* (hereafter *Upper Canada Journal*), I (April, 1851): 28–29.

41 "Meeting of the Profession," *ibid.,* I (May, 1851): 67.

42 A draft of the bill is reprinted in "The Proposed Bill," *ibid.,* I (May, 1851): 69–72.

43 A letter of protest, signed by twenty-nine physicians, and dated May 7, 1851, appeared in the *Upper Canada Journal,* I (May, 1851): 68.

44 "The Medical Bill," *ibid.,* I (June, 1851): 113–114.

45 The proposed act is reprinted in the *Upper Canada Journal,* I (June, 1851): 115. The act is entitled "An Act to Amend the Law of Upper Canada Relative to the Practice of Physic and Surgery," and has as its opening paragraph the following:
"Whereas past experience has shewn that penal enactments have not deterred unqualified persons from practising Physic, Surgery, and Midwifery, but, on the contrary, such enactments have often had the effect of preventing benevolent persons, well qualified, from lending their aid to relieve physical suffering, and it is therefore expedient and proper to repeal such penal clauses as may exist in any Acts now in force in Upper Canada in relation to the practice of Physic, Surgery, and Midwifery: Be it therefore enacted, &c., That [the penal provisions of the 1827 statute] shall be and they are hereby repealed."

46 "The Medical Bill," *ibid.,* I (June, 1851): 114.

47 *Ibid.,* 112–113.

48 "Medical Politics," *ibid.,* I (June, 1851): 158–168. The *Journal*'s reply is of sufficient interest as a synopsis of the major arguments most commonly offered in favor of restrictive legislation in the area of medical practice

that it merits quotations in full in this study. It appears as an appendix to this chapter.

⁴⁹ "The Fate of the Bill," *ibid.,* I (September, 1851): 248–249.

⁵⁰ Political developments during the period following the victory of the reform elements in Canada in the winter elections of 1847–1848 are covered in J. M. S. Careless, *The Union of the Canadas: The Growth of Canadian Institutions, 1841–1857* (Toronto: McClelland and Stewart Ltd., 1967): 113–149.

⁵¹ "The Medical Board, Canada West," *Upper Canada Journal,* I (February, 1852): 471–472.

⁵² "Incorporation of the Profession in C. W.," *Medical Chronicle,* I (April, 1854): 347.

⁵³ The *Canada Medical Journal* attempted to minimize the prevalence of homeopathy in Canada beyond all reason when it wrote that "the regular profession of this Province have little cause, from present appearances, to apprehend any wide spread adoption by the people, of the absurdities of globulism. Canada, although geographically in juxtaposition to a country where hydra-headed Quackery reigns rampant, and rapidly multiplies its heads even without excision of a previously existing one; where homeopathy, soon after its first promulgation, found a sure footing; and where Homeopathic Colleges yearly send forth numbers of manufactured globulists to dispense sugar of milk pilules to every willing dupe, can boast of but four homeopathic practitioners." "Reviews and Bibliographical Notices: *On the Fallacies of Homeopathy,*" *Canada Medical Journal,* I (August, 1852): 347.

⁵⁴ "Homoeopathy," *Upper Canada Journal,* I (November, 1851): 341.

⁵⁵ "Reviews and Bibliographical Notices: *On the Fallacies of Homeopathy,*" *Canada Medical Journal,* I (August, 1852): 347–348, quoting the *British and Foreign Medico-Chirurgical Review.*

⁵⁶ "Eclectic Medicine," *Upper Canada Journal,* I (December, 1851): 385.

⁵⁷ *Ibid.,* 386–387. The same issue of the *Journal* carried a notice that a reputable British medical publisher would no longer publish any homeopathic works, to which the *Journal* commented: "This is the true way to meet the evils of quackery: instead of declaiming against it, however well merited the language used may be, nothing will so surely arrest its progress as a combined opposition to its interests, and a determination to discountenance it by every act which will interfere with the pecuniary gains derivable from it by these parasitical impostors." "A Medical Evil Corrected," *ibid.,* I (December, 1851): 387.

⁵⁸ "The Eclectics," *ibid.,* I (January, 1852): 427–428.

⁵⁹ "A Recreant McGillite," *Medical Chronicle,* IV (March, 1857): 392.

⁶⁰ 22 Vic., c. 47 (Canada). The preamble to the act states: "Whereas the system of Medicine called Homoeopathy is much approved and extensively practised in many countries of Europe, in the United States and also

in Canada; And whereas it is expedient to extend to duly qualified practitioners of this system privileges similar to those enjoyed by licentiates of medicine under the laws in force in this Province..."

61 24 Vic., c. 110 (Canada).

62 The sole exceptions were the original members of the boards of examiners, designated by name in the acts creating these boards.

63 28 Vic., c. 59 (Canada).

64 No homeopathic college was, in fact, ever established in Lower Canada. The educational requirements of the 1847 and subsequent acts made it unlikely that students would pursue their medical studies in the United States, where homeopathic medical schools abounded. As a result, the act creating a homeopathic board of examiners had little practical effect on the medical profession in Canada East. Its existence, however, was a constant irritant to regular physicians, who were no longer the only medical group legally recognized by provincial law.

65 It is interesting, in the light of modern medical therapeutics, that of the two systems, the materia medica of eclecticism was probably more advanced than that of homeopathy.

66 "Legislative Action 'Pro' and 'Con' Legitimate Medicine," *British American Medical and Physical Journal,* N.S. II (July, 1861): 326.

The *British American Medical and Physical Journal* succeeded the *British American Journal of Medical & Physical Science,* and began publication in May, 1850, the month following the last issue of its predecessor. Both periodicals were under the editorship of Archibald Hall and were published in Montreal.

67 *Ibid.*

68 29 Vic., c. 34 (Canada).

69 There were five degree-granting institutions listed in the act: the Toronto School of Medicine; the University of Trinity College, Toronto (whose medical faculty succeeded that of the Upper Canada School of Medicine in 1852); the University of Victoria College (whose medical faculty was created in 1856); the University of Queen's College (whose medical faculty was established in 1854); and the University of Toronto. The University of Toronto did not possess a medical faculty, having been reduced solely to an examining body in medicine by the Hincks Act in 1853. The prevailing view at that time was that medical schools should be proprietary and there was strong sentiment against state support for the education of professionals whose training would lead to lucrative practices.

The 1865 act provided for representation on the Council of "every other college or body in Upper Canada, by law authorized or hereafter to be authorized to grant Medical or Surgical Degrees or Certificates of qualification to practise Medicine, Surgery and Midwifery."

70 21 & 22 Vic., c. 90 (1858). Under the terms of the 1858 act, a single governing board, the General Council of Medical Education and Regis-

tration, was created for the various branches of medicine — physicians, surgeons, and apothecaries — in the United Kingdom. The General Medical Council consisted of representatives of the various universities and medical corporations, together with six appointees of the Crown. It was empowered to supervise the course of study and qualifications required of the graduates and licentiates of the several universities and medical corporations in the United Kingdom, and to register all legally qualified applicants. Only registered practitioners were eligible for certain appointments, could sign legal certificates, could sue for the recovery of fees, or could indicate by the use of any title or designation that they were registered under the act. The Medical Act of 1858 and its replacement, the Medical Act of 1886, together with their amendments, are discussed in *Halsbury's Laws of England* (2d ed.; London: Butterworth and Co., 1936), XXII:291-323. See, also, *Encyclopedia of the Laws of England* (2d ed.; London: Sweet & Maxwell, Ltd., 1908), IX: 171-178, *s.v* "Medicine; Medical Practitioner."

71 In 1857, the dollar was adopted as the unit of currency in Canada by the provincial parliament, effective January 1, 1858.

72 "Medical Education," *Canada Medical Journal,* III (October, 1866): 188. The educational requirements exacted by Canadian medical schools at the time of the act's passage are described as comprising "six months' lectures on each branch [of study] constituting a full course, and two full courses, except in the case of Medical Jurisprudence, extending over four years."

73 It appears that of the six Kingston physicians originally appointed as the new medical faculty of Queen's University, one of them, a Dr. L. P. Litchfield, did not hold a medical degree, although he laid claim to one. Hilda Neatby, *Queen's University,* Vol. I: *1841-1917* (Montreal: McGill-Queen's University Press, 1978): 72.

Such lack of attention to formalistic niceties led, in 1855, to Queen's University being reproached by the medical fraternity for holding terms of five months' duration only, and for not including in its curriculum for a medical degree either the "Institutes of Medicine" or "Medical Jurisprudence." Equally damning in the eyes of the profession was the fact that its tuition charges were lower than those of the other universities in Canada and in the better schools of the United States. Given this state of affairs, the *Medical Chronicle* concluded, "we are not, therefore, surprised that by inducements cogent like these, students should be seduced from other schools as is proudly asserted from New York and other Universities. The temptations of cheapness and laxity are not always irresistible. Want often compels the highway to be deserted for the by-path, and when possession is facilitated the indolent will be drawn into its pursuit. It is, however, obvious that degrees thus procured at inferior price, by less study and upon defective information are not entitled to the estimation enjoyed by others against which these objections do not hold." "Queen's College, Medicinae, Doctores Primitivi," *Medical Chronicle,* III (June, 1855): 25.

See also, "Veritas Praevalebit," *ibid.,* III (October, 1855): 188–193.

[74] It is remarkable that MacNab overlooks the revolutionary direction taken by the 1865 act. In summarizing the statute, she does not once mention that unlicensed practice was not prohibited under its provisions. Indeed, her comments imply the very opposite. "The Act," she observes, "launched a new attack against unauthorized practitioners by setting out the privileges that only those registered were entitled to exercise. The most important privilege was *the right to practise and prescribe,* and to charge fees for these services. The Act made it clear that unregistered men could not use the courts to recover fees for such services. Further, only those on the Register were entitled to an appointment as a medical officer in the provincial service, or in any hospital or the militia, and only they could give a certificate that was required to be signed by a doctor." *Legal History of Health Professions,* 11–12 (italics mine). In point of fact, the statute did not proscribe the right to practice and prescribe to any person, nor did it prevent unregistered practitioners from being appointed to any hospital or other charitable institution wholly supported by voluntary contributions, but only disallowed suits for the recovery of fees for medical services.

[75] Section thirty-two of the act provided that: "Any person who shall wilfully and falsely pretend to be or take or use any name, title, addition or description implying that he is registered under this Act, shall upon prosecution and conviction in any Court of competent jurisdiction, forfeit and pay a penalty not exceeding one hundred dollars."

[76] Kalbach and McVey, *Demographic Bases,* 24–25.

[77] Heagerty, *Four Centuries of Medical History,* I:256.

[78] *Ibid.*

[79] *Ibid.,* 288.

[80] *Ibid.* The committee's report noted: "With regard to the improper treatment of bills presented of late years to the legislature, your committee are of opinion that the only alternative now left by which an effectual resistance may be offered to the unjust procedure of the committees of Assembly appointed to investigate the petitions of medical men, is an union of the profession throughout the province." D. A. Campbell, "Medical Legislation in Nova Scotia; Past, Present and Future," *Maritime Medical News,* I (July, 1889): 97.

[81] Heagerty, *Four Centuries of Medical History,* I:289.

[82] 19 Vic., c. 22 (Nova Scotia). The act was reworded in 1857 [20 Vic., c. 18 (Nova Scotia)].

[83] The population of New Brunswick had made significant gains in the first sixty years of the century. In 1824, it stood at about 74,000 and had more than doubled by 1840, to 156,000. The population of the colony was estimated to be slightly less than 194,000 in 1851 and at over 252,000 ten years later. Kalbach and McVey, *Demographic Bases,* 24–25.

84 W. S. MacNutt remarks on the mobility of the population in both New Brunswick and Nova Scotia during this period, in *The Atlantic Provinces: The Emergence of Colonial Society, 1712-1857* (Toronto: McClelland and Stewart Ltd., 1965): 214-215.

85 22 Vic., c. 18 (New Brunswick).

86 In 1860 [23 Vic., c. 23 (New Brunswick)], the act was amended to provide that holders of degrees from homeopathic medical schools were entitled to registration on the same basis as regular physicians.

87 26 Vic., c. 11 (New Brunswick).

88 *British Colonist*, June 14, 1860, quoted in T. F. Rose, *From Shaman to Modern Medicine: A Century of the Healing Arts in British Columbia* (Vancouver: Mitchell Press Ltd., 1972): 19-20.

89 Estimates of the population of British Columbia during this period differ markedly. E. E. Rich reports that British Columbia had a population of about 11,000 when it was created a colony in 1858. *The Fur Trade and the Northwest to 1857* (Toronto: McClelland and Stewart Ltd., 1967): 286. Kalbach and McVey's figures, taken from the 1941 Census of Canada (Vol. I, p. 5), indicate the population of British Columbia (including Vancouver Island) as 55,000 in 1851, 51,500 in 1861, and 36,250 in 1871. They observe that "there has not been much agreement as to the correct estimates for the population of British Columbia. However, between 1851 and 1861 there seems to be sufficient evidence to indicate that its population fluctuated considerably as a result of the Fraser River gold discoveries in 1856, and that in 1861 after the 'gold rush' its population was estimated to be 52,000." *Demographic Bases*, 24-25, 28.

90 30 Vic., no. 31 (British Columbia).

91 It is clear what policy considerations lay behind disallowing the British Columbia ordinance while the Canada West Medical Act of 1865 was permitted to stand. The ordinance placed certain educational requirements on all prospective practitioners, irrespective of where they obtained their degrees or licenses. The Upper Canada act, on the other hand, provided for the automatic registration of all licentiates in Great Britain, on payment of the required fee.

92 33 Vic., no. 3 (British Columbia).

93 American Medical Association figures show 65 medical schools in operation in 1860 and 75 in 1870. "Medical Education in the United States," *Journal of the American Medical Association*, LXXV (August 7, 1920): 383.

94 Rothstein, *American Physicians*, 282.

95 "Unlicensed Practitioners," *Medical Chronicle*, V (February, 1858): 420.

96 *Ibid.*

97 "Encouragement of the Unlicensed," *ibid.*, V (April, 1858): 507-509.

98 "The Indian Herb Doctor," *ibid.*, V (June, 1857): 39. The *Canada Medical*

Journal noted that "in Lower Canada we had to contend, in some parts, with uneducated and unlicensed practitioners, but the worst of them was superior to the horde of root doctors, steamers, and quacks, that are flocking into every village in Upper Canada, and dividing with the regularly qualified physician, the scanty subsistence the practice of the neighbourhood is capable of affording. These impostors ingratiate themselves into the good opinion of the farmers and country shop-keepers, and descend to familiarities with the lower classes, to which the educated gentleman cannot stoop, and soon the latter finds, that his ignorant and low competitor is preferred to himself, or, at least, divides, pretty equally, public confidence. These fellows have hitherto been allowed to go on unmolested, and have been fostered and encouraged in their proceedings, even by those who should be the protectors of the lawful practitioner, and who, from the position they have been elevated to by the suffrages of the people, should have taken advantage of that position to protect them from fraud and deception. But no! the quacks are numerous, and exercise a baneful influence at all elections; the well educated practitioner must be sacrificed to elevate the village attorney to a place in Parliament." "Medical Convention to be Held at Toronto," *Canada Medical Journal,* I (July, 1852): 313.

[99] 21 & 22 Vic., c. 90 (1858). The identical phrase appears in the preamble to the New Brunswick Medical Act of 1859, the Medical Act for Upper Canada of 1865, and the British Columbia Medical Ordinance of 1867.

[100] Hansard, CXLIX (1858), col. 648, quoted in David L. Cowen, "Liberty, Laissez-Faire and Licensure in Nineteenth Century Britain," *Bulletin of the History of Medicine,* XLIII (1969): 38.

[101] Toronto *Globe,* November 23, 1868, quoted in MacNab, *Legal History of Health Professions,* 12, fn. 50.

[102] Sir William Osler, "The Growth of a Profession," *Canada Medical and Surgical Journal,* XIV (October, 1885): 131.

[103] By certification I mean the endorsement, either through examination or by some other method, of medical practitioners by some semi-public or private body that is not legally empowered to restrict entry into the profession nor to prevent the practice of uncertified physicians.

[104] These findings, together with an extensive bibliography on the subject of licensing, are summarized in Simon Rottenberg, "A Review of the Professional Literature on Occupational Licensing," (mimeographed; Amherst, Mass.: University of Massachusetts, April 28, 1978).

[105] "Analysis of the Ontario Medical Register," *Canada Medical Journal,* VII (July, 1870): 17. Godfrey's estimate of the number of unlicensed practitioners is substantially higher. He observes that at the time of Confederation there were about 760 licensed physicians in Ontario and at least twice that number of unlicensed practitioners. *Medicine for Ontario,* 83. If Godfrey's figures are accurate, then the ratio of licensed physicians to the

province's population was approximately 1:2,010, while the ratio of all practitioners to residents was 1:670.

106 "Degradation of the Medical Profession," *Upper Canada Journal,* III (July, 1854): 557-561.

CHAPTER 3
FIRST STEPS TOWARDS THE PROFESSIONALIZATION
OF MEDICINE, 1867-1887

1 Earlier attempts to form a national association are discussed in H. E. MacDermot, *History of the Canadian Medical Association* (2 vols.; Toronto: Murray Printing Co., 1935-1958), I:16-25. The objects of such an organization seem always to have been the same, the protection of the profession against competition. The *Montreal Medical Gazette,* in supporting a scheme to establish a medical society spanning both Upper and Lower Canada in 1844, noted that "the medical profession in Canada is yearly, nay monthly, increasing in numbers to such an extent, that it almost claims to be a corporate body, and from the influence of its members it would be entitled to obtain by respectful representation of its wants, those legislative protections to which it may become entitled." Quoted in MacDermot, *ibid.,* 16-17. And in 1845, the Montreal Medico-Chirurgical Society proposed the formation of a national organization of licensed practitioners that would have among its objects "the protection of the interests of the qualified and licensed practitioners against the inroads and usurpations of the unlicensed." Quoted in MacDermot, *ibid.,* 18.

2 MacDermot, *ibid.,* 26. At its Cincinnati meeting, the AMA endorsed a resolution calling upon "the members of the profession in the different States to use all their influence in securing such immediate and positive legislation as will require all persons, whether graduates or not, desiring to practice medicine, to be examined by a State Board of Medical Examiners, in order to become licensed for that purpose," and further recommending that "said board be selected from members of the State Medical Society, who are not at the same time members of college faculties." *Transactions of the American Medical Association,* XVIII (1867): 30. The 1867 meeting marked a turning point in the lobbying efforts of the AMA, away from appeals to medical schools to voluntarily raise their standards, to the state legislatures to enact legislation that would limit the production of physicians.

3 "The Canadian Medical Association," *Canada Medical Journal,* IV (October, 1867): 168.

4 "The Approaching Medical Convention at Quebec," *Canada Medical Journal,* IV (September, 1867): 140.

5 *Ibid.,* 142.

⁶ "The Profession," *Upper Canada Journal of Medical, Surgical and Physical Science* (hereafter *Upper Canada Journal*), I (October, 1851): 294.

⁷ MacDermot, *Canadian Medical Association,* I:28.

⁸ "The Canadian Medical Association," *Canada Medical Journal,* IV (October, 1867): 174–175.

⁹ The fact that the new association was politically oriented from its inception is unmistakably clear from its selection of Charles Tupper, perhaps the most politically powerful physician in Canada, as its first president. Tupper, of course, was a political figure of some abilities and had succeeded in bringing Nova Scotia into Confederation despite substantial opposition to the union within the colony. His political acumen made him an especially suitable choice as head of the new nationwide medical organization.

¹⁰ Quoted in "The Canadian Medical Association," *Canada Medical Journal,* IV (October, 1867): 175. The report of Tupper's speech is reported in the third person and has been here transposed into the first person. Mac-Dermot's account (*Canadian Medical Association,* I:34) is taken almost verbatim from the report of the convention carried in the *Canada Medical Journal.*

Soon after the creation of the CMA, one physician went so far as to suggest that the Association itself should act as the nation's sole licensing authority. His scheme called for:

"The Incorporation of the Canadian Medical Association, by an act of the General Parliament, with the following powers.

"The C.M.A. shall prescribe a course of preliminary education, and no person shall be allowed to enter on the study of medicine until he has obtained the Degree of Bachelor of Arts, or pass an examination before the Medical Council. In either case he must present himself before said Council, obtain their certificate of qualification, and register the same before the General Secretary of the C.M.A. and it shall be lawful for the Medical Council to refuse all recognition of any candidate for a license to practise Physic, Surgery or Midwifery, who has not fulfilled the above requirements.

"The C.M.A. shall establish a Curriculum of Medical Study, which shall be adopted by all the Universities, or schools of medicine affiliated to Universities, which Curriculum shall be that, say of the University of Edinburgh, and every person must give satisfactory proof of having fulfilled that Curriculum before he can under any circumstances present himself for a license to practice.

"The Medical Council of the C.M.A. alone shall have the power to grant licenses to practice Physic, Surgery or Midwifery, in the Dominion of Canada." Letter from E. D. Worthington, dated October 22, 1867, *Canada Medical Journal,* IV (November, 1867): 202.

¹¹ "The Canadian Medical Association," *ibid.,* IV (October, 1867): 178–180.

¹² MacDermot, *Canadian Medical Association,* I:39. MacDermot's extensive

quotation from the *Canada Medical Journal* in connection with the recommendations of the 1868 meeting is misleading; the quotation is not a summation of the report of the committee on medical registration but an editorial underscoring the desirability of a uniform law respecting the practice of medicine throughout Canada. The method of presentation, however, would lead the reader to infer the former. The full editorial is contained in "The Canadian Medical Association," *Canada Medical Journal,* V (September, 1868): 141–143.

[13] MacDermot, *Canadian Medical Association,* I:41.

[14] The AMA Code provided that "no one can be considered as a regular practitioner, or a fit associate in consultation, whose practice is based on an exclusive dogma, to the rejection of the accumulated experience of the profession and of the aids actually furnished by anatomy, physiology, pathology, and organic chemistry." The full text of the code of ethics as adopted by the American Medical Association appears in "Code of Medical Ethics," *New York Journal of Medicine,* IX (September, 1847): 258–265.

One of the provisions of the Canadian code, the violation of which led to a call for the resignation of one of the members of the CMA's committee on ethics in 1869, was the following: "It is derogatory to the dignity of the Profession to resort to public advertisements, or private cards, or hand-bills, inviting the attention of individuals affected with particular diseases – publicly offering advice and medicine to the poor gratis, or promising radical cures: or to publish cases and operations in the daily prints, or suffer such publications to be made." "Canadian Medical Association," *Canada Medical Journal,* VI (September, 1869): 117–118.

The code, as adopted by the CMA, is reprinted in full in "Code of Medical Ethics," *Canada Lancet,* XII (May, 1880): 257–264.

[15] A full report of the meeting appears in "Canadian Medical Association," *Canada Medical Journal,* VI (September, 1869): 97–123.

[16] *Ibid.,* 109.

[17] *Ibid.,* 110.

[18] *Ibid.,* 111–112.

[19] *Ibid.,* 117.

[20] A draft bill was presented at the third annual meeting of the CMA held in Ottawa in September, 1870. The bill provided for the creation of a "College of Physicians and Surgeons of the Dominion of Canada," comprising all licensed physicians throughout the country, together with all new registrants. The College was to be directed by a General Council, on which sat representatives of certain designated universities and medical schools, plus twelve representatives elected by the profession. The preliminary and professional educational requirements to be exacted of all prospective practitioners throughout the Dominion were similar to those recommended by the CMA's committees that had earlier reported on these

subjects. The bill required that all new registrants possess the requisite diploma in medicine from a Canadian university "or from any other University or College whose general and professional requirements may be accepted by the General Council as equivalent to its own," and a qualifying examination administered by the Council's board of examiners.

Lest these requirements not curtail the entry of new physicians into the profession at a pace sufficiently fast to satisfy established practitioners, the bill contained the following clause: "XXIX. No Medical School, other than those now in actual operation, shall be established after the passing of this Act, in any part of the Dominion of Canada, unless with the consent and approval of the General Medical Council." Finally, the bill empowered the General Council to remove from the Dominion medical register the name of any physician it judged to "have been guilty of infamous conduct in any professional respect." The provision would thus have effectively legislated the code of ethics of the profession.

The full text of the bill is contained in "Canadian Medical Association," *Canada Medical Journal,* VII (September, 1870): 110–123, and is reprinted in MacDermot, *Canadian Medical Association,* I:182–197.

The Association spent considerable time at its 1870 and 1872 meetings discussing the measure, clause by clause. Although a number of changes were made respecting the structure and organization of the proposed College and Council, the general outlines of the bill remained much the same as in the original draft. See "Canadian Medical Association," *Canada Medical Journal,* VII (September, 1870): 124–142, and "Canadian Medical Association," *Canada Medical and Surgical Journal,* I (October, 1872): 170–177, for the discussions on the bill at these two meetings.

21 Section 93 of the British North America Act [30 & 31 Vic., c. 3 (1867)] provided that legislation pertaining to education was an exclusively provincial matter. The courts have held that provincial statutes requiring the registration of physicians before permitting them to practice in the province are within the power of the provincial legislatures. *Lafferty v. Lincoln* (1907), 38 S.C.R. 620, *rev'g* 5 W.L.R. 301 *(sub nom. R. v. Lincoln).*

22 "Address of William Marsden," *Canada Medical Record,* III (August, 1874): 334; that portion of Marsden's address dealing with the Dominion medical bill is reprinted in Robert B. Kerr, *History of the Medical Council of Canada* (Ottawa: The Medical Council of Canada, 1979): 5–6.

23 Between 1859 and 1869, the province's homeopathic board had licensed 72 homeopathic practitioners. The eclectic medical board, which began issuing licenses in 1862, had licensed 132 eclectic physicians before the board was abolished by the 1869 act. William Marsden, "Analysis of the Ontario Medical Act, with Observations," *Canada Medical Journal,* VI (November, 1869): 196.

24 "Ontario Medical Council," [Proceedings of its first meeting, July, 1869], *Dominion Medical Journal,* I (August, 1869): 236.

25 "The Duties of the Government to Our Profession," *ibid.,* I (November, 1868): 49.

26 The following clause was submitted to the legislature: "Every person desirous of being registered under. . . this Act. . . shall, before being entitled to registration, present himself for examination as to his knowledge and skill for the efficient practice of his profession, before the Committee of Examination. . . and upon passing the examination required, and proving to the satisfaction of the Committee of Examination that he possesses [the requisite preliminary and educational qualifications set by the Council], and that he has otherwise complied with the rules and regulations made by the General Council may on the payment of such fees as the Council may determine, . . . be registered. . . to practice medicine, surgery and midwifery in the Province of Ontario." "Ontario Medical Act," *ibid.,* I (December, 1868): 69.

27 "Medical Legislation," *ibid.,* II (July, 1870): 193.

28 "Ontario Medical Act," *ibid.,* I (December, 1868): 69.

29 Toronto *Globe,* November 27, 1868, quoted in Elizabeth MacNab, *A Legal History of Health Professions in Ontario* (A Study for the Committee on the Healing Arts [Toronto: Queen's Printer, 1970)]: 13.

30 At the first meeting of the new Medical Council, Dr. Duncan Campbell, one of the homeopathic representatives, offered a brief history of why the provincial legislature felt it necessary to include the irregular sects under the new act. His remarks included the following: "Those members of Parliament more particularly interested in the matter, seeing that the preamble of the rule recommended the incorporation of the 'Medical Profession,' demanded that the Homoeopathists and Eclectics should be made to come in also, as they could understand no definition of the words 'Medical Profession,' that would not include all practitioners of medicine legally authorized. We objected that we were properly satisfied with our portion as it was, that our rights were fully guaranteed, and that we wanted no more. They insisted, and we consented on condition that we should have the same number of representatives in this Council as we have in the Homoeopathic Medical Board." "Ontario Medical Council," *Dominion Medical Journal,* I (August, 1869): 238.

Earlier, Dr. William Clarke had reported to the last meeting of the Medical Council under the 1865 act that "it was a fact that nearly half of the members of the Legislature were Homoeopathists; and it was folly to attempt to eliminate the clause [respecting the inclusion of homeopathy and eclecticism in the new act] without destroying the whole Bill." "Ontario Medical Council," [Proceedings of the Medical Council, April, 1869], *Canada Medical Journal,* V (April, 1869): 472.

31 32 Vic., c. 45 (Ontario).

32 "The Ontario Medical Bill," *Canada Medical Journal,* V (December,

1868): 273–274. The *Journal's* attack on the bill also contained the rather peculiar charge that "if a central board of examiners is established before whom all persons desirous of registration must appear for examination, within ten years, medical schools will become as numerous in Ontario as they are in the United States, and few of them will possess the means of affording even an elementary education. This must and will be followed by the addition to the ranks of the profession in the Province, of a legion of men indifferently educated as it will be in the interest of the several schools to ensure the success of their student." *Ibid.,* 275.

The *Journal* had earlier taken exception to the resolution of the Quebec Medical Society for similar reasons. Its resolution, put before the first meeting of the Canadian Medical Association in 1867, had called for a Dominion-wide medical act supervised by a licensing board empowered not only to set the educational standards necessary for licensure, but also to examine all prospective practitioners. "Canada Medical Society," *ibid.,* IV (August, 1867): 93–95.

The debate with the *Dominion Medical Journal* spanned several issues of each periodical. See "Ontario Medical Act," *Dominion Medical Journal,* I (December, 1868): 68–70; "The Ontario Medical Bill," *Dominion Medical Journal,* I (January, 1869): 88; and, "The Ontario Medical Bill," *Canada Medical Journal,* V (January, 1869): 330–331.

33 "Ontario Medical Council," [Proceedings of the Medical Council, April, 1869], *Dominion Medical Journal,* I (April, 1869): 159.

34 George W. Campbell, "Introductory Lecture— Delivered at the Opening of McGill University Session 1869–1870," *Canada Medical Journal,* VI (October, 1869): 149. In commenting on the history of the bill, Dr. Campbell remarked: "Twelve months ago the present Ontario Medical Bill was secretly prepared by a few members of the late Medical Council, was privately printed but was never published, nor was the general opinion of the Profession in Ontario ever pronounced upon it, until at an advanced period of last session of the Ontario Parliament it was attempted to be quietly introduced and smuggled through the house. A copy of the Bill was at length procured by the Faculty of this University, who published a protest against its being passed, and subsequently sent two of their members to Toronto, Drs. Scott and Craik, authorising them to use their best endeavours to have it amended in committee or thrown out altogether. The protest and the zealous efforts of our delegates were of no avail." *Ibid.,* 147.

35 "Ontario Medical Council, *Dominion Medical Journal,* I (April, 1869): 161; and, "Ontario Medical Council," *Canada Medical Journal,* V (April, 1869): 476–477.

36 "Ontario Medical Council, *Dominion Medical Journal,* I (April, 1869): 161; and, "Ontario Medical Council," *Canada Medical Journal,* V (April, 1869): 472. The resolution of the medical section of the Canadian Institute is carried in full in "The Ontario Medical Act and the Medical Section of

the Canadian Institute," *Canada Medical Journal,* V (May, 1869): 497-502. The same article contains several letters and petitions from Ontario physicians similar in nature to the Institute's petition. For the *Journal's* response to the action of the Medical Council in tabling the Institute's petition, see "The 'Medical Council of Ontario' and the 'Canadian Institute' of Toronto," *Canada Medical Journal,* V (May, 1869): 515-517.

37 "Ontario Medical Council," [Proceedings of the Medical Council, July, 1869], *Dominion Medical Journal,* I (August, 1869): 233-234; and "Ontario Medical Council," [Proceedings of the Medical Council, July, 1869], *Canada Medical Journal,* VI (July, 1869): 21.

38 "Ontario Medical Council," *Dominion Medical Journal,* I (August, 1869): 235-240; and, "Ontario Medical Council," *Canada Medical Journal,* VI (July, 1869): 24-33. The accounts of Council meetings that appeared in the two journals were taken from two sets of notes and frequently differ; material contained in one account is often absent from the other.

39 "Ontario Medical Council," *Dominion Medical Journal,* I (August, 1869): 235-240; and, "Ontario Medical Council," *Canada Medical Journal,* VI (July, 1869): 31.

40 "Canadian Medical Association," *Canada Medical Journal,* VI (September, 1869): 100-101.

41 "Adverting to the New Medical Law of Ontario, he [Tupper] was of opinion that the Profession was not to be benefitted by spurious liberality such as that granted here. They could not allow a retrograde step of that kind without injuring themselves in the eyes of the Profession in the rest of the world. He strongly animadverted on the conduct of those gentlemen who had endeavoured to amalgamate the different ideas . . . under the mistaken idea that they were benefiting the public. He asked if the very Board who had sent out the licentiate did not give him his *imprimatur,* one half believing his knowledge was worse than worthless." *Ibid.,* 103.

42 Letter of Dr. Horatio Yates, dated July 30, 1869, *Dominion Medical Journal,* I (August, 1869): 229-230. The following issue of the *Journal* carried a reply from Dr. G. C. Field, one of the homeopathic representatives on the new Council, who pointed out that the import of Dr. Yates' letter was not to deal evenhandedly with irregular practitioners but to wipe them out. He notes of Yates' remarks: "We might suppose him to be a fair and just man, and we would be happy in the belief, but he quickly undeceives us by declaring that his policy is not to deal out evenhanded justice to all, but is one of annihilation—nothing short of the utter demolition of the seceding sections of the profession, alias, in the pithy Saxon, and chastely elegant dicta of the Professor—'Knaves, fools, bastards, base coins, and rascals!'" Letter of Dr. G. C. Fields, dated August 27, 1869, *ibid.,* II (September, 1869): 7.

43 "Medical Legislation," *ibid.,* II (July, 1870): 192.

44 "The Medical Act—Will It Elevate the Profession?" *ibid.,* II (November,

1869): 50. The Council required that all medical students pass an examination on general education before commencing the study of medicine, that medical studies extend continuously over at least four years, such time to date from the passing of the preliminary examination, and that it comprise three sessions of at least six months each in an approved school or college of medicine, twelves months in the office of a qualified practitioner, and attendance at some hospital for a period of twelve months. Additionally, the applicant was to have assisted in at least six cases of midwifery. Finally, prospective licensees were required to submit to two sets of examinations, a primary examination comprising descriptive anatomy, physiology, theoretical chemistry, toxicology, pathology, medical diagnosis, and botany, generally undertaken at the end of the third year of study, and a final examination consisting of surgical anatomy, practical chemistry, medical jurisprudence, sanitary science, midwifery, surgery, materia medica and therapeutics, and theory and practice of medicine. *Ibid.,* and "Ontario Medical Council," [Proceedings of the Medical Council, July, 1869], *ibid.,* I (August, 1869): 241.

45 William Marsden, "Analysis of the 'Ontario Medical Act,'" *Canada Medical Journal,* VI (November, 1869): 193. Not all physicians agreed with Dr. Marsden. See David Mackintosh's speech before the Hamilton Medical and Surgical Society, February, 1870, printed in "Address on Medical Legislation," *ibid.,* VI (April, 1870): 450–469. Dr. Mackintosh observed that "the only argument that I have ever heard, even by its most strenuous supporters, in favour of taking these two nonentities [homeopathy and eclecticism] under our wing is that it will in the course of time annihilate them, that it is in fact giving them 'such protection as vultures give to lambs, covering, and devouring them.' And this is predicted by the *shrewd* men in our Medical Council as an unavoidable sequence from the action of their Bill. Now, we will all admit that this is a 'consummation most devoutly to be wished for;' but are we to do evil that good may abound, or are we by silently acquiescing in the felony, to become accomplices after the fact—not of the crime, of stamping out Homoeopaths and Eclectics, but of the unhallowed association of our names with them? It would indeed be very pleasing to look forward to the happy state of our profession, 50 years hence, and with prophetic eye to view the medical millenium which our successors will enjoy somewhere about the year 1920. But have we any guarantee that matters will remain as they are for five months, far less 50 years?" *Ibid.,* 458–459.

46 William Marsden, "Analysis of the 'Ontario Medical Act,'" *ibid.,* VI (November, 1869): 197.

47 "Report of an Act to Amend the Ontario Medical Act," *ibid.,* VI (February, 1870): 346–352.

48 "Ontario Medical Council," [Proceedings of the Medical Council, April, 1870], *Dominion Medical Journal,* II (April, 1870): 144–145; and, "Ontario Medical Council," [Proceedings of the Medical Council, April, 1870], *Canada Medical Journal,* VI (May, 1870): 501.

49 "Ontario Medical Council," *Dominion Medical Journal,* II (April, 1870): 152; and "Ontario Medical Council," *Canada Medical Journal,* VI (May, 1870): 512–513.

50 "We, the Homoeopathic and Eclectic members of the Council, protest against the action of Committee of the Council in nominating an Executive Committee, in which our members are not fairly represented; and that the said Committee should not be composed of more than six members, and that the Eclectic and Homoeopathic members of the Council ought to have the privilege of naming their representatives upon said Committee." "Ontario Medical Council," *Dominion Medical Journal,* II (April, 1870): 152; and, "Ontario Medical Council," *Canada Medical Journal,* VI (May, 1870): 514.

51 "The Medical Council," *Canada Lancet,* III (July, 1871): 490.

52 "College of Physicians and Surgeons of Ontario," [Proceedings of the Medical Council, June, 1871], *ibid.,* III (July, 1871): 483.

53 *Ibid.,* 484.

54 Letter from Duncan Campbell to Henry Strange, Registrar of the College of Physicians and Surgeons of Ontario, dated October 3, 1871, quoted in full in *Canada Lancet,* IV (November, 1871): 117–118.

55 The address of the President of the Council, Dr. C. W. Covernton, appears in "College of Physicians and Surgeons, Ont.," *Canada Lancet,* IV (January, 1872): 202–209.

56 "College of Physicians and Surgeons, Ontario," [Proceedings of the Medical Council, July, 1872], *ibid.,* IV (August, 1872): 549.

57 J. A. Grant, "Address Delivered Before the Canadian Medical Association, at St. John, New Brunswick," *Canada Medical Record,* II (August, 1873): 25.

58 Data on the number of licentiates in homeopathic and eclectic medicine to 1869 appear in William Marsden, "Analysis of the 'Ontario Medical Act,'" *Canada Medical Journal,* VI (November, 1869): 196.

59 "Meeting of the Medical Council," *Canada Lancet,* IV (August, 1872): 579.

60 "The Ontario College of Physicians and Surgeons and the Students of Medicine," *Canada Medical and Surgical Journal,* I (January, 1873): 330.

61 *Ibid.,* 328.

62 MacNab, *Legal History of Health Professions,* 17.

63 Their letter of resignation, dated December 10, 1873, is contained in "Minutes and Proceedings of the Ontario Medical Council," [June, 1874], *Canada Lancet,* VI (July, 1874): 358.

64 Letter to the Secretary of the College of Physicians and Surgeons of Ontario, dated June 2, 1874, contained in "Minutes and Proceedings of the Ontario Medical Council," *ibid.,* V (July, 1874): 358.

65 MacNab, *Legal History of Health Professions,* 17; and "The Profession in Ontario," *Canada Medical and Surgical Journal,* II (January, 1874): 334.

[66] 37 Vic., c. 30 (Ontario).

[67] "Minutes and Proceedings of the Ontario Medical Council," [July, 1875], *Canada Lancet,* VII (August, 1875): 355–362.

[68] 32 Vic., c. 45 (Ontario). The act is reprinted in the *Dominion Medical Journal,* I (March, 1869): 129–134.

[69] "Ontario Medical Council," *Canada Medical Journal,* VI (May, 1870): 504.

[70] *Ibid.*

[71] "Ontario Medical Council," *Dominion Medical Journal,* II (April 1870): 147; and, "Ontario Medical Council," *Canada Medical Journal,* VI (May, 1870): 504.

[72] "College of Physicians and Surgeons of Ontario," [Proceedings of the Medical Council, June, 1871], *Canada Lancet,* III (July, 1871): 457.

[73] *Ibid.,* 463. The Council attempted to strengthen the punitive provisions of the 1869 act in 1869, 1872, and again in 1873, before proving successful in 1874. MacNab, *Legal History of Health Professions,* 19, fn. 88. For one example, see, "Bill: 'An Act to Amend the Ontario Medical Act,'" *Canada Medical and Surgical Journal,* I (March, 1873): 426–430.

[74] "The Ontario College of Physicians and Surgeons and the Students of Medicine," *Canada Medical and Surgical Journal,* I (January, 1873): 326–327. It was felt by some members of the Council that the authority to enact a suitable penal clause in any provincial medical act was beyond the power of the provincial legislature under the terms of the British North America Act. Dr. Campbell, in responding to the students' demands, noted "that on this very same question of the penal clause he had conferred with both the present and preceding Attorney General of this Province, who had informed him that a certain difficulty lay in the way of enacting such a clause. This was that the power of passing a criminal law does not lie in the hands of the Ontario Government. Mr. Mowat would not give a decided answer on this point. Doubtless several laws of this kind had been enacted, but these gentlemen seemed themselves to have their doubts as to their legality." *Ibid.,* 330.

[75] Lest such contamination inadvertently occur, the *Canada Lancet* took the occasion to carry an abstract of an attack on homeopathy, noting that "after the recent struggle in the Legislature for the passage of the Medical Bill, it may, perhaps, be considered an opportune moment for taking up the more striking fallacies that are urged by these new school men in favour of themselves and in disparagement of us." "Allopathy v. Homoeopathy," *Canada Lancet,* VI (August, 1874): 390.

[76] Walter B. Geikie, "A Defence of the Medical Bill," *ibid.,* VI (April, 1874): 247.

[77] *Ibid.,* 248.

[78] "Minutes and Proceedings of the Ontario Medical Council," [July, 1875] *ibid.,* VII (August, 1875): 358.

79 *Ibid.*

80 *Ibid.*

81 "Prosecutions Under the Ontario Medical Act," *Canada Lancet,* VII (September, 1875): 24. The following issue of the *Lancet* contains a bitter attack on the *Globe*'s defense of unlicensed practitioners in the form of a letter from a Dr. P. P. Burrows, dated September, 14, 1875, under the title "Medical Monopoly," *ibid.,* VIII (October, 1875): 46–47.

82 "The Non-Suppression of Quackery," *ibid.,* VIII (May, 1876): 281–282.

83 "Minutes and Proceedings of the Ontario Medical Council," [July, 1876], *ibid.,* VIII (July, 1876): 334.

84 *Ibid.,* 338.

85 *Ibid.* Soon after the enactment of the 1874 law, a member of the Council had complained of the assessment clause contained in the act and remarked that he would consider it legitimate only if coupled with a stiff penalty provision against unlicensed physicians. William Allison, "The Ontario Medical Act," *ibid.,* VII (July, 1875): 325–328.

86 "Charlatanism," *Canadian Journal of Medical Science,* I (December, 1876): 438.

87 MacNab, *Legal History of Health Professions,* 19. See also, Charles M. Godfrey, *Medicine for Ontario: A History* (Belleville, Ont.: Mika Publishing Co., 1979): 224.

88 MacNab, *Legal History of Health Professions,* 20.

89 See, for example, the *Ontario Medical Register, 1887* (Toronto: College of Physicians and Surgeons of Ontario, June, 1887): xxxviii-xliii. Under the section entitled "How to Proceed to Procure a Conviction," the physician is advised to "go to the nearest or most intelligent Magistrate and lay information . . . (See forms appended.)," whereupon a summons will be issued, and so on.

90 MacNab, *Legal History of Health Professions,* 19, fn. 91.

91 "Medical Act vs. Quackery," *Canada Lancet,* XVIII (October, 1885): 55.

92 The discovery and spread of modern anesthesia in the United States is discussed in William G. Rothstein, *American Physicians in the Nineteenth Century: From Sects to Science* (Baltimore: Johns Hopkins Press, 1972): 250–253; and, Courtney R. Hall, "The Rise of Professional Surgery in the United States: 1800-1865," *Bulletin of the History of Medicine,* XXVI (1952): 231–262.

The literature on surgical antisepsis, or "Listerism," is vast. The reception given to Lister's ideas by the profession in North America, and particularly in the United States, is dealt with in Gert H. Brieger, "American Surgery and the Germ Theory of Disease," *Bulletin of the History of Medicine,* XL (1966): 135–145. See also, Fritz Linder and Hugh Forrest, "The Propagation of Lister's Ideas," *British Journal of Surgery,* LIV (1957): 419–421; and, Astley Paston Cooper Ashhurst, "The Centenary of Lister

(1827-1927): A Tale of Sepsis and Antisepsis," *Annals of Medical History,* IX (Fall, 1927): 205-221. The introduction of Listerism in Canada is covered in Charles G. Roland, "The Early Years of Antiseptic Surgery in Canada," in S. E. D. Shortt, ed., *Medicine in Canadian Society: Historical Perspectives* (Montreal: McGill-Queen's University Press, 1981): 237-251. Opposition to antiseptic surgery in Canada was led by William Canniff— who, besides writing the standard medical history of Upper Canada, was one of the nation's leading surgeons and the first Canadian to author a textbook in medical science. Canniff commented that he could see no reason why it was necessary "to summon the aid of minute germs to account for degeneration and death and decomposition of organic matter in connection with bruised and lacerated tissues." See William Canniff, "An Examination of the Merits of Carbolic Acid as a Remedial Agent in the Practice of Surgery, with a Glance at its History," *Canada Medical Journal,* VI (January, 1870): 295-304. Roland points out that there is no evidence that Canniff, who lived until 1910, "ever accepted the principles of antiseptic surgery." "Antiseptic Surgery in Canada," 245.

It should be noted that no poorly qualified physician, licensed or not, attempted to perform major surgery, either before or after the introduction of effective anesthetics. As one practitioner noted in 1851, surgery was an area of medicine in which "the well-instructed aspirant treads on certain ground, and has nothing to fear from the rivalry or impertinent interference of quackery." "Senex," "Past and Present State of the Medical Profession—Homoeopathy," *Boston Medical and Surgical Journal,* XLIV (1851): 339, quoted in William G. Rothstein, *American Physicians, in the Nineteenth Century: From Sects to Science* (Baltimore: The Johns Hopkins University Press, 1972): 250. Less qualified practitioners, particularly unlicensed practitioners, tended to confine themselves to diagnosing illnesses and prescribing medications.

[93] See Rothstein, *American Physicians,* 262. A detailed analysis of the causes for the dramatic drop in mortality rates in England from the mid-nineteenth century to the early twentieth century and the very limited contribution that medical therapeutics made to this decline appears in Thomas McKeown, *The Role of Medicine: Dream, Mirage, or Nemesis?* (2d ed.; Princeton: Princeton University Press, 1979): 29-113, and *idem, Medicine in Modern Society: Medical Planning Based on Evaluation of Medical Achievement* (London: George Allen & Unwin Ltd., 1965): 41-58. McKeown's conclusions, of course, are equally applicable to Canada.

[94] "College of Physicians and Surgeons of Ontario," [Proceedings of the Medical Council, June, 1871], *Canada Lancet,* III (July, 1871): 462.

[95] "Ontario Medical Council, Minutes and Proceedings," [June, 1878], *ibid.,* X (July, 1878): 346-347.

[96] "Ontario Medical Council, Minutes and Proceedings," [July, 1877], *ibid.,* IX (August, 1877): 363; and, MacNab, *Legal History of Health Professions,* 20-21.

⁹⁷ A.M. Cooke, *A History of the Royal College of Physicians,* Vol. III (Oxford: Clarendon Press for the Royal College of Physicians, 1972): 854-856.

⁹⁸ MacNab, *Legal History of Health Professions,* 21.

⁹⁹ *Ibid.*

¹⁰⁰ "College of Physicians and Surgeons of Ontario," *Canada Medical and Surgical Journal,* VII (May, 1879): 476-477. In the following year, the Council was informed by the Under-Secretary of State of "the steps which are being taken in the matter of the proposed change in the Imperial Medical Act. The letter [from the Under-Secretary] stated that correspondence was going on between the Dominion and the Imperial Government on the subject." "Ontario Medical Council, Minutes and Proceeedings," [July, 1880], *Canada Lancet,* XII (August 1880): 372.

¹⁰¹ "Ontario Medical Council, Minutes and Proceedings," [June, 1878], *ibid.,* X (July, 1878): 349. Even though each academic session lasted only six months, the educational requirements of the Ontario medical board could not be met unless each session were taken in a separate calendar year.

¹⁰² "Ontario Medical Council, Minutes and Proceedings," [July, 1880], *ibid.,* XII (August, 1880): 367-368.

¹⁰³ *Ibid.,* 368. Many physicians felt that the Council had not gone far enough in increasing the preliminary educational requirements. The *Canada Lancet* had seriously proposed a university degree as the prerequisite for medical study as early as 1875. "It is a point that now may be fairly agitated in Ontario and in all the older Provinces of Canada," it noted, "whether a collegiate course in Arts ought not to be exacted as preliminary to the medical courses or as essential to an academical degree in medicine." "Preliminary Medical Education," *ibid.,* VII (July, 1875): 344.

¹⁰⁴ "The Ontario Medical Act and American Graduates," *ibid.,* XIII (February, 1881): 186-187.

¹⁰⁵ *Ibid.,* 187.

¹⁰⁶ "Ontario Medical Council," [Proceedings of the Medical Council, April, 1870], *Canada Medical Journal,* VI (May, 1870): 507.

¹⁰⁷ Michael Sullivan, "Presidental Address, Canada Medical Association," *Canada Medical and Surgical Journal,* XIII (September, 1884): 94.

¹⁰⁸ Sir William Osler, "The Growth of a Profession," *ibid.,* XIV (October, 1885): 133.

¹⁰⁹ *Ibid.,* 138. Osler was one of the strongest supporters of protective legislation for physicians in the United States, his adopted home between leaving the chair of clinical medicine at McGill in 1885, at the age of 36, and his appointment as Regius Professor at Oxford in 1906. Although Osler's contributions to medicine were by no means negligible, they were rarely seminal and have become magnified by some over time. There is, of course, no excuse for the bombastic sentiment which marks Maude

Abbott's description of him. In writing of Osler's connection with McGill, Dr. Abbott remarked with all seriousness: "The exact niche which he will occupy in History's Temple we may not yet appraise. It is enough for us to know that to our graduate roll belongs the name, and to our University the nurture, of one who is already numbered among those Masters of human thought, whom Carlyle has rightly named the Heroes of the race, and whose appearing marks the epochs of this world's spiritual advance." Maude E. Abbott, *McGill's Heroic Past, 1821-1921* (McGill University Publications, Series VI [History and Economics], No. 1, October 12, 1921 [Montreal: McGill University Press, 1921]): 27. See also Donald Jack's preposterous description of Osler as "perhaps the most influential physician since Hippocrates." *Rogues, Rebels, and Geniuses: The Story of Canadian Medicine* (Toronto: Doubleday Canada Ltd., 1981): 639.

[110] The draft is reprinted in full in the *Canada Medical Record,* IV (December, 1875): 68-70.

[111] "Medical Bills," *ibid.,* IV (January, 1876): 94-95.

[112] "Medical Legislation in Quebec," *Canada Lancet,* VIII (January, 1876): 153-154.

[113] *Ibid.,* 154.

[114] The draft is reprinted in full in "Bill: An Act concerning the Medical Profession of the Province of Quebec," *Canada Medical and Surgical Journal,* IV (December, 1875): 276-288.

[115] *Ibid.,* 276.

[116] "Medical Bills," *Canada Medical Record,* IV (January, 1876): 94.

[117] See, for example, "Medical Legislation," *Canada Medical Record,* IV (March, 1876): 141-143, containing an attack on the *Record* by Dr. A. Dagenais, a member of the Montreal Medical Society, reprinted and translated from *l'Union Médicale du Canada,* together with the *Record*'s editorial reply: "The Medical Bill and 'The *Canada Medical Record,*'" *Canada Medical Record,* V (April, 1876): 153-156, reprinting an editorial attacking the *Record* for its stand on the Chapleau bill, translated from *l'Union Médicale du Canada,* V (February, 1876): 87 ff., and the *Record*'s response; and, "College of Physicians and Surgeons, L. C.," *Canada Medical and Surgical Journal,* IV (June, 1876): 574-575.

[118] The amendments appear in full in the *Canada Medical and Surgical Journal,* IV (May, 1876): 522-524. For a synopsis of the proceedings of the meeting, see "Semi-Annual Meeting of the College of Physicians and Surgeons, C. E.," *Canada Medical and Surgical Journal,* V (October, 1876): 188-190.

[119] "Medical Legislation," *Canada Medical Record,* V (December, 1876): 63.

[120] The delegation consisted of Dr. Russell and Dr. Fenwick of Montreal, representing the College of Physicians and Surgeons of Lower Canada; Dr. Howard of McGill University: Dr. F. W. Campbell of Bishop's University; Dr. Larue of Laval University; Dr. Rottot of Victoria College; Dr. Dage-

nais, representing the promoters of Mr. Chapleau's bill; and, Dr. Marsden, representing the medical profession in Quebec City. *Ibid.,* 64.

121 40 Vic., c. 26 (Quebec). The act is reprinted in full in "The New Medical Bill," *Canada Medical Record,* V (January, 1877): 86–90, and, "The Act of Amendment Relating to the Practice of Medicine in the Province of Quebec," *Canada Medical and Surgical Journal,* V (January, 1877): 326–336.

122 "College of Physicians and Surgeons of the Province of Quebec," [Triennial Meeting of the College and Meeting of the Board of Governors, Three Rivers, July, 1877], *Canada Medical and Surgical Journal,* VI (August, 1877): 95.

123 The 1847 act had stipulated that midwives practicing in Montreal, Quebec, and Three Rivers were required to obtain a certificate of competency from the College [10 & 11 Vic., c. 26, sec. 15 (Canada)]. The 1876 law, on the other hand, extended the Medical Board's power to admit females to the practice of midwifery to the entire province. When the act was later amended in 1879, however, it was found expedient to add the following provision:

"Nothing in this section or in the by-laws which may be made, shall prevent as it occurs often, women in the country, from practising midwifery or assisting midwifery without being admitted to the study or the practice of midwifery; but they must obtain a certificate from a duly licensed physician ascertaining that they have the necessary knowledge." [42 & 43 Vic., c. 37, sec. 17 (Quebec)].

124 "College of Physicians and Surgeons of the Province of Quebec," [Meeting of the Board of Governors, Quebec, September, 1877], *Canada Medical Record,* VI (October, 1877): 18.

The profession was outraged that in 1880 the Circuit Court in Montreal found in favor of a licensed midwife who sued for the recovery of fees for services tangential to attendance upon accouchement. The judge in the case agreed with a witness for the plaintiff that midwives were entitled to render services and give advice not only during pregnancy but also before pregnancy "in relation to placing or maintaining the female organs in a fit condition for conception or successful gestation." "A Legal Question," *Canada Medical and Surgical Journal,* VIII (May, 1880): 475–477.

125 "Prosecuting Quacks," *ibid.,* IX (October, 1880): 185.

126 42 & 43 Vic., c. 37 (Quebec).

127 [Triennial Meeting of the College of Physicians and Surgeons, Montreal, July, 1880], *Canada Medical Record,* VIII (July, 1880): 272.

128 *Ibid.*

129 "Prosecuting Quacks," *Canada Medical and Surgical Journal,* IX (October 1880): 185–186.

130 "College of Physicians and Surgeons," *Canada Medical Record,* IX (December, 1880): 69.

[131] "College of Physicians and Surgeons, Province of Quebec," *ibid.,* IX (August, 1881): 287. A listing of successful prosecutions against unauthorized practitioners in Quebec between May, 1881, and July, 1882, appears in "College of Physicians and Surgeons," *ibid.,* X (July, 1882): 239. Seventeen convictions were obtained during the period, of which three were against unlicensed midwives. Twelve practitioners were fined $25 plus costs, and two, $100 plus costs. The three convicted midwives were each fined between $10 and $20. Most judgments provided for 30 days' imprisonment in cases where the monetary penalties were not paid.

[132] 45 Vic., c. 32 (Quebec).

[133] "The Triennial Meeting of the College of Physicians and Surgeons, P.Q.," [Proceedings, Quebec, July, 1883], *Canada Medical Record,* XI (July, 1883): 236.

[134] "McGill University," *Canada Medical and Surgical Journal,* V (June, 1877): 575.

[135] "Medical Education," *ibid.,* VI (December, 1877): 283.

[136] "College of Physicians and Surgeons, P. Q.," *ibid.,* VI (December, 1877): 286.

[137] *Canada Medical Record,* VI (January, 1878): 101.

[138] 42 & 43 Vic., c. 37 (Quebec). Section 11 of the act, dealing with the licensing of graduates of medical schools outside the British Empire, employs language almost identical to that found in the resolution of the Medical Board adopted at its meeting in September, 1877. See "College of Physicians and Surgeons of the Province of Quebec," [Meeting of the Board of Governors, Quebec, September, 1877], *Canada Medical Record,* VI (October, 1877): 18.

[139] "The Triennial Meeting of the College of Physicians and Surgeons, P. Q.," *Canada Medical Record,* XI (July, 1883): 236.

[140] "Address by the President," *Transactions of the Canada Medical Association* (10th Annual Meeting), I (1877): 17.

[141] Data for the Ecole de Médecine during this period, when the school was engaged in a bitter dispute with Laval University, are incomplete, and are not included in the totals shown. The following figures for the Ecole de Médecine, however, are suggestive of the trends in enrollment and number of graduates:

Year	Students	Graduates
1882	111	6
1883	n/a	33
1884	n/a	n/a
1885	155	26
1886	159	24
1887	183	36
1888	177	37
1889	202	36
1890	213	53

Data are from *Medical Education and Medical Colleges in the United States and Canada, 1765–1886* (Springfield, Ill.: Illinois State Board of Health, 1886): 45; and, *Medical Education, Medical Colleges and the Regulation of the Practice of Medicine in the United States and Canada, 1765–1891* (Springfield, Ill.: Illinois State Board of Health, 1891): 16.

For an account of the school's struggle with the Montreal branch of Laval's medical faculty and for an insight into the enormous power of the Vatican over Quebec education during the period, see John J. Heagerty, *Four Centuries of Medical History in Canada* (2 vols.; The Macmillan Company of Canada, Ltd., 1928), II:103–110; and, Charles-Marie Boissonnault, *Histoire de la Faculté de Médecine de Laval* (Quebec: Les Presses Universitaires Laval, 1953): 212–223.

142 "A Central Examining Board," *Canada Medical and Surgical Journal,* XIV (July, 1886): 761.

143 "Changes in Our Medical Act," *ibid.,* XV (August, 1886): 55.

144 *Ibid.,* 57.

145 The text of the proposed amendments to the medical act is reprinted in "Amendments to the Medical Act," *ibid.,* XV (November, 1886): 252–254. A summary of the suggested revisions appears in "College of Physicians and Surgeons, Province of Quebec," *Canada Medical Record,* XIV (September, 1886)): 625–626.

146 The petition of the McGill University medical faculty appears in "The Medical Act," *Montreal Medical Journal,* XVII (July, 1888): 74–76.

147 *Ibid.,* 76.

148 "The New Medical Bill," *Montreal Medical Journal,* XXI (August 1892): 147.

149 "The Medical Bill," *Canada Medical Record,* XXI (Februry, 1893): 118. There is not one whit of evidence to support the contention that medical graduates in either Quebec or Great Britain were unemployed, much less starving, despite adverse economic conditions brought on by the depression of 1893.

150 "The Medical Bill," *ibid.,* XXI (March, 1893): 141.

151 34 Vic., c. 25 (Prince Edward Island).

152 Warren E. Kalbach and Wayne W. McVey, *The Demographic Bases of Canadian Society* (2d ed.; Toronto: McGraw-Hill Ryerson Ltd., 1979): 25.

153 Heagerty, *Four Centuries of Medical History,* I:264.

154 The comparable ratios for New Brunswick and Nova Scotia in 1871 were 1:1,544 and 1:1,480 respectively.

155 Heagerty specifies that "all the *bona fide* physicians of the Island were registered." *Four Centuries of Medical History,* I:264 (italics mine).

156 37 Vic., c. 6 (Prince Edward Island).

157 35 Vic., c. 31 (Nova Scotia).

158 The act originally exempted military physicians from its provisions, but the exemption was removed by amendment in 1880 [43 Vic., c. 6 (Nova Scotia)].

[159] "A Medical Act for Nova Scotia," *Canada Medical and Surgical Journal,* I (February, 1873): 380.

[160] See, for example, *Provincial Board v. Bond* (1890) 22 N.S.R. 153 (C.A.), where an unlicensed practitioner was shown to be treating tumors by the application of plasters. Although the trial court held that the act did not constitute the practice of medicine under the terms of the Nova Scotia statute, the appellate court reversed the judgment and allowed a penalty of $20 for one day's illegal practice plus costs.

[161] D. A. Campbell, "Medical Legislation in Nova Scotia; Past, Present and Future," *Maritime Medical News,* I (July, 1889): 99.

[162] *Ibid.*

[163] "Medical Legislation," *Canada Lancet,* XI (February, 1879): 185.

[164] R. P. Howard, "The President's Address, Delivered Before the Canada Medical Association at its 13th Annual Meeting in Ottawa," *Canada Medical and Surgical Journal,* IX (September, 1880): 67.

[165] 44 Vic., c. 19 (New Brunswick).

[166] The physicians originally comprising the Council, together with its officers, are listed in W. Benton Stewart, *Medicine in New Brunswick* (Moncton, N.B.: New Brunswick Medical Society, 1974): 53.

[167] 45 Vic., c. 30 (New Brunswick).

[168] 47 Vic., c. 17 (New Brunswick).

[169] "New Brunswick Medical Act," [Letter dated August 8, 1885], *Canada Lancet,* XVIII (September, 1885): 12.

[170] 49 Vic., c. 82 (New Brunswick).

[171] Heagerty, *Four Centuries of Medical History,* I:265–266; and, Ross Mitchell, *Medicine in Manitoba: The Story of Its Beginnings* ([Winnipeg]: Manitoba Medical Association, [1954]): 47–55. The population of Manitoba in 1871 was estimated at just over 25,000. Kalbach and McVey, *Demographic Bases,* 25.

[172] 34 Vic., c. 26 (Manitoba).

[173] 40 Vic., c. 13 (Manitoba).

[174] The first register, with the deletion of those physicians who never practiced in Manitoba, is reprinted in Mitchell, *Medicine in Manitoba,* 57–58. One of the three American medical-school graduates was a homeopathic physician. Dr. Charles Whitefield Clark, who received his license in Manitoba in December, 1882, took his degree from the Hahnemann Medical College in Chicago and was licensed by the Ontario Homeopathic Medical Board in 1866. He was later elected to membership on the Council of the Manitoba College as the representative of homeopathic practitioners in the province. *Ibid.,* 61.

[175] 49 Vic., c. 31 (Manitoba).

176 O.N.W.T. 1885, no. 11.

177 Hilda Neatby, "The Medical Profession in the North-West Territories," in Shortt, ed., *Medicine in Canadian Society,* 169.

178 Neatby writes: "At least where professional interests were at stake, doctors reported unlicensed practitioners." *Ibid.,* 170.

179 Quoted in Heber C. Jamieson, *Early Medicine in Alberta: The First Seventy-Five Years* (Edmonton: Canadian Medical Association, Alberta Division, 1947): 43.

180 Quoted in *ibid.,* 44.

181 O.N.W.T. 1888, no. 5.

182 In 1890, the ordinance was amended to provide for the registration of any diplomate of any medical college in Great Britain without examination [O.N.W.T. 1890, no. 14].

183 A. S. Munro, "The Medical History of British Columbia," *canadian Medical Association Journal,* XXVI (1932): 725.
     Munro's history appears in eight parts: Part 1: XXV (1931): 336–342; Part 2: XXV (1931): 470–477; Part 3: XXVI (1932): 88–93; Part 4: XXVI (1932): 225–230; Part 5: XXVI (1932): 345–348; Part 6: XXVI (1932): 601–607; Part 7: XXVI (1932): 725–732; and, Part 8: XXVII (1932): 187–193.

184 Munro, "Medical History of British Columbia," XXVI (1932): 725.

185 49 Vic., c. 13 (British Columbia).

186 Medical Act, 1886 (49 & 50 Vic., c. 48).

187 56 Vic., c. 27 (British Columbia).

188 The 1886 act explicitly applied to homeopathic applicants, who were required to sit the same examinations as were regular candidates. In 1893, an amendment to the law [53 Vic., c. 30 (British Columbia)] provided that homeopathic physicians holding diplomas from authorized schools requiring a three-year course of study "shall be bound to pass the regular examination of the Council, but only in: anatomy, physiology, pathology, chemistry, obstetrics, and surgery."

189 Munro, "Medical History of British Columbia," XXVI (1932): 725.

190 *Ibid.,* XXVI (1932): 230.

191 R. L. MacDonnell, "Introductory Address, Delivered at the Opening of the Fifty-Seventh Session of the Medical Faculty of McGill University, October 1, 1889," *Montreal Medical Journal,* XVIII (November, 1889): 324.

192 Thus, under its ordinance of 1885, the Northwest Territories exacted a registration fee of $50 from all new applicants, except in the case of resident practitioners registering for the first time, who were charged only one-tenth as much. Neatby, "Medical Profession in the Territories," 169.

CHAPTER 4
THE TRIUMPH OF THE GUILD SYSTEM, 1887-1912

[1] Canadian census data.

[2] In 1870, there were 75 medical schools operating in the United States. By 1880, this number had increased to 100, and by 1890, to 133. U.S. Department of Commerce, *Historical Statistics of the United States: Colonial Times to 1970* (2 vols.; Washington: Government Printing Office, 1975), I:76 [Series B 275-290].

[3] "Medical Incomes in Canada," *New York Medical Journal,* XLIV (August 7, 1886): 168. The median income is estimated from the following report: "There is only one medical man in the city who last year earned $5,000 from his profession, combined with the interest he received on his previous savings. There is not one man on the list who had $4,000, and only four who touched $3,000. When we come to the comparatively modest and moderate $2,000, we naturally conclude that we shall have a full legion. But no, we have only fourteen all told who come up to this figure. When we come to between $2,000 and $1,000, the number becomes encouragingly large. As many as fifty-one of the best known and greatly-sought-after doctors of our city are put down under their own hands and seals as having last year lived on from $1,000 to $1,800. Some of these are professors. There remains only the unfortunates who worry along with from $800 down almost to zero. Of these, we are sorry to say, there were last year thirty-six."

A section of the original *Globe* report, listing the incomes of 31 physicians and 42 of the leading clergymen of Toronto, is reproduced in Godfrey, *Medicine for Ontario,* 141. The sample shows that of the physicians there mentioned, 23 earned $1,000 or more, while 32 clergymen earned $1,000 or more. The *Globe*'s somewhat sensationalistic headline to the story reads: "The Singular Poverty of the Medical Profession—a Fearful Warning to Medical Students—Keep Out of Such a Poor Business."

[4] "Average weekly hours and wages for males over sixteen years of age, selected occupations, Ontario, 1884 to 1889," *Historical Statistics of Canada,* M. C. Urquhart and K. A. H. Buckley, eds. (Toronto: The Macmillan Company of Canada Ltd., 1965): 93 [Series D 166-167]. The data show printers averaging $8.51 per week, carpenters $9.97 per week, and plumbers $10.91 per week. Assuming a fifty-two week work year, these figures generate average annual incomes of $443, $518 and $567 respectively.

[5] "Range of wages paid in selected occupations as reported by immigration agents, selected areas, 1881 to 1904," *ibid.,* 95 [Series D 196-207].

[6] "The Ontario Medical Council," *Canada Lancet,* XVI (July, 1884): 355.

[7] 50 Vic., c. 24 (Ontario).

[8] The 1874 Ontario act contained the following clause: "Any registered med-

ical practitioner who shall have been convicted of any felony in any court shall thereby forfeit his right to registration, and by the direction of the council his name shall be erased from the register, or in case of a person known to have been convicted of a felony, who shall present himself for registration, the registrar shall have power to refuse such registration." 37 Vic., c. 30 (Ontario). In 1879, the courts ruled that registration could not be denied a convicted felon who had undergone his whole sentence, regardless of the language of this provision of the medical act. It was held that under the Criminal Procedure Act, 1869, (Canada), c. 29, sec. 128, where "an offender convicted of a felony not punishable with death, who had endured the punishment to which he was adjudged, the punishment so endured should, as to the felony, have the like effect as a pardon under the Great Seal." *R. v. College of Physicians and Surgeons: Re McConnell* (1879) 44 U.C.Q.B. 146 (C.A.).

9 "Unprofessional Advertising," *Canada Lancet,* XX (September, 1887): 26–27.

10 Elizabeth McNab, *A Legal History of Health Professions in Ontario* (A Study for the Committee on the Healing Arts [Toronto: Queen's Printer, 1970]): 34. Of the other two cases, Dr. John McEown could not be located and hence could not be served with a summons. "The First Meeting of the Newly Elected Medical Council," [Minutes of the Ontario Medical Council, Toronto, June, 1890], *Canada Lancet,* XXII (July, 1890): 356. The fourth case apparently concerned a Dr. James C. Bright, who had been found guilty of administering an abortifacient by a court of law and whose name was ordered struck from the register. Charles M. Godfrey, *Medicine for Ontario; A History* (Belleville, Ont.: Mika Publishing Co., 1979): 224.

11 "The First Meeting of the Newly Elected Medical Council," *Canada Lancet,* XXII (July, 1890): 356.

12 *Ibid.*

13 MacNab, *Legal History of Health Professions,* 34.

14 "College of Physicians and Surgeons of Ontario," [Proceedings of the Ontario Medical Council, Toronto, June, 1892], *Canada Lancet,* XXIV (August, 1892): 371.

15 Godfrey, *Medicine for Ontario,* 224.

16 *Re Washington* (1893) 23 O.R. 299 (C.A.).

17 Godfrey, *Medicine for Ontario,* 225. It appears that this was not the end of Dr. Washington. Godfrey reports that "Washington must have been a popular physician—so popular that Dr. William E. Bessey was charged in 1898 with impersonating Washington and carrying on in the same manner. The prosecutor alleged that Bessey had represented himself as Washington, had put up one of Washington's cards in a hotel in Kingston and had made improper and fraudulent bargains for the cure of 'numerous patients.'" In his defense, Bessey claimed that his impersonation was purely a

coincidence and that he suffered from a catarrhal condition that had badly affected his eyesight. "The Discipline Committee," continues Godfrey, "voted to erase Dr. Bessey from the Register." *Ibid.*

[18] Quoted in Godfrey, *ibid.,* 227–228.

[19] "The Late Action of the Discipline Committee," *Canada Lancet,* XXV (January, 1893): 178. The same meeting of the disciplinary committee also considered the case of a Dr. Anderson who was charged with "having been connected with a band of itinerant doctors, the 'College of Eminent Physicians and Surgeons'; with entering into conspiracy with one Murray (now in jail in Liverpool for fraud, and illegally practising medicine) for the purpose of deceiving suffering people; allowing his name to be used as a registered practitioner for the purpose of carrying out the fraudulent scheme, and of evading the Ontario Medical Act."

[20] Godfrey, *Medicine for Ontario,* 228.

[21] *Ibid.,* 225–230,

[22] *Allinson v. General Council of Medical Education and Registration* (1894) 1 Q.B. 750, at 754, quoted in MacNab, *Legal History of Health Professions,* 35.

[23] *Re Crichton* (1906) 13 O.L.R. 271 (C.A.).

[24] MacNab, *Legal History of Health Professions,* 35.

[25] *Re Stinson and College of Physicians and Surgeons* (1910) O.L.R. 627 (C.A.).

[26] "The Ontario Medical Council," *Canada Lancet,* XVI (July, 1884): 356. There is some indication that as the Ontario licensing law became more restrictive and the incomes of physicians practicing in the province rose, medicine became an increasingly attractive profession for the children of wealthier parents, who could afford to underwrite the costs of a university education before their sons settled on a future occupation.

[27] For example, Dr. T. Aikins, speaking at the convocation of the University of Toronto medical faculty in 1889, noted that terms of nine months' duration would "do away with the need for 'cramming' for examinations as at present." "Is a Six Months' Session Not Quite Long Enough for Both Professors and Students, in the Medical Colleges?" *Canada Lancet,* XXI (May, 1889): 281.

[28] "The Summer Session," *Canadian Practitioner,* XV (June 1890): 288.

[29] 54 Vic., c. 26 (Ontario).

[30] "College of Physicians and Surgeons of Ontario," [Proceedings of the Ontario Medical Council, Toronto, June, 1892], *Canada Lancet,* XXIV (July, 1892): 343.

[31] "The Ontario Medical Council," *ibid.,* XXIII (July, 1891): 347–348.

[32] "The Ontario Medical Council," *Canadian Practitioner,* XVI (June, 1891): 281.

[33] Editorial, *Maritime Medical News,* III (November, 1891): 199.

34 "The Overcrowding of the Medical Profession," *Canada Lancet,* XXV (January, 1893): 177–178.

35 "Over-Production of Medical Men," letter from "Medicus," dated November, 1891, *ibid.,* XXIV (December, 1891): 123.

36 R. L. MacDonnell, "Introductory Address, Delivered at the Opening of the Fifty-Seventh Session of the Medical Faculty of McGill University, October 1, 1889," *Montreal Medical Journal,* XVIII (November, 1889): 323.

37 "Provincial Medical Boards," letter from William Osler, dated December 2, 1889, *Montreal Medical Journal,* XVIII (December, 1889): 479. See, also, a second letter from Osler, dated January 2, 1890, in which he remarks that "the Boards have done splendid service for the profession and for the public in the Canadian Provinces. They form permanent organizations which are not likely to be disturbed, and it is of the utmost importance that the Colleges work harmoniously with them." *ibid.,* XVIII (February, 1890): 612. Osler's second letter replies to a series of queries put to him by Dr. MacDonnell in a letter appearing in the same number of the *Journal; ibid.,* 610–611.

38 "State Control of Medical Schools," *Canada Medical Record,* XVIII (January, 1890): 95. The same article notes that physicians visiting Montreal from the United States "take away about $30,000 of fees from the honest practitioners of Montreal alone per annum." *Ibid.*

39 "The Ontario Medical Council," [Proceedings of the Ontario Medical Council, Toronto, June, 1895], *Canadian Practitioner,* XX (July, 1895): 531–532.

40 "The fact seems to be that a *specific certificate* is required; that equivalents are totally ignored, and that no matter how well a man may be educated, nor what proof he may present of a good training, evidenced by his having passed certain examinations, he cannot enter the sacred fold of the active medical profession without presenting to the registrar one, and one only, specific Departmental certificate. The single exception made is in favor of graduates in arts, who are entitled to register by statute." "Matriculation in Medicine in Ontario," *Canada Lancet,* XXVIII (November, 1895): 99.

41 *Ibid.,* 100.

42 "Matriculation in Medicine in Ontario," *ibid.,* XXVIII (December, 1895): 134.

43 *Ibid.*

44 The *Lancet* noted in 1895 that nearly half the students at one American medical college were from Ontario. *Ibid.*

45 Originating in Michigan, the Patrons of Industry established themselves in Ontario in 1890. Primarily a farmers' party, the Patrons espoused the elimination of protective tariffs and railway grants, the reservation of public lands for settlers only, an end to legislation establishing or encouraging the establishment of business and professional cartels, and the provincial taxing of corporation stocks and mortgages. At one point, the party toyed

with the notion of allying itself with the temperance movement but, although a majority of its membership favored prohibitory legislation, the Patrons went no further than issuing a declaration sympathetic to prohibition.

The organization's first political success came with the election of one of its members to the provincial legislature in a by-election preceding the general election of 1894. In the provincial general election of June, 1894, 17 Patrons were elected to Ontario's 94-member House of Assembly, making them the third-largest party in the province. The Patrons' popularity seems to have quickly dissipated, however, inasmuch as four years later, the party managed to elect only one member to the provincial legislature. The movement is discussed at some length in Louis Aubrey Wood, *A History of Farmers' Movements in Canada: The Origins and Development of Agrarian Protest, 1872–1924* (Toronto: Ryerson Press, 1924; reprint ed., Toronto: University of Toronto Press, 1975): 109–146. See, also, John David Smart, *The Patrons of Industry in Ontario* (unpublished M.A. dissertation, Carlton University, 1969).

[46] MacNab, *Legal History of Health Professions,* 32.

[47] *Ibid.,* 32–33.

[48] "The Medical Curriculum," *Canadian Practitioner,* XXI (April, 1896): 291–292.

[49] MacNab, *Legal History of Health Professions,* 33.

[50] The University of Toronto medical faculty, re-established in 1887, extended its formal course to five years in 1908, following the lead of McGill University. "A Degree in Arts," *Montreal Medical Journal,* XXXVI (December, 1907): 849.

[51] "Ontario Medical Council, Special Meeting, November 17th and 18th," [1908], *Canada Lancet,* XLII (January, 1909): 383–385. See also, "The Ontario Medical Council," *ibid.,* XLII (March, 1909): 488.

[52] "Overcrowded Professions," *Canada Medical Record,* XXIII (March, 1895): 142.

[53] "An Overcrowded Profession," *Canada Lancet,* XXVIII (September, 1895): 29.

[54] See the excellent studies by Thomas McKeown evaluating the effects of clinical medicine on mortality and morbidity rates in Britain: *The Role of Medicine: Dream, Mirage, or Nemesis?* (2d ed.; Princeton: Princeton University Press, 1979): 29–113; and, *Medicine in Modern Society: Medical Planning Based on Evaluation of Medical Achievement* (London: George Allen & Unwin Ltd., 1965): 38–58.

[55] Irving H. Cameron, "The Overcrowding and the Decadence of Scholarship in the Profession," *Montreal Medical Journal,* XXVIII (September, 1899): 651.

[56] *Ibid.,* 657. Banks' claim that all students who had passed their preliminary examinations were bound to pass their professional examinations was

totally without foundation. Indeed, in Ontario, the failure rate was extremely high. For example, at the June, 1904, meeting of the Medical Council, it was reported that of 142 candidates taking the final professional examination that spring, only 93 had passed. "The Ontario Medical Council Convention," [Proceedings, Toronto, June, 1904], *Canada Lancet,* XXXVII (August, 1904): 1141. See, also, "Ontario Medical Council Meeting," [Proceedings, Toronto, July, 1908], *Canada Lancet,* XLI (August, 1908): 955, where it was noted that between 60% and 65% of all those taking the Council's intermediate examinations that year had failed.

57 Irving H. Cameron, "The Overcrowding and the Decadence of Scholarship in the Profession," *Montreal Medical Journal,* XXVIII (September, 1899): 659. Dr. Cameron's remarks are heavily sprinkled with Latin phrases and sentences, no doubt to indicate that his own erudition was no lower than that demanded of future practitioners. That the greater part of his audience probably did not understand a word not uttered in plain English does not appear to have detracted from the popularity of his address.

58 "Medical Education," *Martime Medical News,* XII (August, 1900): 279.

59 "The State and the Medical Profession," *Canada Lancet,* XL (December, 1906): 363–364.

60 "The Ontario Medical Council," [Proceedings, Toronto, June, 1895], *Canadian Practitioner,* XX (July, 1895): 538. The prosecutor's report for 1897 is reproduced in Godfrey, *Medicine for Ontario,* 142. It indicates that in the previous twelve months, 34 persons were successfully prosecuted for illegal practice in the province and fined a total of $1,413.

61 "College of Physicians and Surgeons of Ontario," [Proceedings of the Medical Council, Toronto, June, 1892], *Canada Lancet,* XXV (October, 1892): 61.

62 *Ibid.*

63 24 O.R. 561 (C.A.).

64 *R. v. Valleau* (1900) 3 C.C.C. 435 (Ont.). Earlier, in *R. v. Stewart* [(1880) 17 O.R. 4], the defendant was acquitted on a charge of practicing medicine without license on the grounds that he prescribed no drugs, claiming that he could cure solely by looking intently at the patient.

65 "Christian Science Wins," *Canada Lancet,* XXX (April, 1898): 422.

66 "President's Address, Ontario Medical Association," *ibid.,* XXXIV (July, 1901): 573–574.

67 "Christian Scientists in Court," *ibid.,* XXXVIII (March, 1905): 660.

68 "The Ontario Medical Council Convention," [Proceedings, Toronto, June, 1904], *ibid.,* XXXVII (August, 1904): 1141.

69 "Christian Scientists in Court," *ibid.,* XXXVIII (March, 1905): 660.

70 "Annual Meeting of the Ontario Medical Council," [Proceedings,

Toronto, July, 1905], *ibid.*, XXXVIII (July, 1905): 1086.

71 *Ibid.*, 1087. The Council noted in its minutes that "the words 'or any other method of healing,' are supposed to cover the case of the Christian Scientists and other faith healers. As brought down in the report of the Legislative Committee, read by Dr. Robertson, the words read 'art of healing.' 'Art' was changed to 'method,' as the Council did not wish to admit that Christian Science was an art." *Ibid.*

72 MacNab, *Legal History of Health Professions,* 37.

73 The decision is quoted in full in "The Ontario Medical Act — An Important Judgment," *Canada Lancet,* XL (January, 1907): 457–459.

74 *Re Ontario Medical Act* (1906) 13 O.L.R. 501, at 508 (C.A.).

75 13 O.L.R. 501, at 511–512.

76 "The Ontario Medical Act — An Important Judgment," *Canada Lancet,* XL (January, 1907): 457.

77 The bill is reprinted in full in "Proposed Osteopath Bill," *ibid.,* XL (April, 1907): 753–757.

78 "The Osteopath Bill," *ibid.,* XL (April, 1907): 728.

79 "Osteopathy," *ibid.,* XL (July, 1907): 1047–1048.

80 MacNab, *Legal History of Health Professions,* 38.

81 "Osteopathy Again," *Canada Lancet,* XLIII (November, 1909): 162.

82 "The Osteopath Bill," *ibid.,* XLIII (April, 1910): 564–565. At the same time, the regular profession was confronted with a new challenge in the form of the incorporation of the provincial Optometrists Association. All attempts by the Medical Council to have the Association's charter annulled met with failure. MacNab, *Legal History of Health Professions,* 38.

83 MacNab, *Legal History of Health Professions,* 38.

84 "The Ontario Medical Council and Osteopathy," *Canadian Medical Association Journal,* II (June, 1912): 514.

85 MacNab, *Legal History of Health Professions,* 47. Legal tolerance of drugless practitioners received a serious setback in 1917, with the release of the *Hodgins Report on Medical Education in Ontario* (Toronto: King's Printer, 1917). Mr. Justice Frank E. Hodgins of the Ontario Supreme Court had been appointed to head a commission of inquiry regarding osteopaths and other drugless healers in 1915. The report not only condemned chiropractic — "Their repudiation of all modern scientific knowledge and methods is such that it would be impossible to recommend any way in which they could be allowed to practice and by which the public could be safeguarded." — but also concluded that "no concessions" be made in the province's medical laws to accommodate osteopaths. With respect to Christian Scientists, the report concluded: "Their rights should be carefully restricted to the bona fide exercise of the tenets of their religion, and they should possess no other or different right or immunity from that enjoyed by the clergyman or minister who is called in for the spiritual

benefit of a member of his communion and whose ministrations often react beneficially on physical suffering." And further, where Christian Science practitioners "come in contact with disease it seems hardly fair or reasonable... that there should not be required a sufficient knowledge of elementary medicine or of health and disease to prevent contagious and infectious diseases being unrecognized," and "to insist on this knowledge would not take away the right of the individual to trust himself to the efficacy of the treatment, absent or present, which depends in large measure on the mental and spiritual." Excerpts from the report appear in an article lauding the Commission's findings: "Medical Education in Ontario," *Journal of the American Medical Association,* LXXI (July 6, 1918): 42–43.

The definition of the practice of medicine recommended by the Commission for inclusion in the provincial medical act was taken almost verbatim from that formulated by a special committee of the Ontario Medical Council in 1914.

"The term 'practice of medicine' shall mean and include:

"(1) The use of any science, plan, method, system or treatment with or without the use of drugs or appliances for diagnosing, alleviating, treating, curing, prescribing or operating for any human disorder, illness, ailment, pain, wound, infirmity, injury, defect or deformity or physical or mental condition.

"(2) Diagnosing, alleviating, treating, curing, prescribing or operating for any human disorder, illness, disease, ailment, pain, wound, infirmity, injury, defect or deformity or physical or mental condition, and the holding out, offering or undertaking by any means or method to do any of the foregoing and including midwifery and the administration of anaesthetics.

"(3) Any manipulative or other kind of physical or mental treatment whatsoever, suggested, prescribed or advised, for body or mind, administered to or operated upon or intended to be followed by the patient himself or herself, intended or professing immediately or ultimately to benefit the patient, and the holding out, offering or undertaking by any means or method to use the same or to diagnose." *Hodgins Report,* 66, quoted in MacNab, *Legal History of Health Professions,* 46, fn. 287.

Thus, every conceivable ministration to the sick and infirm, or to those seeking any improvement in their physical or mental condition, from holding exercise classes, to teaching disturbed children, to giving confession, was to fall under the rubric of medical practice!

86 13 & 14 Geo. V., c. 35 (Ontario).

87 15 Geo. V., c. 49 (Ontario).

88 Under the act, not only could a well-trained osteopathic physician not use the title "Doctor" nor issue prescriptions or death certificates, but he was unable to treat his patients in public hospitals or use provincial laboratories. MacNab, *Legal History of Health Professions,* 49. The result of

this treatment by the authorities is evidenced by the fact that only 74 osteopaths were practicing in Ontario in 1962. Donald L. Mills, *Study of Chiropractors, Osteopaths and Naturopaths in Canada* (Royal Commission on Health Services [Ottawa: Queen's Printer, 1966]): 17.

[89] Mills, *Chiropractors, Osteopaths and Naturopaths*, 208, 221, 265.

[90] The following observations respecting the forms of medical care available to low-income Americans at the turn of the century are applicable, to a somewhat lesser degree, to Canada:

"For much of the population struggling through the depression of the 1890s, *private* medical services were an unnecessary luxury. As alternatives to paying private practitioners, the poor and newly arrived immigrants often sought care from one of a number of cheaper sources: the outpatient clinics of hospitals (known then as Hospital Dispensaries) where general practitioner and specialist care was available; from the public, medical school or city dispensaries, where medical care was also gratis to the consumer and from the 'lodge' or 'club' where, for a relatively small cost, a physician's services were guaranteed for a specified period of time. To the private practitioner, consumers using these alternative services were viewed as lost clients. The services themselves were viewed as a type of competition which was stealing away potential income. Furthermore, the private practitioner saw the specialist and the young, newly graduated physicians who were staffing the alternative care facilities as the precipitators of the crisis." Gerald E. Markowitz and David Karl Rosner, "Doctors in Crisis: A Study of the Use of Medical Education Reform to Establish Modern Professional Elitism in Medicine," *American Quarterly,* XXV (1973): 91.

[91] "Improvement in the Character of the Medical Profession," *Canada Lancet,* XXIII (April, 1891): 249.

[92] "The Ontario Medical Council," *ibid.,* XXVI (July, 1894): 345-346.

[93] Quoted in Godfrey, *Medicine for Ontario,* 204.

[94] "The 'Lodge Doctor' in Relation to Medical Ethics," *Montreal Medical Journal,* XXVIII (May, 1899): 390.

[95] Dr. Goodwin's remarks read like the testimony of a reformed sinner. He confesses at one point: "Years ago I offered to give them [club practice] up if no one else would take them. Now I have given them up and shall do what I can do to induce others to forego them. Finally I wish to say that I have set down naught in malice. I have been a sinner against the code in some respects, but I have taken frequent opportunities of speaking well of the brethren. Seldom have I spoken against any. When I have done so it has been by way of retaliation, but I am aware that even this, according to highest ethical standards, cannot be defended." F. W. Goodwin, "Medical Ethics," *Maritime Medical News,* XIV (June, 1902): 198-199.

[96] *Ibid.,* 197.

[97] "The Business Side of the Profession," *Canada Lancet,* XXXIX (October, 1905): 170.

The *Lancet* chose the occasion to add an attack on "the abuse of hospital charity," which, it noted, was partly accounted for by the "need for clinical material" for educational purposes. But, "much as the student's side of the case has to be considered," it continued, "the side of the general practitioner must not be overlooked. He was once a student, and therefore not unreasonable; but he is now a qualified practitioner, and must make a living. It is quite plain that the more the public is pauperized to the advantage of the student of medicine, the worse will it be for him when he passes from the college halls and hospital wards into the realities of his professional life. Whether for clinical material or for any other reason, no hospital has the right to do anything that would cheat a member of the profession out of a fee. The law society gives no legal advice, nor are there any law hospitals. The only persons who should receive free attendance are those who can establish their claim to be ranked as paupers, and can show that they are unable to pay for medical attendance. The test should in no case be the fact that he selects a public ward, and is willing to become the subject of clinical study as a means of obtaining free medical or surgical advice. The length to which this pauperizing process is being carried on in the large cities where there are medical colleges is alarming. But it is felt throughout the entire country. People of means are leaving their own localities constantly and betaking themselves to the large cities where they can secure cheap hospital rates, and free attendance. We think the time is not far off when the profession will take some action in this matter. The profession can be protected, and, yet, the interests of medical colleges not be made to suffer in the least." *Ibid.,* 171.

98 In 1907, the *Lancet* felt the need once again to refer to lodge practice as a "great and growing evil." "The Medical Profession," *ibid.,* XL (June, 1907): 937.

99 Editorial, *Canada Medical Journal,* I (June, 1852): 244–245.

100 *Facett v. Mothersell* (1864) 14 U.C.C.P. 104.

101 *Jackson v. Hyde* (1869) 28 U.C.Q.B. 294 (C.A.).

102 John Ordronaux, *The Jurisprudence of Medicine* (Philadelphia: T. & J. W. Johnson & Co., 1869), sec. 54, quoted in Robert Vashon Rogers, *Law and Medical Men* (Toronto: Carswell & Co., 1884): 77.

103 *Kempffer v. Conerty* (1899) 2 O.L.R. 658n. (C.A.).

104 *McNulty v. Morris* (1901) 2 O.L.R. 656 (C.A.).

105 *Town v. Archer* (1902) 4 O.L.R. 383.

106 *Gerbracht v. Bingham* (1912) 23 O.W.R. 82, 4 O.W.N. 117, 7 D.L.R. 259. There appears to be a possibility of this changing. In October, 1983, the Ontario Supreme Court, in *Soldwisch v. Toronto Western Hospital,* held that denying the plaintiff the right to a jury trial in medical malpractice suits was "legally insupportable." The Court ruled that the practice of permitting judges alone to hear such cases "must be held to be wrong in principle and must no longer be followed, no matter its antiquity, no matter the stature of those who developed and followed it." How effective this

ruling will in fact prove in reversing a tradition of such long standing has yet to be seen, especially since the Court held that the very case before it was of such complexity that it was beyond the abilities of any jury to reach a competent verdict! The case is reported in "Juries ruled competent to judge malpractice," *The Globe and Mail,* October 13, 1983: 1, 2.

107 At least this is the view of one leading authority. See Earl A. Cherniak, "Statutory Enactments Relating to Hospitals, Doctors, Dentists and Pharmacists," *Special Lectures of the Law Society of Upper Canada* (1963): 123.

108 MacNab, *Legal History of Health Professions,* 23.

109 50 Vic., c. 24, sec. 2 (Ontario).

110 Dates of first passage of similar legislation are: Manitoba: 51 Vic., c. 36, sec. 9 (1888); Prince Edward Island: 55 Vic., c. 42, sec. 27 (1892); British Columbia: 61 Vic., c. 9, sec. 61 (1898); New Brunswick: 3 Edw. VII, c. 118 (1903); Alberta: 6 Edw. VII, c. 28, sec. 59 (1906); Saskatchewan: 6 Edw. VII, c. 28, sec. 55 (1906); Newfoundland: 7 Eliz. II, no. 11 (1959). Nova Scotia enacted a limitation period of three years in 1930 [20 Geo. V, c. 34 (Nova Scotia)], but, in 1933, the period was altered to one year [23 & 24 Geo. V, c. 37 (Nova Scotia)].

111 With respect to the statute of limitations on negligence suits in the United States, Prosser summarizes the courts' treatment of medical malpractice as follows: "The obvious and flagrant injustice of such cases [in which there was a literal application of the limitation period] has led to the adoption of a series of transparent devices to get around the rule. Thus the negligent treatment, or at least the defendant's duty, is held to continue until the relation of physician and patient has ended; ... or the failure to recover and remove the sponge or other foreign object left in the plaintiff's body is held to be 'continuing' negligence. Quite recently [1969] there have been a wave of decisions meeting the issue head-on, and holding that the statute will no longer be construed as intended to run until the plaintiff has in fact discovered that he has suffered injury, or by the exercise of reasonable diligence should have discovered it." William L. Prosser, *Handbook of the Law of Torts* (4th ed.; St. Paul, Minn.: West Publishing Co., 1971): 144.

112 "It has always been held that the date that the patient learns of the negligent act is of no materiality and the limitation period runs without reference to the knowledge of the patient." Cherniak, "Statutory Enactments Relating to Doctors," 111.

113 (1892) 22 O.R. 369 (C.A.).

114 *Ibid.,* at 373.

115 *Town v. Archer* (1902) 4 O.L.R. 383.

116 R.W. Powell, "The President's Address," *Montreal Medical Journal,* XXIX (September, 1900): 646–647.

117 *Ibid.,* 647.

118 "Medical Defence," *Montreal Medical Journal,* XXX (October, 1900):

795–796. See also, Dr. W. S. Muir's address before the Maritime Medical Association in July, 1901, which refers to the pressing need for such an association. "Presidential Address," *Maritime Medical News,* XII (July, 1901): 288.

119 "A Medical Defence Union," *Canada Lancet,* XXXIV (February, 1901): 325.

120 See the *Lancet*'s editorial, "A Dominion Medical Defence Union," *Canada Lancet,* XXXIV (August, 1901): 682–683.

121 George Elliot, "The Winnipeg Meeting of the Canadian Medical Association," *Canada Lancet,* XXXV (September, 1901): 7–9.

122 In 1905, the fee was raised to $5.00. In 1932, the Association expanded its coverage to members to include medical malpractice liability insurance, insuring its risk with Lloyd's of London; the rates charged its members naturally reflected this coverage. Canadian Medical Protective Association, *Eightieth Annual Report* (Ottawa: Canada Medical Protective Association, 1981); 13. In 1983, the annual fee stood at $500.00. *Eighty-second Annual Report* (1983): 42. At the end of 1983, the Association, in its *Introductory Booklet for New Members,* announced that its fees for 1984 would be staggered, depending on the physician's area of specialization. These fees range from $250.00/year for interns to $1950/year for obstetricians, anesthesiologists, and certain types of surgeons. The fee for practitioners of family medicine was set at $1200/year.

123 Editorial, *Canada Lancet,* XXXVI (December, 1902), reprinted in Canadian Medical Protective Association, *Eightieth Annual Report,* 34.

124 *Ibid.,* 35–37.

125 Membership figures, by province, from 1902 to 1907 appear in "The Canadian Medical Protective Association," *Canada Lancet,* XLI (October, 1907): 169.

126 "The Canadian Medical Protective Association," *Maritime Medical News,* XXI (December, 1909): 435.

127 *Ibid.*

128 Gilbert Sharpe and Glenn Sawyer, *Doctors and the Law* (Toronto: Butterworths, 1978): 245–246.

129 "The Protection of Quacks," *Canada Medical Record,* XVII (March, 1889): 141.

130 The code adopted by the Quebec College in September, 1878, is reprinted in full in "Code d'Ethique Médicale," *Union Médicale du Canada,* VII (November, 1878): 514–525.

131 "Medical Society Proceedings," [Provincial Medical Board, Quebec, September, 1897], *Canada Medical Record,* XXV (October, 1897): 717.

132 61 Vic., c. 30 (Quebec).

133 "Electoral Reform Committee," *Canada Medical Record,* XXVI (April, 1898): 200–207.

[134] "The College of Physicians and Surgeons of Quebec," *Montreal Medical Journal,* XXVII (March, 1898): 231–232.

One minor but recurring problem with which English-speaking physicians had to contend was the lack of decent English translations of the College's minutes and of its rules and regulations. Indeed, at the meeting of the Board of Governors in October, 1896, Dr. J. B. O'Connell felt compelled to remonstrate against the inadequate translation of the College's regulations. "College of Physicians and Surgeons of the Province of Quebec," *Canada Medical Record,* XXV (November, 1896): 103. The situation does not appear to have improved over the years. In commenting on the July, 1903, meeting of the full College, the *Montreal Medical Journal* noted: "The new rules and regulations were of course drawn up in French and then translated into English. But as it is hard enough for a person whose business it is to write, to write clearly, when his expression has passed through the mind of a translator, it is easy to see what lucidity there will be, and therefore, many of the regulations are hard to understand. One example will serve. Under the heading of 'duties of assessors' it is stated: 'every candidate who shall fail in any course, shall be obliged to repair this bad note at the final examination in following September; because every candidate failing in the primary examination cannot be admitted to follow the final course before repairing his failure with success.'" "The College of Physicians and Surgeons," *Montreal Medical Journal,* XXXII (August, 1903): 591–592.

[135] "District Electoral Committee of the Members of the Montreal Medico-Chirurgical Society," *Montreal Medical Journal,* (March, 1898): 237–239.

[136] "Electoral Reform Committee," *Canada Medical Record,* XXVI (April, 1898): 201–202.

[137] See the report of the meeting of the Board of Governors at Laval University in July, 1898, at which the reform candidates took their seats. *Canada Medical Record,* XXVI (July, 1898): 352–355.

[138] 63 Vic., c. 26 (Quebec.)

[139] 61 Vic., c. 31 (Quebec).

[140] 4 Edw. VII, c. 27 (Quebec); 8 Edw. VII, c. 59 (Quebec); 1 Geo. V (2d), c. 37 (Quebec).

[141] 63 Vic., c. 27 (Quebec).

[142] E. P. Benoit, "Matters of Paramount Importance to the Profession—The College of Physicians and the Pineault and Roy Laws," *Montreal Medical Journal,* XXX (July, 1901): 558–560.

[143] The 1904, 1908, and 1911 laws were similarly worded.

[144] E. P. Benoit, "Matters of Paramount Importance to the Profession—The College of Physicians and the Pineault and Roy Laws," *Montreal Medical Journal,* XXX (July, 1901): 561.

[145] *Ibid.*

[146] *Ibid.,* 562. Dr. Benoit's account notes that: "The very same day that Mr.

Gosselin won his case against the College in the Court of Revision (thus confirming definitely this judgment as far as Mr. Gosselin is concerned), Messrs. Chabot, Bernard, Brunet, Paradis, Filon and Millette applied in turn to Judge Caron [the trial judge in the Gosselin case], laying a claim not only to their license, but also to $1,000.00 damages each. The Judge granted to each of them $100.00 and their licenses." *Ibid.*, 562-563.

147 *Ibid.*, 563.

148 "The Judgment Against the College of Physicians and Surgeons of the Province of Quebec," *Montreal Medical Journal*, XXX (July, 1901): 565. See also, the *Journal*'s attack on the practice of the provincial legislature of occasionally passing a private bill by which a practitioner was licensed to practice in the province despite his having failed to be granted registration through the College. "Admission to Practice by Grace of Legislature," *ibid.*, XXXII (April, 1903): 306-308.

149 See "The College of Physicians and Surgeons," *ibid.*, XXXII (August, 1903): 591-594; and, "The College of Physicians and Surgeons Again," *ibid.*, XXXII (October, 1903): 740-743.

In 1907, the College succeeded in amending the medical act to provide that the professional curriculum be broadened and that every applicant complete four years of nine months each of formal training [7 Edw. VII, c. 43 (Quebec)].

150 Charles-Marie Boissonnault, *Histoire de la Faculté de Médecine de Laval* (Quebec: Les Presses Universitaires Laval, 1953): 295-300.

151 *Ibid.*, 296.

152 *Ibid.*, 300.

153 9 Edw. VII, c. 55 (Quebec).

154 The relevant section of the new law provided that: "Without limiting the meaning of the words 'practice of medicine', the attending of confinements, treating habitually and continuously following the treatment of diseases or surgical affections, either by giving medicine or by making use of mechanical, physical or chemical processes or of radiotherapy or of X rays, shall constitute the practice of medicine."

In 1918 [8 Geo. V. c. 56 (Quebec)], the definition was extended to include "the giving of medical consultations."

155 53 Vic., c. 10 (Prince Edward Island).

156 "The Medical profession of Prince Edward Island finding that the Medical Act in force was not suited to their wants, and at the same time being deficient in a great many ways, introduced before the Legislature at its last session and secured the passage of a Bill that is superior in a great many respects to the old one.... Prince Edward Island, although the last to swing into line in matters legislative, now occupies no inferior position, and is ready to extend offers of inter-provincial reciprocity." *Maritime Medical News*, IV (July, 1892): 134-135.

157 55 Vic., c. 42 (Prince Edward Island).

[158] 57 Vic., c. 19 (Prince Edward Island).

[159] "Maritime Medical Reciprocity and Medical Legislation in P.E. Island," *Maritime Medical News,* VI (May, 1894): 291–292.

[160] "Medical 'Free Trade,'" [Letter from Dr. R. MacNeill of Stanley Bridge, P.E.I., dated 25 April, 1893, to the editors of the *Presbyterian Witness*], *Maritime Medical News,* V (June, 1893): 88–89.

[161] 62 Vic., c. 24 (Prince Edward Island).

[162] 1 Geo. V, c. 22 (Prince Edward Island).

[163] The one exception concerned the practice of midwifery by females, which continued to remain exempt from the provisions of the medical act. See, for example, R.S.P.E.I. 1951, c. 94, sec. 37.

[164] 58 Vic., c. 35 (New Brunswick); and, 62 Vic., c. 23 (New Brunswick).

[165] 58 Vic., c. 35, sec. 2 (New Brunswick).

[166] 10 Geo. V, c. 52 (New Brunswick).

[167] 10 Geo. V, c. 52, sec. 53 (New Brunswick).

[168] Mills, *Chiropractors, Osteopaths and Naturopaths,* 223.

[169] 7 Eliz. II, c. 74, sec. 28 (New Brunswick).

[170] 62 Vic., c. 32, sec. 16(d) (Nova Scotia).

[171] 18 Eliz. II, c. 15 (Nova Scotia).

[172] "Professional Examinations of the Provincial Medical Board," *Maritime Medical News,* XV (June, 1903): 213. In a curious *volte-face,* the *News,* which had earlier celebrated the actions of the profession in Prince Edward Island as an example to the rest of the Maritimes for securing enactment of a statute providing for compulsory professional examinations before its Medical Council, now felt the need to apologize for a similar provision in the Nova Scotia law. "At first glance," it observed, "it seems decidedly unfair to compel men who have obtained qualifications from reputable schools of medicine to submit to the worry and additional expense of another examination before obtaining authority to practice.

"Not one substantial argument could be brought forward to support the change were the Medical Board of Nova Scotia taking the initiative on this question, but when we find the principle of a state examination in operation in all of the other provinces of the Dominion of Canada the matter assumes a different aspect. As a matter of simple justice to its own licentiates the Medical Board should not allow Nova Scotia to be a dumping ground for men who have failed to qualify for practice in the other provinces of Canada." *Ibid.,* 214.

[173] *Ibid.,* 213.

[174] Data are taken from medical directories for 1904, 1906, 1909, 1912, 1914, 1916, and 1918.

[175] Colin D. Howell, "Reform and the Monopolistic Impulse: The Professionalization of Medicine in the Maritimes," *Acadiensis,* XI (1981): 13.

Howell's informative article is, unfortunately, marred by too heavy a reliance on the medical journals themselves for his view of the actual status of the profession at the end of the nineteenth century. His conclusions that "irregular practitioners and quacks" were rampant and that the courts showed unusual sympathy to the plaintiffs in malpractice suits are based solely on the complaints of physicians in the medical press. *Ibid.,* 7.

In addition, there is some question respecting the assumption underlying much of the article. "It should be noted," Howell comments, "that the impulse towards professional reorganization was strongest among the elite members of the profession — those attached to hospitals, medical colleges, and the public health bureaucracy — and weakest among the rank and file." *Ibid.,* 5. Indeed, it is more likely that the opposite is true, as rank and file physicians sought to obtain the respectability, deference, and honoraria previously accorded only the profession's elite.

Despite these shortcomings, however, Howell's essay contains much useful information on the profession in the Maritimes from the 1880s to World War I.

176 The totals for 1910 are not good indicators of the number of physicians actually practicing in Nova Scotia in that year since many practitioners from the Maritimes registered in more than one province. This process was facilitated during the period from 1894 to 1898, when the Maritimes effected reciprocal registration.

177 Fortunately these effects proved only temporary, and gradually disappeared after Dominion reciprocity was introduced in 1912.

178 John Stewart, "Presidential Address," [Nova Scotia Medical Association, July, 1908], *Maritime Medical News,* XX (October, 1908): 391.

179 7 Edw. VII, c. 52 (Nova Scotia).

180 The incident is recounted in John Stewart, "Presidential Address," *Maritime Medical News,* XX (October, 1908): 393; and, Howell, "Professionization of Medicine," 17, fn. 56. Under the new provision, Dyas appealed to the courts, where the Board's decision to erase Dyas' name was upheld.

181 11 & 12 Geo. V, c. 29 (Nova Scotia).

182 Female midwives were exempt from the provisions of Nova Scotia's medical acts until recently, but had been required to prove their competence to the Medical Board and to obtain a certificate to that effect when practicing within the city of Halifax. [See, for example, the medical act of 1954, 3 Eliz. II, c. 4, sec. 2 (Nova Scotia).] In 1969 [18 Eliz. II, c. 15 (Nova Scotia)], all provisions exempting female midwives were deleted from the medical act.

183 John Stewart, "Presidential Address," *Maritime Medical News,* XX (October, 1908): 394. The problem of charitable medical care had been a long-standing irritant to the profession in Nova Scotia. In 1890, the *News* strongly supported the idea of a means test for users of hospital dispensaries. "Of all the plans so far adopted with a view to preventing the abuse

of dispensaries and other medical charities," it editorialized, "that of having a wage limit seems to have yielded the best results. Under this plan a single man who receives more than a certain weekly sum must pay something for medical attendance. The wage limit is of course a larger sum for a married man, and in addtiion so much is allowed per child. This method of selection by no means altogether precludes the possibility of unequal and indeed undesirable pressure in individual cases, chiefly because the wage that means enough and contentment to one man is associated with debt, embarrassment and unhappiness in another.

"The number and equipment of the hospitals in most civilized countries is a credit both to their civilization and to their charity. Perhaps no service is so deserving of public and private support as a competent and adequate hospital service. But into this noble service may creep and has crept, such an indiscriminateness of charity, and so *ready* a dispensation of its advantages as we believe to be neither due nor morally healthful to the receivers of the charity, nor right to the public and profession who provide it." *Maritime Medical News,* II (May, 1890): 46.

[184] One legal writer has observed of this provision: "Through this comprehensive definition the Board, comprised entirely of physicians, could restrict developments that may compete with their notions about treatment of disease. In fact this has already happened with regard to acupuncture. The Board on February 21, 1976 made it an official policy that acupuncture be deemed to be a medical procedure and/or treatment modality within the [act's] definition [of medical practice]." Duncan Beaveridge, "Regulation of the Medical Profession in Nova Scotia," *Dalhousie Law Journal,* V (1979): 520–521.

[185] The provision in the 1921 act originally referred to "homeopathy, osteopathy or *optometry* or other system different than that taught in the so-called 'regular schools of medicine.'" (Italics mine.) In 1923 [13 Geo. V, c. 21, sec. 3 (Nova Scotia)], the provincial legislature, obviously made aware that they had, by this provision, required of optometrists the same level of preliminary and professional study required of physicians, deleted the reference to optometry.

[186] John J. Heagerty, *Four Centuries of Medical History in Canada* (2 vols.; Toronto: The Macmillan Company of Canada, Ltd., 1928), II:305–306, 309.

[187] 56 Vic., c. 12 (Newfoundland).

[188] 60 Vic., c. 9 (Newfoundland).

[189] 6 Edw. II, c. 8 (Newfoundland).

[190] The practice of midwifery by females was exempt from the provisions of the Newfoundland medical acts. However, in 1920 [11 Geo. V, c. 18 (Newfoundland)], with the enactment of the Midwives' Act, the Governor-in-Council was empowered to make rules and regulations governing the training, qualifications, and registration of midwives in the colony and to fix penalties for their violation. With passage of the Health and Public

Welfare Act of 1931 [22 Geo. V, c. 12, secs. 347 to 372 (Newfoundland)], a Midwifery Board was created to examine, license, and register female midwives in the colony. The provisions of the Health and Public Welfare Act respecting midwifery were somewhat revised with enactment of the Midwifery Act of 1936 [1 Edw. VIII, no. 22 (Newfoundland)] and, with minor alterations, remain in force currently.

191 49 Vic., c. 31 (Manitoba).

192 In 1882, Dr. Charles Whitefield Clark, a graduate of the Hahnemann Medical College and a registrant of the Ontario Homeopathic Board, was entered upon the Manitoba medical register. Clark practiced in Winnipeg and appears to have been particularly popular. For many years he represented the homeopathic practitioners of the province on the Council of the College. Ross Mitchell, *Medicine in Manitoba: The Story of its Beginnings* ([Winnipeg]: Manitoba Medical Association, [1954]): 61.

193 51 Vic., c. 36 (Manitoba).

194 The revisions respecting homeopathy appear to have made no real difference to the composition of the profession in Manitoba, since homeopathic representation on the Council never increased beyond one member. These provisions were finally repealed and the following substituted in 1953 [2 Eliz. II (2d), c. 35, sec. 11 (Manitoba)]: "The council may admit to registration . . . any person who is a graduate of any homeopathic medical school or college that is approved by the University of Manitoba, and who has satisfactorily completed not less than twelve months' service in a resident medical capacity in one or more approved hospitals."

In 1964 [13 Eliz. II, c. 29 (Manitoba)], all references to homeopathy were removed from the province's medical act.

195 3 & 4 Edw. VII, c. 33 (Manitoba).

196 Heagerty, *Four Centuries of Medical History,* II:137.

197 Mills, *Chiropractors, Osteopaths and Naturopaths,* 225. Mills also reports that a number of chiropractors had begun operating in Manitoba at the beginning of the century. *Ibid.,* 211.

198 5 & 6 Edw. VII, c. 43 (Manitoba).

199 Thus, a chiropractor who had employed the title "Doctor," without being registered under the Manitoba act was held to be in violation of the act's provision against using a title implying that one were a registered practitioner. "The theory of chiropractic, being to cure a patient of disease or human ailment, has the same purpose as the practise of medicine, irrespective of the different methods used, and before this title can be used registration under the Act is necessary." *McDiarmid v. Elliot* (1934) 1 W.W.R. 722, 41 Man.R. 665.

200 9 Geo. VI, c. 43 (Manitoba).

201 9 Geo. VI, c. 5 (Manitoba.

202 O.N.W.T. 1894, no. 34. The provision appears to have also exempted from the Council's professional examinations physicians previously regis-

tered in another province, but the Council apparently disregarded this clause. In 1900, the legislature, in an attempt to encourage practitioners to enter the area, amended the medical statute [O.N.W.T. 1900, c. 15] to make clear that registrants from the other provinces within the Dominion need not sit the College's examinations. This action was taken without first consulting the College and was directly opposed to the policies of the College's Council. Despite the 1900 ordinance, the Council continued to require that all applicants other than British licentiates take their professional examinations before the College's own examiners. As a consequence, in 1903 [O.N.W.T. 1903 (2d), c. 15], the legislature once again amended the medical statute, permitting a rejected applicant to sue in the courts. The matter was finally settled in 1904, in *Re Sinclair*. Sinclair, a member of the Manitoba College, was refused registration by the Territories Council unless he first underwent its professional examinations. On a reference to the Supreme Court *en banc,* it was held that, under the terms of the Territories ordinance, Sinclair's name be entered upon the register of the Territorial College [7 Terr.L.R. 178 (C.A.)].

In any case, as Heagerty notes, "from the year 1900 onward, during which immigration was at its height, there was a steady influx of physicians into the Northwest Territories... [but] the demand was always greater than the supply." *Four Centuries of Medical History,* 1:266.

203 Hilda Neatby, "The Medical Profession in the North-West Territories," in S. E. D. Shortt, ed., *Medicine in Canadian Society: Historical Perspectives* (Montreal: McGill-Queen's University Press, 1981): 179.

204 *Ibid.,* 180. Neatby's account of the attempt to prosecute unlicensed practitioners operating in the Yukon during the gold rush is of some interest, if for no other reason than that it reveals the attitude of mind of the members of the Territories' Medical Council. "At the council meeting of January 1898," she writes, "the registrar reported much correspondence on medical practice there. It was agreed that Dr. N. J. Lindsay, a member of the council, who was planning to go to the Yukon, whether in a professional or other capacity is not clear, should be empowered to conduct examinations and accept registrations in order that what was later termed 'the very deplorable state of affairs' might be remedied. Dr. Lindsay paid his visit during 1898. He was unable to conduct examinations as the papers did not arrive. He did accept thirteen registrations, four of which were later invalidated. He also organized some sort of body, termed by him a college of physicians and surgeons, later referred to as the 'Yukon Medical Council,' about which nothing is very clear except that it seems to have been a kind of stepchild to the college of the Territories. It seems fair to assume from the addresses in the register that, in addition to nine fees from the Yukon, the council collected at least fifteen others from men planning to go there, a total of $1,200. Dr. Lindsay's expenses amounted to something over $100. Yet when the Yukon organization requested,

through Dr. Lindsay, financial aid in conducting prosecutions, the answer was that such fines as came in from the Yukon would be turned over to them, but that, as Dr. Lindsay had already contributed $10, nothing more should be asked." *Ibid.,* 180-181. By what authority the Territories Council assumed the right to collect an additional "registration" fee from physicians intending to practice in the Klondike, we are not told. Certainly the actions of Dr. Lindsay would be difficult to justify in law.

205 *Ibid.,* 179-180.

206 O.N.W.T. 1892, no. 24.

207 O.N.W.T. 1898, no. 22.

208 Neatby, "Medical Profession in the Territories," 182-183.

209 In light of this, Neatby's conclusion is striking. "There seems to have been a feeling," she observes, "that the cause of discipline suffered somewhat from the fact that the only punishment authorized was the extremely severe one of expulsion from the profession. No doubt, however, official censures were sufficient to warn those members of the public who were willing to be warned." *Ibid.,* 183.

Consider also her summary of the activities of the organized profession in the Territories: "The limited sources available make it very difficult to pass any judgment on the activities of the early leaders of the medical profession on the prairies. Like other newcomers they had to establish themselves and their families; and in order to do so, they had to exploit the professional training and the professional monopoly that was theirs. They were impatient at opposition, and they may sometimes too narrowly have assumed that what benefited the profession would benefit the public. But the Legislative Assembly and public opinion were well able to correct this tendency, and the constant stress on professional privileges of these able and energetic men was invaluable in modern pioneer communities whose insistence on medical services of some kind could make them an easy prey to any glib practitioner." *Ibid.,* 184.

210 *Ibid.*

211 6 Edw. VII, c. 28 (Saskatchewan).

212 *R. v. McSloy* (1917) 1 W.W.R. 112, 9 Sask.L.R. 265, 26 C.C.C. 381, 31 D.L.R. 725 (C.A.).

213 8 Geo. V (2d), c. 35 (Saskatchewan).

214 4 Geo. V, c. 54 (Saskatchewan).

215 Mills, *Chiropractors, Osteopaths and Naturopaths,* 224.

216 8 Geo. V (2d), c. 67 (Saskatchewan).

217 1926 [16 Geo. V, c. 38 (Saskatchewan)]; 1927 [17 Geo. V, c. 47 (Saskatchewan)]; 1929 [19 Geo. V, c. 56 (Saskatchewan)].

218 Mills, *Chiropractors, Osteopaths and Naturopaths,* 224.

219 "Drugless Practitioners in Saskatchewan," *Canadian Medical Association Journal,* XX (March, 1929): 318.

220 *Ibid.*

221 6 Geo. VI, c. 68 (Saskatchewan).

222 Mills, *Chiropractors, Osteopaths and Naturopaths,* 17.

223 6 Edw. VII, c. 28 (Alberta).

224 Unlike the Saskatchewan act, however, Alberta's 1906 statute applied to the practice of midwifery only in incorporated villages, towns, and cities having a resident physician. This exemption appears in all subsequent provincial medical acts.

225 Heber C. Jamieson, *Early Medicine in Alberta: The First Seventy-Five Years* (Edmonton: Canadian Medical Association, Alberta Divison, 1947): 54.

In 1909, the College received a minor setback in the courts. On an appeal from a physician who had had his name erased for unethical conduct by the College's disciplinary committee, the court ruled: "The section of the Act [dealing with the disciplining of physicians]... shows plainly... that the unbecoming or improper conduct referred to is of the same nature, though perhaps not of the same degree, as the criminal conduct mentioned in the same paragraph, and was intended primarily to deal with the relation of physicians with their patients, and their conduct as it might affect their patients, especially as criminal conduct as it affected other people was dealt with by the previous paragraph, and not for the purpose of regulating quarrels between physicians which might be grounds for civil actions in Court, much less for the purpose of regulating and enforcing that somewhat elastic doctrine known as professional ethics." *Re Bechtel* (1909) 10 W.L.R. 473 (Alta.).

Needless to say, nothing could have been further from the intentions of the profession when the bill was originally drafted. Physicians were fortunate that the medical act had been written in such a way as to permit a appeal from the College to the courts only in cases where a practitioner was punished by erasure of his name from the register, and not where a lesser punishment, such as suspension, was involved.

226 Assuming a constant growth rate between 1901 and 1911, the population of the province increased by 17.8% annually. The rate of increase in the number of physicians between 1906 and 1912 was approximately 19.4% per year.

227 *American Medical Directory* (Chicago: American Medical Association), 1906 and 1912. Jamieson's appendix of Alberta practitioners lists 202 registrants in 1906, of which all but one were previously registered in the North-West Territories, but these figures almost certainly over-estimate the number of physicians actually operating in the province in that year. The total number of registrants in Alberta through 1910, according to Jamieson, was 325. *Early Medicine in Alberta,* 141-198.

228 2 & 3 Geo. V, c. 27 (Alberta).

229 The original reading of the 1911 law contained a contradiction. One clause explicitly provided that "the examination of candidates for admission to practise medicine, surgery, midwifery, osteopathy or homeopathy in the Province of Alberta shall be under the control of the University of Alberta." The following section, however, specified that "the subjects of all examinations under this Act shall be such as are prescribed by the Senate of the University of Alberta except as to osteopaths and homeopaths." In 1913 [4 Geo. V (2d), c. 2 (Alberta)], the exemption accorded osteopaths and homeopaths was repealed.

All provisions respecting homeopathy were finally deleted from the province's medical act of 1975 [24 Eliz. II (2d), c. 26 (Alberta)].

230 It was not until 1926 [16 & 17 Geo. V, c. 19 (Alberta)] that the following provision was inserted into the medical statute: "Nothing in this Act contained shall apply to or affect those who practice the religious tenets of their church without pretending a knowledge of medicine or surgery." Until passage of this amendment, even the practice of Christian Science was held to violate the medical act.

231 10 & 11 Geo. V, c. 21, sec. 4 (Alberta).

232 Mills, *Chiropractors, Osteopaths and Naturopaths,* 224.

233 In the period 1891 to 1901, British Columbia had the highest rate of increase in population of any province and this growth rate was eclipsed only by the prairie provinces during the following decade. See Warren E. Kalbach and Wayne W. McVey, *Demographic Bases of Canadian Society* (2d ed.; McGraw-Hill Ryerson Ltd., 1979); 31, 34.

234 A. S. Munro, "The Medical History of British Columbia," *Canadian Medical Association Journal,* XXVI (1932): 725. Munro reports that thirty-nine physicians registered under the new medical act in 1886.

235 T. F. Rose, *From Shaman to Modern Medicine: A Century of the Healing Arts in British Columbia* (Vancouver: Mitchell Press Ltd., 1972): 54.

236 *Ibid.,* 93.

237 56 Vic., c. 30 (British Columbia). The 1886 act had stipulated that "homoeopathic physicians may be registered under this Act, on complying with the terms [respecting regular applicants]." 49 Vic., c. 13, sec. 53 (British Columbia).

238 61 Vic., c. 9 (British Columbia). It was with the enactment of this statute that all licensed physicians in the province were formally incorporated into the College of Physicians and Surgeons of British Columbia, under the direction of the Medical Council established by the 1886 act.

239 The Vancouver Medical Association was founded in 1886 and immediately took up the question of a tariff of fees and "other matters of material interest to the medical profession," including the problem of lodge practice. After a stormy beginning, the Association became firmly established

as the spokesman for physicians in the city and was successful in gaining enactment of a number of municipal by-laws insinuating the profession into the community, including the medical inspection of schools and the testing of the city's milk supply. The Victoria Medical Society, established in 1899 as successor to the Victoria Medico-Chirurgical Society, also appears to have concerned itself primarily with the economic status of the profession. Rose reports that the main subject of discussion at its early meetings centered on the propriety of contract practice, which it soon condemned as inimical to the interests of physicians. In 1900, the British Columbia Medical Association was formed. Although apparently neither as powerful nor as influential as the Vancouver Medical Association, it, too, added its voice to the need for more restrictive legislation. For a brief overview of these organizations, see Rose, *From Shaman to Modern Medicine,* 92–107.

[240] Mills, *Chiropractors, Osteopaths and Naturopaths,* 223.

[241] 9 Edw. VII, c. 6 (British Columbia).

[242] In 1921 [11 Geo. V, c. 38 (British Columbia)], provision for the examination of chiropractors and drugless practitioners who had satisfied certain educational requirements was included in the province's medical act. In both cases, graduation from a college offering instruction in the particular system of practice whose course was at least three years of six months each was required. In addition, candidates had to pass the Council's examinations in all the usual subjects, except in the principles and practice of medicine, where, instead, they were examined in their own system of treatment.

[243] This practice seems to have been fairly common among many physicians. In 1922 [12 Geo. V, c. 4 (British Columbia)], the medical act was once again amended to enlarge the sanctions available to the Council in dealing with practitioners found guilty of unprofessional conduct. Henceforth, the Council could simply suspend members of the College if it found erasure too severe a punishment.

The 1898 and subsequent acts permitted the Council to hear complaints against physicians charged with infamous or unprofessional conduct on the application of any three registered practitioners. However, a British Columbia court has held that the Council was not obligated to hold an inquiry unless it so chose since, according to the ruling, the power was a purely discretionary one. The specific case involved a physician charged with gross negligence, which the Council refused to consider on the ground that it was not its province to deal with an issue which might be the subject of an action at law. *Ex Parte Inverarity* (1903) 10 B.C.R. 268. The Council appears to have almost never used its powers of discipline, even in instances of the grossest malpractice. Rose reports that "in the whole history of organized medicine in the province to date [1968] only two doctors have been struck from the register for 'grossly unethical conduct', both of whom achieved reinstatement within a year or two." *From Shaman to Modern Medicine,* 93.

[244] 2 & 3 Geo. V, c. 27, sec. 3 (Alberta). As in Alberta, the law was so broadly worded that it included the practice of Christian Science. In 1930 [20 Geo. V, c. 42 (British Columbia)], the provincial legislature of British Columbia finally exempted religious practitioners by adding the following provision to the law: "Nothing in this Act contained shall apply to or affect those who practice the religious tenets of their church without pretending a knowledge of medicine or surgery, provided that the laws and regulations relating to contagious diseases and sanitary matters are not violated."

[245] *R. v. Barnfield (Sequah)* (1895) 4 B.C.R. 305.

[246] *R. v. Evans* (1916) 23 B.C.R. 128 (C.A.).

[247] *R. v. Telford* (1921) 2 W.W.R. 225, 29 B.C.R. 452. 36 C.C.C. 195, 58 D.L.R. 593 (C.A.).

[248] An analysis of the figures in table 1 of Margaret Andrews' article on medical practice in Vancouver between 1898 and 1920 shows that over 75% of the physicians practicing in the city were graduated from Canadian medical schools and that this proportion did not change over the course of the twenty years under study.

Location of Medical School	1898–1909 (%)	1910–1920 (%)
Canada	77.4	76.2
United States	12.8	10.9
Great Britain	9.2	9.5
Other or No Degree Indicated	.5	3.4

Data appear in Margaret W. Andrews, "Medical Attendance in Vancouver, 1886–1920," in Shortt, ed., *Medicine in Canadian Society,* 420.

[249] *Ibid.,* 419. Andrews' article is flawed by her misleading statement — belied by her own raw data — that the doctor-resident ratio in Vancouver showed a steady improvement between 1898 and 1920. She then states: "A ratio of five doctors per 10,000 of population was asserted as desirable by Abraham Flexner in his influential report of 1910 on medical education in the United States and Canada, and it is tempting to conclude immediately from this assertion that Vancouver had an overabundance of doctors." *Ibid.,* 418–420. Few historians of the medical profession would regard invoking Flexner on the desirable ratio of doctors to the population as of any real value. Current scholarship has shown the Flexner Report, which was written in consultation with Dr. Nathan P. Colwell, secretary of the Council on Medical Education of the American Medical Association, to have been little more than the most powerful salvo in the AMA's campaign to reduce the number of medical schools operating in the United States. On the Flexner Report, see, for example, James G. Burrow, who notes that "Flexner sought to reduce physician supply and to raise the standards of medical education, and the former goal was not incidental to the latter." *Organized Medicine in the Progressive Era: The Move Toward Monopoly*

(Baltimore: The Johns Hopkins University Press, 1977): 47. And Paul Starr has observed of Flexner: "His report more successfully legitimated the profession's interest in limiting the number of medical schools and the supply of physicians than anything the AMA might have put out on its own." *The Social Transformation of American Medicine* (New York· Basic Books, Inc., 1982): 120. Andrews' apparent unfamiliarity with the historical literature on the Flexner Report — and with the concurrent work done by economists, who have reached similar conclusions — casts serious doubt on the value of her own discussion.

250 "To-day there are about ninety full specialists or near-specialists in Greater Vancouver with its 300,000 population and three hundred registered practitioners." A. S. Munro, "The Medical History of British Columbia," *Canadian Medical Association Journal,* XXVII (1932): 192.

251 "Canadian Medical Association," [Proceedings of the Twenty-sixth Annual Meeting, London, Ontario, September, 1893], *Canada Lancet (Supplement),* XXVI (October, 1893): 12.

252 *Ibid.*

253 "Report of the Committee on Interprovincial Registration," *Montreal Medical Journal,* XXVII (August, 1898): 642.

254 "Dominion Registration," *ibid.,* XXVII (August, 1898): 638.

255 Editorial, *Manitoba and West Canada Lancet,* VI (January, 1899): 130. The Manitoba Medical College, the only medical school west of Ontario, was at that time turning out between fifteen and twenty graduates per year. Meanwhile, the population of western Canada was increasing at approximately 30,000 per year. Yet the *Manitoba Lancet* felt it necessary to note that "the standard of examination in Manitoba Medical College has been very considerably advanced and the period of study lengthened, mainly with the object of not overloading the profession." *Ibid.*

256 T. G. Roddick, "Abstract of an Address on a Proposed Scheme for a Dominion Medical Council," *Montreal Medical Journal,* XXVIII (May, 1899): 323–324.

257 *Ibid.,* 326. The only historian who appears to have taken notice of these motives is Lloyd G. Stevenson, chairman of the department of the history of science and medicine at Yale University. In a round-table discussion on Canadian medical history held in 1966, Dr. Stevenson remarked of Roddick's objectives in working for a dominion-wide medical council that Sir Thomas "was convinced that the medical schools were over-producing; Canada was going to have too many doctors and couldn't absorb them all. He thought that a national standard would receive international recognition and that the surplus of doctors could then go and work in the Indian Medical Service, the merchant marine, and elsewhere." *Physicians' Panel on Canadian Medical History* (Round-table Discussion on Canadian Medical History, held October 7, 1966) ([Toronto]: Schering Corporation, 1967): [6–7].

²⁵⁸ Roddick's first draft is reprinted in full in "Draft of Proposed Act to Incorporate the Medical Council of Canada," *Montreal Medical Journal,* XXIX (March, 1900): 234–240.

²⁵⁹ "On the Dominion Registration Bill," *ibid.,* XXIX (March, 1900): 231.

²⁶⁰ *Ibid.,* 229.

²⁶¹ *Ibid.,* 230.

²⁶² Historical accounts of the passage of the Canada Medical Acts of 1902 and 1911 appear in H. E. MacDermot, *Sir Thomas Roddick: His Work in Medicine and Public Life* (Toronto: Macmillan Company of Canada, 1938): 84–112; and, Robert B. Kerr, *History of the Medical Council of Canada* (Ottawa: Medical Council of Canada, 1979): 15–23. For a brief history of Roddick's efforts to gain enactment of the acts, see Major-General J. W. B. Barr, "The Medical Council of Canada," *Canadian Medical Association Journal,* CXI (1974): 185, 193, 267. Unfortunately, Barr's account is too abbreviated to prove of more than limited value.

²⁶³ Extensive excerpts from Roddick's speech introducing his bill appear in MacDermot, *Sir Thomas Roddick,* 95–101.

²⁶⁴ "Dr. Roddick's Medical Council Bill," *Canada Medical Record,* XXX (June, 1902): 282–283. Roddick's remarks moving second reading of the bill appear in full on pp. 278–286.

²⁶⁵ In referring to the difficulties Roddick confronted in gaining passage of his measure, one newspaper is reported to have commented in 1902: "You seldom meet a man who really likes doctors' bills." Quoted in MacDermot, *Sir Thomas Roddick,* 102.

²⁶⁶ Quoted in Kerr, *Medical Council of Canada,* 18; and, MacDermot, *Sir Thomas Roddick,* 101.

²⁶⁷ Although both MacDermot and Kerr noted that Laurier withdrew his opposition to the bill during the 1902 session of Parliament, neither provides a satisfactory account of the reasons for the Prime Minister's change of mind.

²⁶⁸ 2 Edw. VII, c. 20 (Canada). The act is reprinted in "Roddick Bill," *Canada Lancet,* XLIII (January, 1910): 362–370; and, in the version that appeared in the Revised Statues 1906, as Appendix A of Kerr's *Medical Council of Canada.*

²⁶⁹ 2 Edw. VII, c. 20, sec. 10(h) (iii) (Canada).

²⁷⁰ "Dominion Medical Registration," *Canada Lancet,* XXXVI (May, 1903): 749.

²⁷¹ *Ibid.,* 751. It is perhaps unnecessary to add that the *Lancet* did not consider the possibility of altering the Ontario medical act so that graduates in medicine from Ontario's universities intending to take the Medical Council of Canada examinations would be exempt from sitting the provincial board's examinations. Such a change would, of course, have removed the objections Ontario physicians had to amending the federal act along the lines suggested by Quebec practitioners.

272 "Quebec and the Dominion Registration Bill," *Canada Lancet,* XXXVI (November, 1902): 199–200.

273 *Ibid.,* 199.

274 The act stipulated that, to give effect to the statute, each province would first have to pass legislation to the effect "that registration by the Council shall be accepted as equivalent to registration for the like purpose under the laws of the province." 2 Edw. VII, c. 20, sec. 6(3) (Canada).

275 "The Establishment of a Medical Council for Canada," *Montreal Medical Journal,* XXXI (May, 1902): 376.

276 *Ibid.,* 374–375.

277 "The Canadian Medical Act, 1902," *Maritime Medical News,* XIV (June, 1902): 216. The *News* hailed the act as "the most noteworthy legislation passed by the Parliament of Canada during the recent session," and predicted that the statute would prove to be "of inestimable value to the medical profession of Canada." *Ibid.,* 215–216.

278 3 Edw. VII, c. 63 (Nova Scotia); 3 Edw. VII, c. 16 (Prince Edward Island).

279 3 Edw. VII, c. 23 (Manitoba).

280 Both acts were passed in 1906: 6 Edw. VII, c. 28 (Alberta), and 6 Edw. VII, c. 28 (Saskatchewan).

281 MacNab, *Legal History of Health Professions,* 40.

282 MacDermot, *Sir Thomas Roddick,* 104.

283 *Ibid.*

284 2 Edw. VII, c. 20, sec. 2(a) (Canada).

285 Quoted in Kerr, *Medical Council of Canada,* 19. Kerr points out that the definition was provided despite the view of H. S. Osler, the College's solicitor, that it was probably best that no exhaustive definition be included in the federal act. Indeed, no such definition would have been necessary once the Ontario profession succeeded in changing the provincial law to include an adequately restrictive definition of medical practice. In the wake of several failures to so amend the provincial medical statute, however, a strict definition in the federal law was thought crucial. In any case, despite the College's recommendation, the suggested definition was not included in the 1911 amendments to the Roddick bill.

286 2 Edw. VII, c. 20 sec. 10(h) (Canada).

287 The federal law was viewed as "un empiétement sur l'autonomie des provinces en matière d'éducation." In addition, the French-speaking profession felt that passage of the Roddick bill would provoke conflicts "non seulement entre les bureaux provinciaux de médecine et ce bureau central, à pouvoirs quasi-illimités, mais même entre les deux principaux groupes de nationalité qui ont, chacune, leurs idées, leurs aspirations et leurs méthodes au sujet de la haute éducation." "Entendons-nous," *Bulletin Médical de Québec,* II (April, 1901): 452, quoted in Claudine Pierre-Deschênes, "Santé Publique et Organisation de la Profession Médicale au Québec,

1870–1918," *Revue d'Histoire de l'Amérique Française,* XXXV (1981): 359.

288 "A Dominion Medical Council," *Canada Lancet,* XXXIX (October, 1905): 164–165.

289 J. P. McInerney, "Is the Medical Profession of New Brunswick Making Good on Its Own Behalf?" *Maritime Medical News,* XX (December, 1908): 27.

290 "Dominion Registration," *Canada Lancet,* XLIV (November, 1910): 162.

291 T. G. Roddick to H.W. Powell, letter dated 26 January 1910, reprinted in Kerr, *Medical Council of Canada,* 100.

292 Kerr, *Medical Council of Canada,* 20. In October, 1910, the *Canada Lancet* editorialized:

"In season and out of season we have urged the claims of this question. We are not at all discouraged. Progress is being made. Gradually those who oppose Dominion registration are lessening in numbers and in the keenness of their opposition. On the other hand those in its support are increasing in numbers and influence. . . .

"We have much pleasure in giving the following resolution adopted at the August meeting of the Alberta Medical Association. Here it is: 'Your committee on legislation beg leave to recommend that in the opinion of this Association it would be in the best interests of the medical profession, not only of this province, but of the whole Dominion, that Dominion registration be brought about as soon as possible by the adoption of the Canada Medical Act, 1910.' This was carried.

"Other provinces should fall in line. We would like to see the concurrence of British Columbia and Quebec. In Quebec the course is now a five-year one. This removes any real difficulty in the way so far as that province is concerned. The standard in it so far as time is concerned is as high as in any other province. The colleges should therefore accept the principle of Dominion registration. Just think of how this would read, 'A National Medical Profession.'" "Dominion Registration," *Canada Lancet,* XLIV (October, 1910): 85–86.

293 Kerr, *Medical Council of Canada,* 21. MacDermot notes of the delay caused by British Columbia's request: "This last-minute check was extremely disheartening, and Roddick was wont to refer to it as the one that tried his patience more severely than any other." *Sir Thomas Roddick,* 107–108.

294 Quoted in MacDermot, *Sir Thomas Roddick,* 108. Roddick himself could not offer the amended bill to the House since he ceased holding a seat in Parliament in 1904.

295 1 & 2 Geo. V, c. 16 (Canada). It is instructive to examine the state of medical education at one of the best schools in North America in the first decade of the century, when Roddick's bill was enacted. Apparently the single most important aspects of proper medical training at that time were

the unlearning of the therapeutics of the preceding century and the ability to properly diagnose. Lewis Thomas, the chancellor of the Memorial Sloan-Kettering Cancer Center, describes the nature of medical training and practice at the College of Physicians and Surgeons of Columbia University at the beginning of the twentieth century in the following terms: "Education," he writes, "was already influenced by the school of therapeutic nihilism for which Sir William Osler and his colleagues at Johns Hopkins had been chiefly responsible. This was in reaction to the kind of medicine taught and practiced in the early part of the nineteenth century, when anything that happened to pop into the doctor's mind was tried out for the treatment of illness. The medical literature of those years recounts the benefits of bleeding, cupping, violent purging, the raising of blisters by vesicant ointments, the immersion of the body in either ice water or intolerably hot water, endless lists of botanical extracts cooked up and mixed together under the influence of nothing more than pure whim, and all these things were drilled into the heads of medical students—most of whom learned their trade as apprentices in the offices of older, established doctors. Osler and his colleagues introduced a revolution in medicine. They pointed out that most of the remedies in common use were more likely to do harm than good, that there were only a small number of genuine therapeutic drugs—digitalis and morphine the best of all, and they laid out a new, highly conservative curriculum for training medical students.... The principal concern of the faculty of medicine was the teaching of diagnosis. The recognition of specific illnesses, based on what had been learned about the natural history of disease and about the pathologic changes in each illness, was the real task of the doctor. If he could make an accurate diagnosis, he could forecast from this information what the likely outcome was to be for each of his patients' illnesses....

"[The medical student] would explain what had happened and what was likely to happen. [This] art of prediction needed education, and was the sole contribution of the medical school; good medical schools produced doctors who could make an accurate diagnosis and knew enough of the details of the natural history of disease to be able to make a reliable prognosis. This was all there was to science in medicine, and the store of information which made diagnosis and prognosis possible... was something quite new in the early part of the twentieth century." Lewis Thomas, *The Youngest Science: Notes of a Medicine-Watcher* (New York: Viking Press, 1983): 19–21.

[296] New Brunswick: 1 Geo. V, c. 20 (1911); British Columbia: 2 Geo. V, c 23 (1912); Quebec: 2 Geo. V, c. 38 (1912); Ontario: 2 Geo. V, c. 29 (1912). Upon its entry into confederation, Newfoundland enacted the necessary legislation to bring its medical act into conformity with those of the other provinces: 13 Geo. VI, no. 57 (1949).

[297] The Canadian Medical Association still hoped that the matriculation standards of the various provinces would, over time, become standardized. In

his presidential address before the Association in 1911, Dr. G. E. Armstrong, speaking of the Medical Act, commented: "The amended bill leaves preliminary education to the provincial boards, but it is hoped that very soon the councils of the English-speaking provinces will unite on a uniform standard of matriculation, that of the province of Quebec remaining somewhat different on account of the educational methods of the province, although to have one door of entrance to the study of medicine for the entire Dominion would be most desirable." G. E. Armstrong, "Canadian Medical Association: President's Address," *Canadian Medical Association Journal,* I (July, 1911): 594.

298 A list of the orginal members of the Medical Council appears in Kerr, *Medical Council of Canada,* 101–102.

299 The date fixed as that of the legal establishment of the Medical Council of Canada was November 7, 1912, the date of its inaugural meeting in Ottawa. *Ibid.,* 22.

300 For a brief history of the Council during the period from 1912 to 1920, see Kerr, *Medical Council of Canada,* 24–30.

301 *Canadian Medical Association Journal,* III (July, 1913): 993–994. Fourteen of the seventy-one applicants took their examinations in French.

302 Kerr, *Medical Council of Canada,* 27.

303 *Ibid.,* 30.

304 49 & 50 Vic., c. 48, sec. 27 (1886).

305 5 Edw. VII, c. 14, sec. 1 (1905).

306 In 1906, Nova Scotia became the first province to enter into reciprocity with Great Britain. The provincial medical board had been required to admit to registration without examination all British registrants as early as 1899 [62 Vic., c. 32, sec. 17 (1)]. When Britian enacted the 1905 amendments to its medical act, Nova Scotia applied for recognition of the province's registrants, which was established by the requisite Order-in-Council [Stat. R. & O. 1906, no. 383].

Quebec was next to act, apparently by a provincial Order-in-Council at the beginning of 1908 which amended the province's medical act of 1907 [7 Edw. VII, c. 43, sec. 4] that had required applicants from Great Britain to undergo the province's professional examinations. Reciprocity was effected by a British Order-in-Council in February, 1908 [Stat. R. & O. 1908, no. 203] and the province's extension of recognition to British registrants was formalized by a Quebec statute of 1909 [9 Edw. VII, c. 55, sec. 1].
£216 Like Nova Scotia, Prince Edward Island had been required to license all British registrants without examination since passage of its 1899 medical act [62 Vic., c. 24, sec. 9]. In 1910 the province applied for and was granted recognition of its registrants by Great Britain under a British Order-in-Council [Stat. R. & O. 1910, no. 71].

Three years later, in 1913, New Brunswick amended its medical act to admit British registrants to practice without examination [3 Geo., c. 33].

Reciprocity was formalized by a British Order-in-Council of the same year [Stat. R. & O. 1913, no. 1116].

These four provinces were joined by four others after the outbreak of the war. In 1915, Saskatchewan altered its medical statute to provide for reciprocity [6 Geo. V, c. 26, sec. 2] and the necessary British Order-in-Council was passed in the same year [Stat. R. & O. 1915, no. 586]. 1915 also saw the Ontario medical act amended to empower the provincial Medical Council to enter into reciprocity agreements on such terms as it deemed expedient [5 Geo. V, c. 27, sec. 2]. As a result, the province established reciprocity with Great Britain almost immediately, the agreement being brought into force in that year by a British Order-in-Council [Stat. R. & O. 1915, no. 507]. Manitoba's legislature acted in March, 1916 [6 Geo. V, c. 67], with passage of the necessary British Order-in-Council recognizing Manitoba registrants coming late in the same year [Stat. R. & O. 1916, no. 384]. Lastly, in 1917, Alberta altered its medical act to extend registration without examination to all applicants whose names were entered on the British register [7 Geo. V, c. 3, sec. 26]. The same privilege was extended to Alberta registrants by a British Order-in-Council in 1919 [Stat. R. & O. 1919, no. 1897].

Of all the provinces, British Columbia was alone in not entering into reciprocity with Great Britain. The province's medical act had been amended in 1916 [6 Geo. V, c. 40, sec. 2] to empower the British Columbia Medical Council to set "such terms and conditions as the Council may deem expedient" respecting reciprocity with British registrants. However, the Council never used this authority and applicants whose names were entered on the British register were required to meet the same conditions and sit the same examinations as were all other candidates for licensure in the province.

As a separate British possession, Newfoundland was legally in a position to institute reciprocal registration with Great Britain as early as 1886. However, inasmuch as the colony had not even established a medical register until 1893, no action was taken by Newfoundland until 1913, when its medical board requested that Great Britain recognize the colony's registrants. This was effectuated by a British Order-in-Council of that year [Stat. R. & O. 1913, no. 1364]. The colony itself had licensed holders of British medical degrees without examination under the provisions of its medical act of 1906 [6 Edw. VII, c. 8, sec. 3].

307 Jas. M. MacCullum, "Medical Licensure," [from the Report of the Conference on the Medical Services in Canada, Dec. 18–20, 1924], *Canadian Medical Association Journal,* XV (March, 1925): 260.

308 Via the following Orders-in-Council: Ceylon, 1887 [Stat. R. & O. Rev. 1904, VIII:2]; Hong Kong, 1913 [Stat. R. & O. 1913, no. 324]; India, 1892 [Stat. R. & O. Rev. 1904, VIII:3].

309 Stat. R. & O. Rev. 1904, VIII:1.

310 Stat. R. & O. 1905, no. 1295.

311 Apparently the Ontario Medical Council was particularly indignant that recognition had been extended to Italian and Japanese physicians. Kerr, *Medical Council of Canada,* 29.

312 14 Geo. V, c. 33, sec. 2 (Saskatchewan).

313 There is some question whether this was the intent of the profession in Saskatchewan when it sought this amendment. In late 1924, Dr. A. M. Young of the Saskatchewan Medical Council, in speaking of the proposed change at the Conference on the Medical Services in Canada, remarked: "At the last meeting of the legislature, we had inserted in our Act the words, 'after examination by said Council'; referring to the Medical Council of Great Britain. We were quite of the opinion that they did not conduct an examination, but had certain assessors or inspectors, and we said that so far as we were concerned we would accept that as coming within the meaning of our Act. In other words, we did not [intend to] exclude British practitioners from reciprocity, but we were in favour of this method of inter-provincial registration." Conference on the Medical Services in Canada, "Discussion," *Canadian Medical Association Journal,* XV (March, 1925): 263.

Regardless of intent, the legal effect of the Saskatchewan amendment was to terminate automatic recognition of British registrants in the province. Consequently, reciprocity was formally broken by Great Britain in 1926 [Stat. R. & O. 1926, no. 557]. In 1949, Saskatchewan once again amended its medical act to grant recognition to British registrants without examination [13 Geo. VI, c. 82, sec. 1]. A British Order-in-Council effectuated reciprocity in the same year [Stat. R. & O. 1949, no. 2392] and is currently still in force.

314 The action of the New Brunswick Council led to revocation of reciprocity by a British Order-in-Council of 1926 [Stat. R. & O. 1926, no. 1415].

315 Recognition of Ontario degrees in Great Britain ceased with passage of an Order-in-Council of 1927 [Stat. R. & O. 1927, no. 1246].

316 Quebec's medical act was amended in 1927 [17 Geo. V, c. 60, sec. 3], but Great Britain's Order-in-Council revoking recognition of Quebec registrants was not passed until the following year [Stat. R. & O. 1928, no. 248].

317 Alberta maintained reciprocity until 1975, when its medical act was amended to remove any provision according special treatment to British registrants [24 Eliz. II (2d), c. 26]. A British Order-in-Council revoking recognition of Alberta registrants was consequently passed later in the same year [Stat. R. & O. 1975, no. 809].

Nova Scotia had altered its medical act in 1969 to empower its medical board to determine the conditions under which agreements respecting reciprocal registration operated [18 Eliz. II, c. 15, sec. 13]. In 1977, in response to the action of the Nova Scotia board in severing reciprocity, a British Order-in-Council revoking recognition of Nova Scotia registrants was passed [Stat. R. & O. 1977, no. 1720].

Newfoundland had entered Confederation under a system of reciprocal registration with Great Britain. In 1974, the province's medical act was amended to allow Newfoundland's medical board to set the terms and conditions governing such agreements [22 Eliz. II, c. 119, sec. 16 (3)]. Consequent to a change in the board's policy respecting automatic registration of British registrants, Great Britain revoked its recognition of Newfoundland registrants in 1978 [Stat. R. & O. 1978, no. 283].

Prince Edward Island amended its medical statute in 1952 [1 Eliz. II, c. 31, sec. 22], and Manitoba in 1981 [29 & 30 Eliz. II, c. 11, sec. 19], in both cases empowering their medical councils to determine the terms and conditions of any reciprocal agreements respecting registration into which the provinces might enter. As of 1984, both provinces appear to have continued their policy of extending provincial registration to British registrants without requiring a professional examination.

[318] Jas. M. MacCallum, "Medical Licensure," *Canadian Medical Association Journal,* XV (March, 1925): 259.

[319] Kerr points out that in 1915 Winnipeg joined Montreal as a site for the Council examinations and that soon after Halifax and Toronto were added as test centers. It was not until 1928, however, that examinations were held across the country, in Halifax, Montreal, Kingston, Toronto, London, Winnipeg, Edmonton, and Vancouver. *Medical Council of Canada,* 55.

[320] Jas. M. MacCallum, "Medical Licensure," *Canadian Medical Association Journal,* XV (March, 1925): 259.

[321] Kerr, *Medical Council of Canada,* 30, and, Conference on the Medical Services in Canada, "Discussion," *Canadian Medical Association Journal,* XV (March, 1925): 262.

[322] 6 Edw. VII, c. 28, sec. 30(c) (Saskatchewan). The law required prospective practitioners to sit an examination before the members of the provincial Medical Council "or examiners appointed by them for that purpose."

[323] 8 Geo. V (2d), c. 35, sec. 3 (1) (Saskatchewan).

[324] 8 Geo. V. (2d), c. 67, sec. 4 (1) (Saskatchewan).

[325] Conference on the Medical Services in Canada, "Discussion," *Canadian Medical Association Journal,* XV (March, 1925): 263. The account here given of the Saskatchewan Medical Council by Dr. A. M. Young erroneously suggests that this amendment was in fact passed by the provincial legislature.

[326] Indeed, it appears that by 1927, for all practical purposes, all candidates seeking licensure in Saskatchewan did so via the mediation of the national Medical Council. At the Second Conference on the Medical Services in Canada, it was reported that Saskatchewan no longer held its own examinations and instead accepted those of the Medical Council of Canada. A. Primrose, "Chairman's Address," *Canadian Medical Association Journal,* XVII (May, 1927): 517.

327 "Report of the Committee on Medical Education," [Sixty-first Annual Meeting of the Canadian Medical Association, August, 1930], *Canadian Medical Association Journal,* XXIII (Supplement): xxvii. The report announced that out of a total of 9,594 physicians in Canada, 2,574, or 26.7% were enrolled with the Medical Council. It was also noted that in 1929, of the 355 graduates of Canadian medical schools, 247, or 69.8%, took the Dominion examinations.

328 *Canadian Medical Association Journal,* XXI (July, 1929): 96; and *Canadian Medical Assocation Journal,* XXIII (September, 1930): 463.

329 *Canadian Medical Association Journal,* XXV (August, 1931): 246.

330 The decision is reported in the *Canadian Medical Association Journal,* XXVI (May, 1932): 688.

331 Kerr, *Medical Council of Canada,* 31.

332 24 Geo. V, c. 29 (Ontario).

333 MacNab, *Legal History of Health Professions,* 44. One further development might be noted: the establishment of conjoint examinations with the nation's medical schools, thus reducing two sets of examinations that graduating medical students were required to sit to one only. At its annual meeting of 1940, held in Ottawa, the Medical Council adopted a scheme whereby any medical school that so wished, could arrange with the Registrar of the Council to hold its final examinations coincidentally with those of the Medical Council. *Canadian Medical Association Journal,* XLIII (October, 1940): 402. These combined examinations were immediately adopted by four of the Dominion's nine schools, the University of Manitoba, Queen's University, the University of Western Ontario, and the University of Toronto. Kerr, *Medical Council of Canada,* 39. They have since been accepted by a majority of medical faculties in Canada.

334 This appears to be the view of, among others, Howard S. Becker, "The Nature of a Profession," in Nelson B. Henry, ed., *Education for the Professions* [The Sixty-first Yearbook of the National Society for the Study of Education (Chicago: The National Society for the Study of Education, 1962)]: Part II, 17–46; Marie Haug, "The Sociological Approach to Self-Regulation," in Roger D. Blair and Stephen Rubin, eds., *Regulating the Professions* (Lexington, Mass.: Lexington Books, D. C. Heath and Company, 1980); 61–80; Jethro K. Lieberman, *The Tyranny of the Experts: How Professionals are Closing the Open Society* (New York: Walker and Company, 1970); and, Wilbert E. Moore, *The Professions: Roles and Rules* (New York: Russell Sage Foundation, 1970).

335 See Thomas McKeown, R. G. Record and R. D. Turner, "An Interpretation of the Decline of Mortality in England and Wales during the Twentieth Century," *Population Studies,* XXIX (1975): 391–422.

336 It should be made clear that the "standards" that are being raised, and to which I am referring, are solely those relating to entry into the profession.

The term is not meant to encompass standards of practice. Indeed, there is good reason to believe that licensing has inhibited innovation and discouraged a high level of competence in medical practice. As one prominent economist has observed: "The point is clear: the result of various professional restrictions has most certainly been to delay, if not prevent, the introduction of new forms of service and to lend support to the inefficient and uninnovative practitioner." Sylvia Ostry, "Competition Policy and the Self-Regulating Professions," in Philip Slayton and Michael J. Trebilcock, eds., *The Professions and Public Policy* (Toronto: University of Toronto Press, 1976): 20. See, also, the following two articles, which analyse the effect of licensure on innovations in medical practice: Edward H. Forgotson and John L. Cook, "Innovations and Experiments in Uses of Health Manpower—The Effect of Licensure Laws," *Law and Contemporary Problems,* XXXII (1967): 731–750; and, Nathan Hershey, "The Inhibiting Effect Upon Innovation of the Prevailing Licensure System," *Annals of the New York Academy of Sciences,* CLXVI (1969): 951–956.

[337] These three attributes of modern guilds are set out in J. A. C. Grant, "The Gild Returns to America," *The Journal of Politics,* IV (August, 1942): 316–317.

[338] Malcolm G. Taylor, "The Role of the Medical Profession in the Formulation and Execution of Public Policy," *Canadian Journal of Economics and Political Science,* XXVI (1960): 127.

STATISTICAL APPENDIX

[1]   J. A. MacFarlane, *Medical Education in Canada* [Royal Commission on Health Services (Ottawa: Queen's Printer, 1965)]: 64.

[2]   Thomas McKeown, *The Role of Medicine: Dream, Mirage, or Nemesis?* (2d ed.; Princeton: Princeton University Press, 1979).

Index

Dominion, 95, 210, 237–249,
251–252, 361, 363, 375
registration, 103–105, 113,
118–120, 122–126, 130–132,
134–141, 147–149, 152–155,
158–159, 168, 170, 178,
212–213, 217, 223, 225, 228,
230, 238, 240, 242, 248,
251–252, 254–256, 259, 326,
349, 351, 361, 374–375, 380
Richardson, Dr. James, 105
Robertson, Dr. William, 30
Roddick, Sir Thomas, 238–245,
249, 251–253, 372–373, 375
Roddick Act, 246–247, 249–250,
252, 254, 374
Rolph, Dr. John, 43, 82, 306, 313,
316
Royal College of Physicians,
London, 19–20, 68, 312
Royal College of Surgeons,
Edinburgh, 20, 38, 43, 70, 312
Royal College of Surgeons,
London, 19–20, 37–38, 68, 300,
312
Royal Faculty of Physicians and
Surgeons, Glasgow, 20, 37, 312
Russell, Lord John, 60–61

St. Francis District Medical
Association, 205
St. John's Medical Society, 225
St. Lawrence School of Medicine,
83
Sangster, Dr. Alexander, 177
Saskatchewan, 229–232, 259, 378,
380
Medical Acts, 229–232, 249, 257,
259, 378–379
See also Education, Saskatchewan
Scott, Dr. James, 16, 85
self-regulation,
See Medical profession, self-
governing body

Sherwood, Henry, 36
ship's surgeons,
See Military surgeons
Simcoe, Colonel John Graves, 13
similia similibus curantur,
See Homeopathic medicine
Sorel Medical Society, 135
special-interest group,
See Medical profession
Strachan, John, 27–28, 306
Sullivan, Dr. Michael, 129
surgeons, 95–96, 109, 118–119, 134,
158, 189, 223, 227, 295, 304,
369
See also Medicine; Midwifery,
midwives
syphilis epidemic, 11–12, 297

Territories Medical Council,
See North-west Territories
Thomson, Samuel, 24–25, 67, 303
See also Eclectic medicine;
Thomsonianism,
See Eclectic medicine
Toronto Medico-Chirurgical
Society, 53
Toronto School of Medicine, 82–83,
314, 317, 324
Town v. Archer, 202
trade, medicine regarded as a,
See Medicine, regarded as a trade
Trinity College,
See University of Trinity College
Tupper, Dr. Charles, 97, 99, 106,
330

United Empire Loyalists, 10, 13,
296–297
in Maritimes, 34, 311
monopoly on professions, 34
unauthorized practice,
See Unlicensed practitioners
University of Alberta, 233, 259–260